AF496518

THE ABC OF
HORSE AND
PONY PROBLEMS

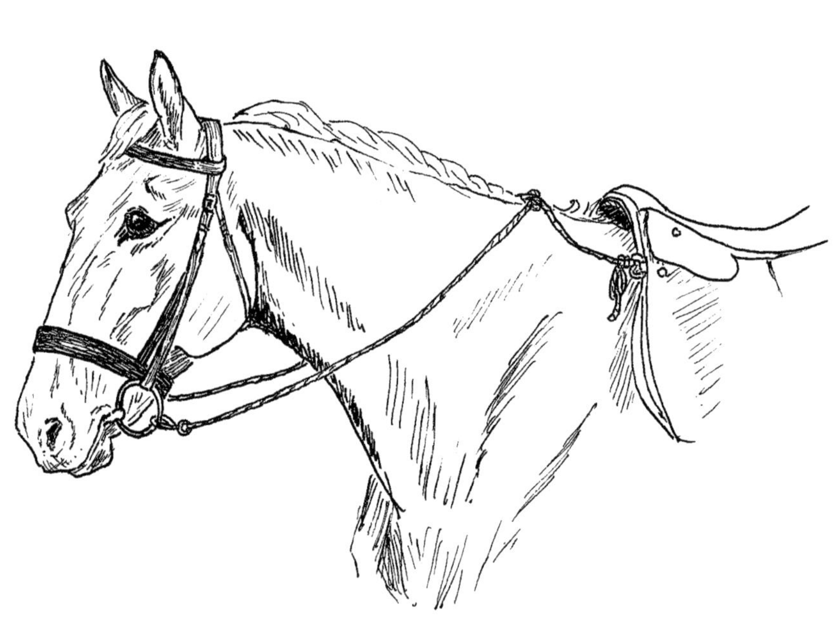

THE ABC OF HORSE AND PONY PROBLEMS

JOSEPHINE KNOWLES FBHS

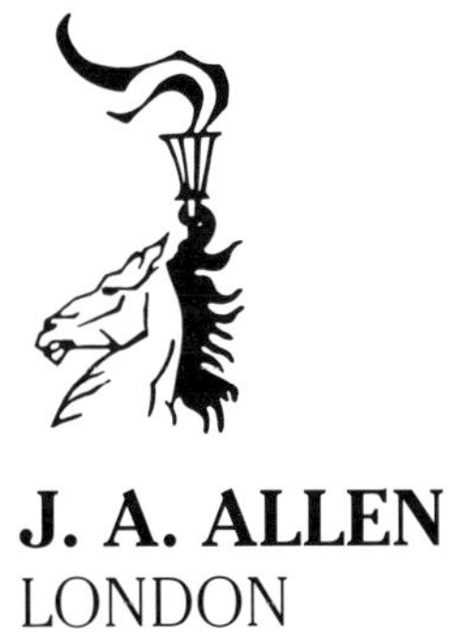

J. A. ALLEN
LONDON

British Library Cataloguing in Publication Data
A catalogue record for this book is available from
the British Library

ISBN 0.85131.691.3

Published in Great Britain by
J. A. Allen & Company Limited
1, Lower Grosvenor Place, Buckingham Palace Road,
London, SW1W 0EL

© J. A. Allen & Co. Limited, 1997

No part of this book may be reproduced or transmitted
in any way or by any means, eletronic, or mechanical,
including photocopy, recording or any information
storage and retrieval system, without permission in
writing from the publishers. All rights reserved.

Text illustrations Ejnar Newcombe-Baker
Design Nancy Lawrence
Edited by Lesley Young
Typeset by Textype Typesetters, Cambridge
Printed by Dah Hua Printing Press Co. Ltd., Hong Kong

CONTENTS

INTRODUCTION

Of all the animals we have domesticated it is the horse whose natural way of life we have changed not. Many horses are kept in a loose box 3.6 x 3.6 m (12 x 12 ft) (or, worse still, tied up in a stall) for 22 or 23 hours out of 24. Few are able to touch another horse and many are kept quite alone in complete isolation from their own species. When the horse is at last allowed out of its confined area for an hour or so, we then expect it to carry us on its back and, without argument, to comply with our every wish and whim willingly and quietly.

In their natural state horses run wild in herds of mixed sexes and ages, continually grazing and moving on. As foals they are disciplined by their mothers, then by their elders or their contemporaries with the strongest characters. They are not confined in a small space. They are never forced to keep still. They are never alone. They are allowd to use their free will and follow their instincts. They are free to play and get rid of excess energy.

The biggest wonder is that there are not more delinquent or completely mentally screwed-up horses! It only shows what wonderfully amenable and amazingly adaptable animals horses are.

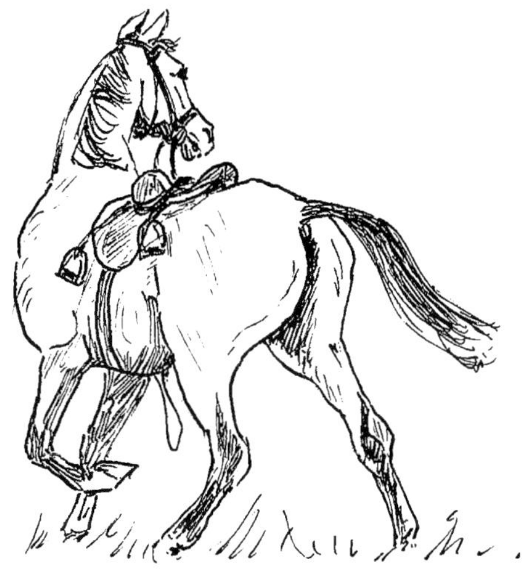

Think for a moment and put yourself in the position of a horse kept in a loose box for months on end – often with no company of your own kind. According to your temperament, you might well become bored and sullen or stressed, irritable, aggressive and anxious to escape from your tiny, confined area. On meeting other horses, might you not refuse to leave them? If your saddlery or rugs were painful or itchy or your rider was rough or unbalanced or gave unintelligible aids and then hit you, might you not try to get rid of them?

All of these reactions are considered to be vices in horses, yet humans lose their tempers, attack each other, drink, take drugs, smoke, bite their nails, go on strike, sulk or refuse to co-operate and none of these actions cause great surprise – just human nature we say.

In my opinion it is the way that horses are kept, treated, fed and worked that is the cause of many problems and so-called vices. A happy, contented, mentally relaxed horse is far less likely to have problems so, if possible:

- Keep your horse within sight and touch of other horses.
- Make sure your horse/pony can see out over an open top door. (Many small ponies are shut in boxes with horse-sized doors, over which they can see nothing at all of the outside world. Imagine how imprisoned you would feel in such circumstances. It is quite easy to improvise a low door with a pallet, a saw and a few extra boards. This will transform a small pony's quality of life.)
- Make the greatest possible effort to turn your horse/pony out for most or at least part of every day.
- If you have a large yard or a paddock with a shed in it, your horse/pony will be far happier and less likely to develop problems or vices when living there than in the confines of a smart loose box or, worse still, a stall.
- Give your horse an occupation – hay or clean straw to nibble at little and often, or a large swede to roll around and chew at.
- Lead the horse out to graze if you can't turn it out.
- Make its exercise enjoyable and, if possible, stress free.
- Discipline your horse so that is respects you but is not frightenend of you.
- Be consistent in what you say 'no' to. Do not stop the horse from doing something one day and allow it to get away with the same thing the next day.
- Use the same actions and tone of voice when asking for obedience.
- Do not forget to praise the horse with your voice and by rubbing or scratching it (as horses do to each other in friendship).
- If you have to punish, it must be short, sharp and instantaneous – even a minute's gap between misdeed and punishment is too long. The horse will not realise why you are punishing it and will become nervous, confused or angry according to its temperament.
- Never punish a horse unless you are one hundred per cent certain it will know why you are doing it.

- Never punish a horse or use stronger aids when riding unless you are one hundred per cent certain that the horse understood what you asked of it the first time.
- Repeat your request clearly and calmly – give your horse a chance before punishing it.
- Many problems are caused by confusion. The handler/rider punishes the horse when they have handled it badly or ridden it incorrectly and the horse has not understood. The horse becomes more stressed and more confused and starts to use its strength. It is then considered dangerous. Yet the same horse, when handled or ridden by a calm, understanding, sympathetic, knowledgeable person, can be a transformed animal within a week (sometimes in only an hour). Because it has been understood and it now knows what is wanted and can trust and rely on its handler/rider, it becomes relaxed, calm and co-operative. I have seen this happen hundreds of times.
- It is nearly always the person handling, feeding or riding the horse who is the cause of problems in the first place.
- Do not just try to stop a stable vice as the horse is likely to seek another outlet for its frustration or stress. Look for the cause. If you catch the problem as it is starting, a simple change of environment/regime may prevent it from becoming a habit.
- Put yourself in the horse's place and try to puzzle out why the problem first occurred and what you can do to prevent it continuing.
- Remember that neurotic, stressed people produce neurotic, stressed, disobedient children, dogs and horses!

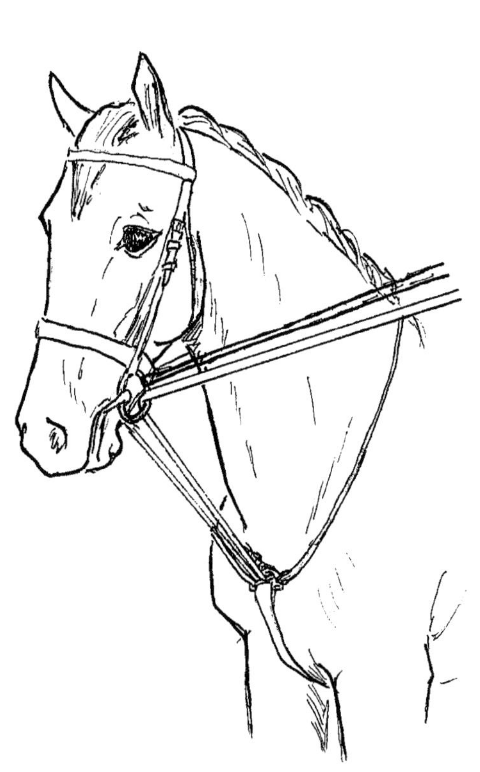

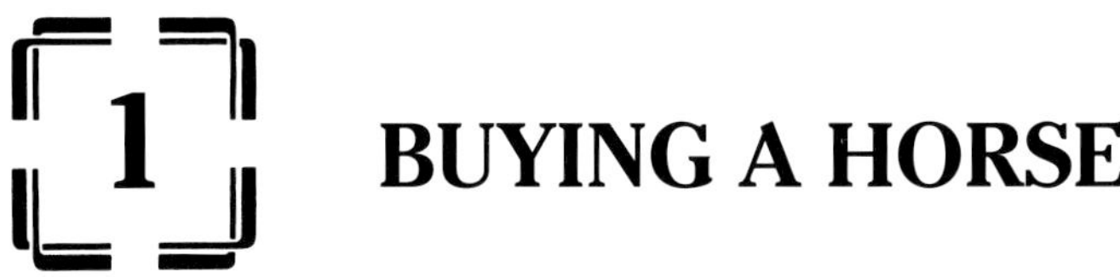

BUYING A HORSE

YOU AS A RIDER

Before you even start looking for a horse you must think hard about several factors.

Above all, be realistic about your riding ability and the time you have free for riding.

Do not buy a young or lively horse or pony if:

- You are nervous.
- You can only ride at weekends.
- You are away at boarding school (unless someone experienced can ride and school the horse or pony regularly for you).
- You have the additional stress of a young family and running a house.
- Think carefully about what you want to get out of riding before you buy your horse or pony.
- If you just want to hack out quietly and use riding to relax your mind, choose something quiet but willing, and traffic proof.
- Realise that nearly all horses and ponies are far more lively in the winter and in cold, windy weather.
- Keeping a horse in at night and out by day in the winter is likely to make it more lively than keeping it out all the time.
- A horse kept in all the time must be exercised every day and may well be extremely lively, especially if it is unused to living in.
- A horse or pony bought from a riding school because it is very quiet and sensible may change completely when ridden only occasionally in a private home.
- Do not buy a great big horse if you are only a little person (unless you are a very capable rider wanting to compete successfully).
- Do not 'overhorse' a small child on a big pony because 'they won't grow out of it so quickly'. They may well not be able to control it either!

BUYING A HORSE IN A SALE

Some genuine horses are put in sales but the majority are there because they have problems, so beware! Take a very experienced person with you, who has bought and sold horses for years and is well used to buying in sales. You may

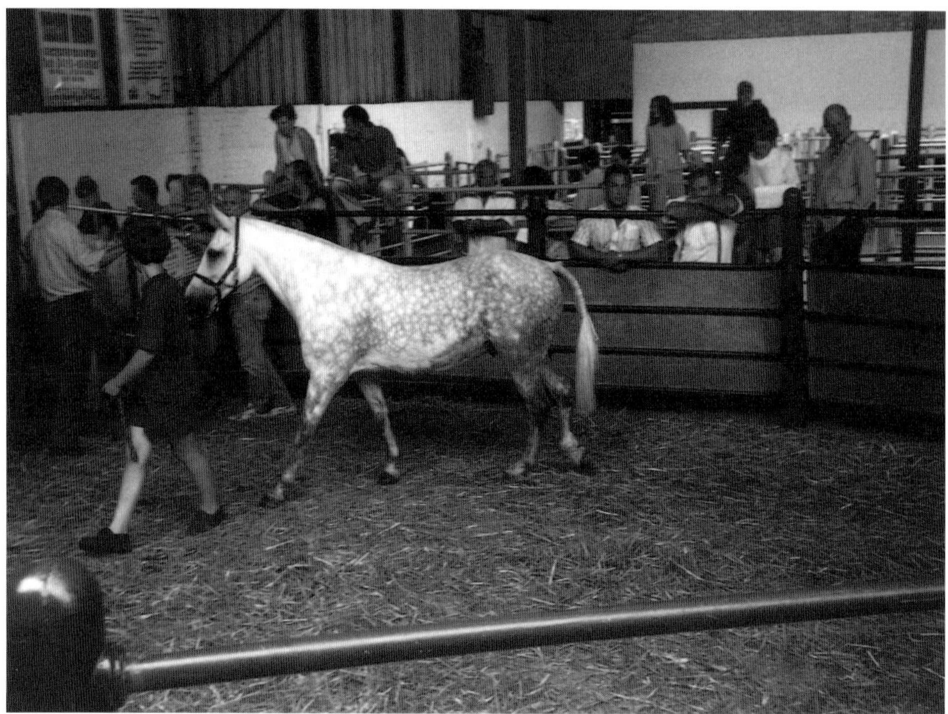

A relaxed, calm pony in the sale ring.

pay less than you would pay privately but you may also buy a horse with big problems or unsoundness or that is difficult to ride, impossible to box, shoe, clip, etc.

Most sales have some form of warranty, either written in the printed catalogue or posted up in the auctioneer's office. Read and check the wording carefully as sales differ as to the length of the warranty and what it covers. Much of the flowery wording used to describe horses in a sale catalogue does not constitute a warranty of any sort. To buy an unwarranted horse in a sale is asking for trouble.

If you do intend to buy in a sale, go somewhere where the horses can be ridden and jumped and do not buy a horse that you have not at least seen ridden even if you have not ridden it youself. Some sales have no facilities for riding other than in the concrete yard of a cattle market.

Note the length of time the warranty covers – normally between 24 hours and 48 hours. If you want the horse vetted before you take it home there is usually a vet in attendance at horse sales. Try the horse as soon as you get it home. See if it trots out level after the journey. Canter it and work it in circles to see if it is sound in its wind.

If you find a problem which is covered by the warranted description of that horse, telephone the auctioneers immediately. If you are even an hour over the time when the warranty expires, that horse, with all its problems, is yours. Sales have different methods of dealing with the problem of horses returned for failing the warranty. Some want them returned to the sale yard immediately, others ask you to keep the horse and await further instructions. If the problem is one of unsoundness a vet appointed by the auctioneers will inspect the horse. If the horse was warranted 'quiet ro ride' and you find that it is not, the auctioneers will arrange for someone of their choice to ride it.

BUYING PRIVATELY

If you are going to see a horse, arrive early. You may find it being lunged or ridden to quieten it down or to get rid of filling in its legs!

Take an experienced person with you to look the horse over for any obvious problems! Always see the horse being tacked up. See the owner ride and jump the horse first so that you can watch how it goes and find out what sort of temperament it has. You and the person you have taken with you should both ride the horse so that you can compare notes on what you both felt about it.

Ask the owner why the horse is being sold. If the answer is evasive, be suspicious.

Don't just try the horse in an indoor school, *manège* or small paddock. Ride it in open fields and out on the road. Go to and fro past the entrance to its stable yard several times to see if it is inclined to nap. If possible, ride it out with another horse and see if it will go away from home when the other horse turns towards home. This is a stiff test and many horses will hesitate and be reluctant to go on away from home and their companions if the other horses are going towards home. With strong legs and the use of a stick, if necessary, you should be able to make the horse obey you, albeit unwillingly. If it is nappy it will almost certainly play up under such circumstances.

Find an excuse to use a stick just once and note the horse's reaction to it. Does it put its ears back, swish its tail and give a little buck? Does it slow down and nearly stop, ears back? All of these are signs of an ungenerous horse which may prove unwilling and argumentative. Does it shoot forwards or sideways in a panic when you hit it? If so, it has probably had a good hiding for something in the past. You would hope that the horse would respond to a smack by going forward confidently and more freely.

In the field, canter towards home up beside another horse and see if yours gets strong and excitable.

Jump towards home and away from home. Rearrange a jump to see if the horse is equally willing to jump a fence it has not been practised over.

If possible, see the horse being caught up from the field and loaded into a trailer or horse box.

If you like the horse and think it will suit you, have it vetted by an experienced *horse* vet.

BUYING FROM A DEALER

The advantage of going to a dealer is that you should find several possible horses to look at. Be very honest about your experience and riding ability. Do not make out that you are more experienced or more confident than you really are. Do not waste the dealer's time by looking at or riding horses which are far more expensive than you can afford. Go to a dealer who will be willing to exchange the horse if you cannot get on with it. This arrangement has a great advantage over buying privately or in a sale. If you do want to exchange the horse you first bought, expect to pay more money for the replacement. After all, the dealer has a living to make and time is money.

CONFORMATION

No matter how low the price is, before you buy a horse have it properly vetted by an experienced horse vet. He or she will note every blemish and conformation defect and will be able to tell you which ones will affect the horse's performance and soundness. You should, however, be able to spot some for yourself.

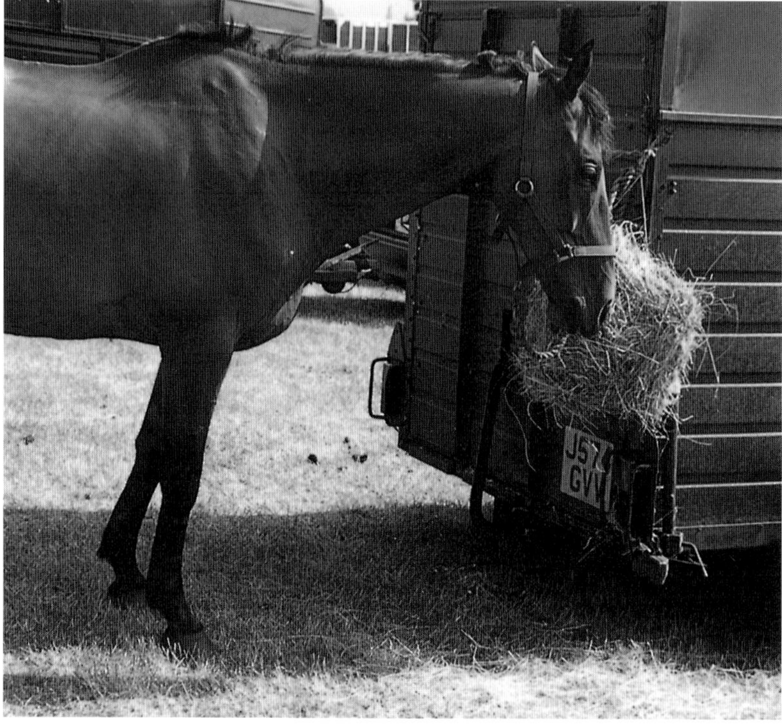

A straight shoulder with the withers directly above the forelegs.

Shoulder

If your horse has a straight shoulder, the saddle is likely to sit closer to its withers. You will feel that you are sitting almost on the horse's withers and nearly over its forelegs and that there is not very much in front of you as you sit on the horse. The horse is likely to have a fairly short stride. All of these things are undesirable in a riding horse. You cannot change the horse's conformation but you can help the situation slightly by getting the horse fit and schooling it correctly. If your saddle keeps sliding forward up its neck, ask a saddler to fit point straps (an extra girth strap attached to each of the two point pockets of the saddle tree, see page 97). If you then attach your girth to the new point strap and what was the front girth strap, this will help to keep the saddle in the correct place. If the back of the saddle moves up and down, use the point strap and the second girth strap. Check that, with the point strap in use, the saddle is still a good, comfortable fit for the horse, well clear of its withers and not putting undue inward pressure on either side of and below the withers.

Choosing a horse with a good shoulder
Take an imaginary line from the highest point of the horse's withers to the ground. This line should come well behind the horse's forelegs.

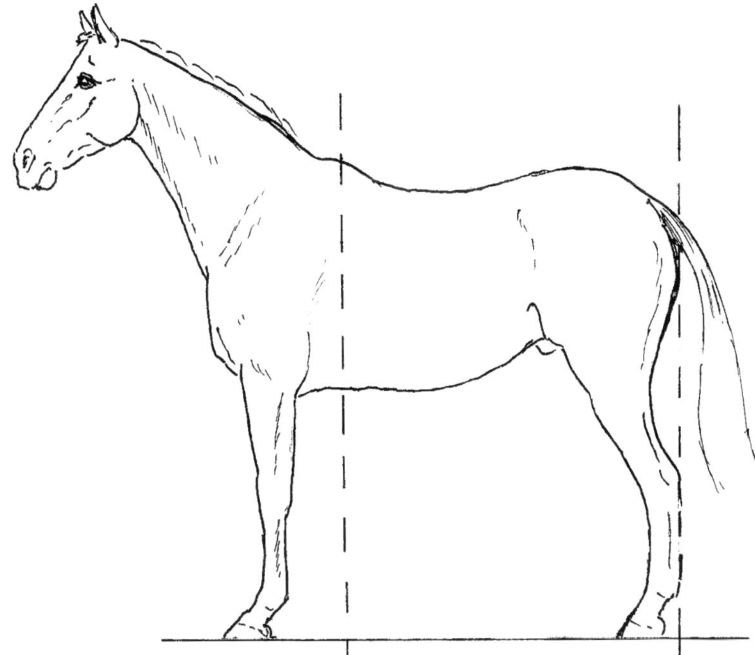

A straight line from the highest point of the withers to the ground should come well behind the foreleg.

The back of the hindquarters, hock and fetlock joint should be in line.

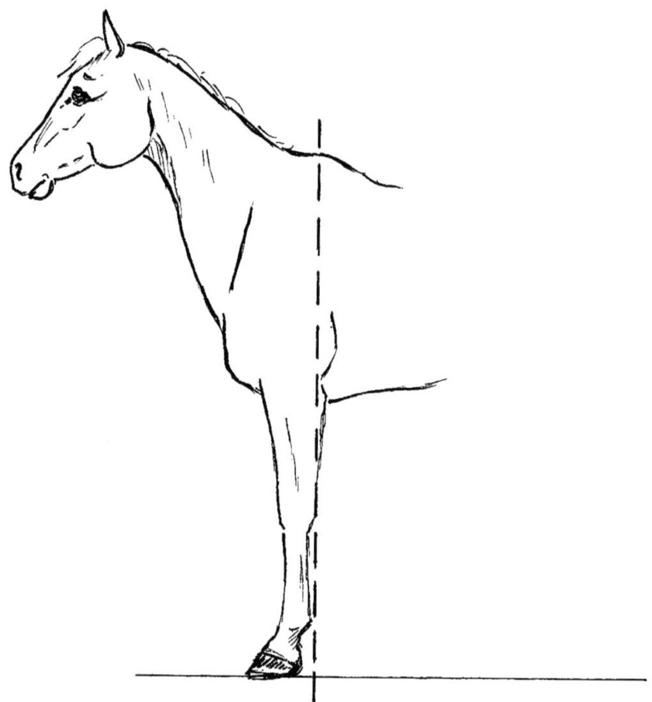

Not a good shoulder. A straight line from the highest point of the wither goes down through the foreleg.

Ewe neck

A horse with an 'upside down' neck will naturally tend to throw its head up to evade the bit and may develop the additional problem of a large bulge of muscle on the lower line of its neck. It will not be easy to ride.

Do not buy a horse with this conformation. If you already own one, the first thing to do is to soften the hard bulge of incorrect muscle by hacking the horse quietly on a loose rein as it cannot go in a correct outline until that muscle has softened somewhat.

The horse can be lunged without side reins to encourage it to lower its head and relax its neck. A young horse will then need working in carefully adjusted side reins (ask for advice from a knowledgeable person) and schooling by being ridden on a light contact, always encouraging it to lengthen the topline of its neck.

Lungeing in a cavesson and with no bit in the horse's mouth may also encourage it to relax.

This type of horse will lean against the noseband to which a **standing martingale** is attached and will continue to develop muscle on the lower neck.

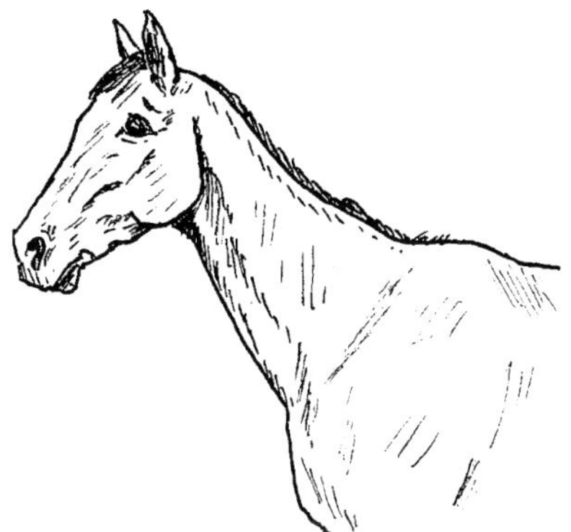

A ewe neck.

When a horse wearing a **running martingale** tries to put its head up, the downward pressure on the rein comes a foot or more behind the bit. The ewe-necked horse is still able to lean against this pressure, bring its head back towards you and thus continue to develop the muscle on its lower neck.

One type of martingale which does encourage the horse to lower its head and lengthen the top of its neck is the **Market Harborough** and this is what I would recommend for a ewe-necked horse. An older horse will probably improve most quickly if ridden in a Market Harborough which encourages the horse not only to lengthen the topline of its neck and lower its head, but also to build up the muscle on top of its neck. This martingale is attached to the girth between the forelegs. After passing through a loop in the neck strap it divides into two narrow pieces of leather which go through the snaffle bit rings from inside to outside before clipping on to the Ds on the reins. The Market Harborough should be fitted so that the ordinary reins come into a straight line contact just before the Market Harborough straps do. It does not force the horse's head down, it just asks the horse to lower its head again if it raises it too high. It may well take two years to break down the muscle underneath the neck and then build up the muscle on top of the neck as the muscle below the neck and the habit of using this muscle have to be corrected first. The build up of muscle on top of the neck will then come very gradually. As things improve the horse may sometimes be ridden in any bridle or bit in which it continues to go calmly with a good head carriage and a long line along the top of its neck. If it is at its best in the Market Harborough, continue with this until you find it will happily keep its correct outline without it. Do not use a running martingale unless you need a neckstrap to hold on to and then adjust the martingale very loosely so that there is never a downward pull on the reins. Never use a standing martingale on a horse which has had this problem.

A horse can safely be jumped or hunted in a Market Harborough as the horse has complete freedom to stretch its neck out downwards. NB: get a horse well used to a Market Harborough on the flat before you jump in it. Ask a knowledgeable person to fit it correctly on your horse. Do remember, however, that you cannot jump a horse in a Market Harbough under the rules of certain competitions – so check before you enter.

Thick in the throat; protruding glands in the throat

Horses with either of these problems will find it difficult, or even impossible, to come down on to the bit and go in a correct outline. There is no cure so if you want a dressage horse do not buy one with these problems.

Hindquarters

Looking at the horse from the side, take an imaginary line from the hindquarters to the ground. In a well-made horse this should also touch the hock and fetlock joint.

Cowhocks

Cowhocks are a weakness. Looking from the rear, the points of the hocks nearly touch and the feet appear to be turned out. A horse with turned-out hind feet is likely to brush (knock) the inner, lower part of the fetlock joint with the shoe of the opposite foot, causing a swelling of the joint or even a small cut.

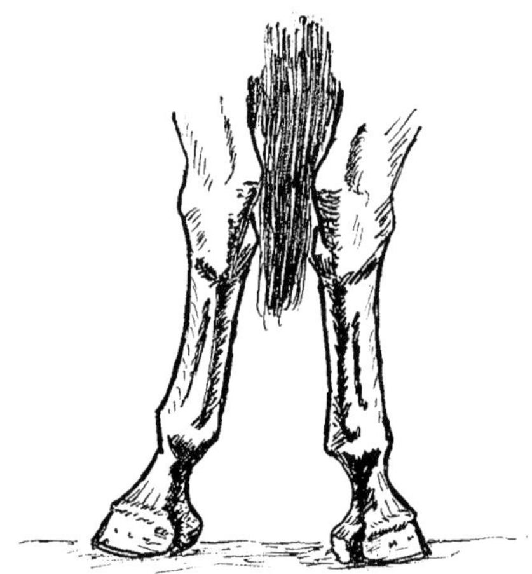

Cow hocks.

Looking from the rear, take an imaginary line straight to the ground through the centre of the hock joint. This line should also pass through the centre of the cannon bone, fetlock, pastern and hoof.

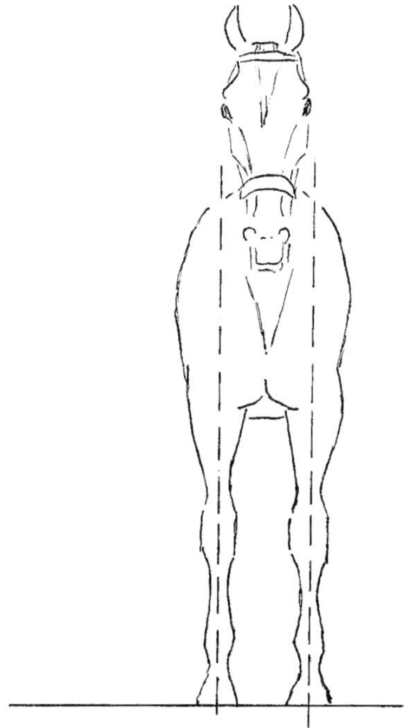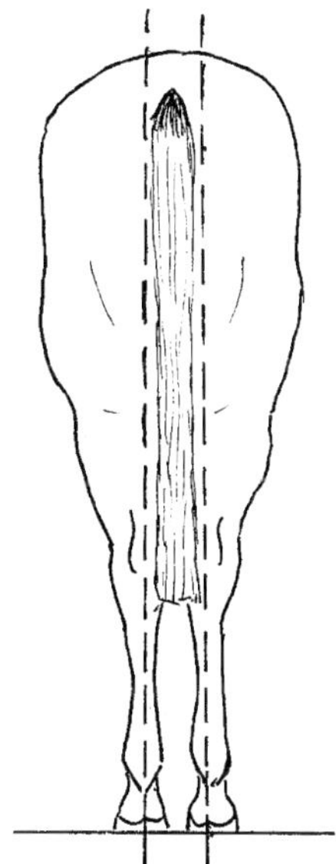

There should be a straight line through:

forearms	*hocks*
cannon bones	*cannon bones*
fetlocks	*fetlocks*
pasterns	*pasterns*
hooves	*hooves*

Sickle hocks

Sickle hocks appear to curve rather than drop straight to the ground. They are a weakness, as are hind legs that look left out behind.

Forefeet turned out

A horse with this conformation will also be likely to brush (see Cowhocks).

Forefeet turned in (pigeon toes)

A horse with this conformation will be likely to dish. (When moving, the horse throws its forelegs outwards from the knee downwards.) Looking at the horse from the front, take an imaginary line to the ground through the centre of the horse's forearm. This line should also pass through the centre of the knee, cannon bone, fetlock, pastern and hoof. The forelegs should not be too close together.

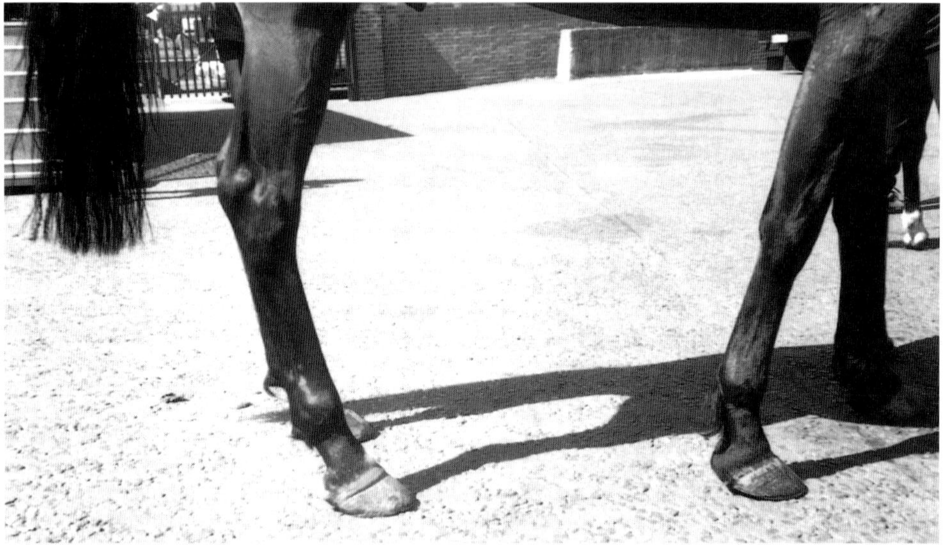

Sickle hocks and long, overgrown feet.

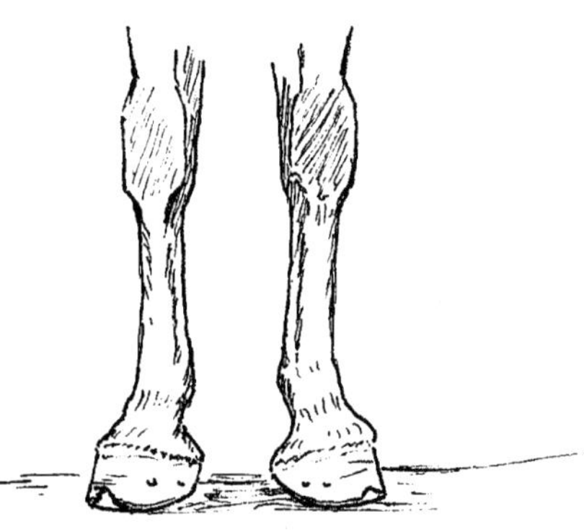

Toes turned out. This horse is likely to brush because the legs will move in an inward arc.

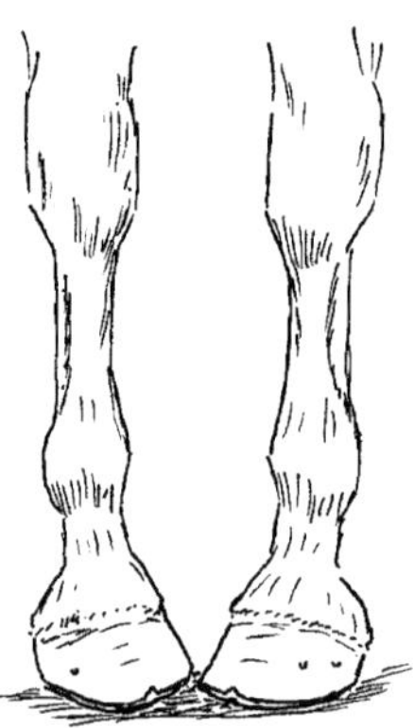

Pigeon toes cause the outward circular swinging action of the forelegs known as dishing.

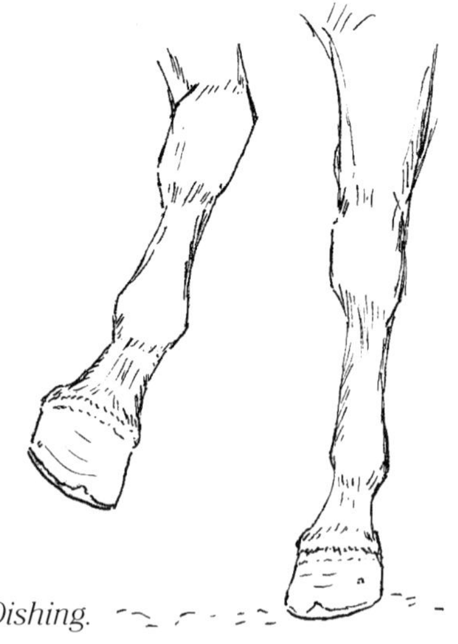

Dishing.

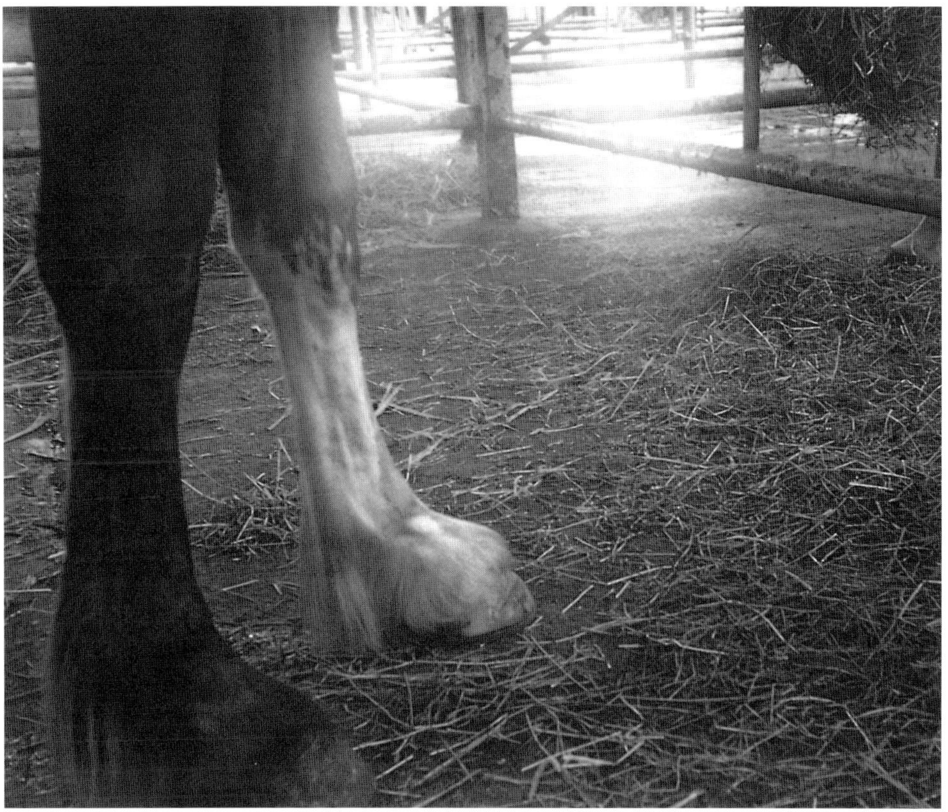

This horse is back at the knee which will put extra strain on the tendons. There is a broken 'line' through the pastern and hoof (see 'C' in the illustration below).

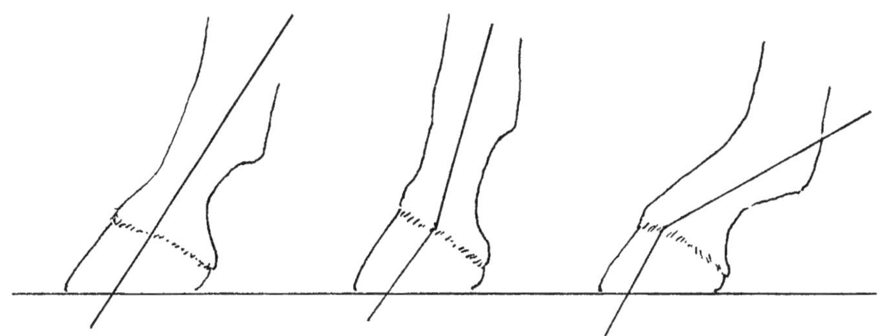

A: correct, unbroken line travelling through pastern and hoof at the same angle.

B: a broken line. The pastern is upright. This horse is probably a 'jolty' ride.

C: a broken line. This is a very sloping pastern. This horse may be a comfortable, 'springy' ride but extra strain is being put on the joints and tendons.

YOUR NEW HORSE

Expect a horse that has just arrived and been put in a new stable to be a bit worried and unsettled at first. If possible, turn it out (in daylight) in a safe field and give it a chance to settle down. (Do not turn it out alone if it has always had company as it may just gallop madly about.) If it has been living out already, this is no problem but if it is clipped and has been kept in, check if it is used to being turned out in a New Zealand rug each day. If it has not been turned out at all for several weeks, do not turn it out as it may gallop madly in this new, strange place and damage itself. If possible, and you know what work it has done previously, lunge or ride it first in a small, enclosed area. Make certain the tack fits well and is properly adjusted. Use tack of the type the horse was accustomed to with its previous owner. If you are going to ride out go with another rider. Do simple things. Do not do anything that might overface the horse until it has settled and learnt to trust you.

Do not give a new horse a lot of hard feed. Overfeeding is the cause of many problems with horses. If it is not overfat, give it as much good, clean hay as it will eat and 450 g (1 lb) of hard food night and morning if it is stabled. If it is out on good grass, it will not at first need any food other than a handful in its manger when you bring it into the stable before riding. This will give it something to look forward to when it comes in and help it to remain calm in the stable.

Realise that:

- A horse kept entirely stabled needs exercising for at least an hour every day.
- A horse which has been used to living out may change completely and become very lively to ride when kept entirely stabled. This will be true even if it is fed only on hay.
- Some horses can be really jumpy and nervous or overexcitable in a new environment. They can take a week or more to settle down.
- A different rider can utterly change a horse's behaviour.
- A very nervous or very noisy, rough person can totally change a horse's behaviour in the stable and when ridden.
- What a horse is fed can change its behaviour. Even if the previous owner says the horse has been having 5.4 kg (12 lb) of hard food a day, start with 900 g (2 lb) (but also give the horse as much good hay as it will eat) and gradually build up the quantity of hard food as you and the horse get to know each other.
- Feed according to the work you intend to give the horse. If it is just doing quiet hacking, it probably only needs 900 g–1.3 kg (2–3 lb) of hard food per day in the winter plus good hay ad lib. Overfeeding of hard food causes very many of the behavioural problems of horses.

- Try to put yourself in your horse's place. Would you be calm and happy living as your horse lives? Would you enjoy and be contented with the sort of work your horse does?
- Would you respect yet trust the person looking after you and riding you?
- Would you understand your rider's aids and obey them calmly and willingly?

Meeting other horses

When a new horse is introduced to others there is almost certain to be some jealously.
- It is advisable to keep a new horse separate from others for a week in case it is carrying any infection.
- Ideally, life is more peaceful if mares and geldings are kept in separate fields and where the two sexes cannot sniff at each other over a dividing fence.
- If the sexes are mixed, you are asking for trouble if you introduce a new gelding into a field where there is already one gelding running with a mare or mares.
- If there is just one mare in with a gelding, she may be jealous of a new mare.

Kicking usually starts within a few seconds of the horses first sniffing each other. This first introduction can be safely conducted by putting the horses that are to be field companions in separate stables and then leading the newcomer up to each door, allowing several seconds for sniffing, squealing and striking out.

At first, put the newcomer out with just one or two horses, then, when they have settled, gradually turn out the others during the day. They should all have settled down before dark.

It is a good idea to lead a new horse round the field boundary and show it where the water is. If there are any through passages or open yards, show it the way in and out so that it will not get lost, trapped or cornered if the others gang up on it. Constantly check what is happening during the first few days. If you are feeding or haying the horses in the field, be aware that your new horse will be very vulnerable at these times and plan accordingly, feeding it separately if necessary.

When riding out, the new horse may kick in self-defence if another horse comes up too close behind it or beside it. The other horses may kick it out of jealously to keep it away from another horse who is their 'friend'. Horses are very possessive and often react in this way to a newcomer.

Remember that if your horse lays its ears back as another horse comes up alongside you when you are riding, you must use the rein and leg *nearer* to the other horse. By doing this you turn its head towards the horse it might want to kick and its hindquarters away from it. All our instincts tell us to turn the horse's head away from the other horse but this turns the horse's hindquarters towards it and into the ideal kicking position!

Strange stables

Some horses and ponies can go absolutely berserk and act totally out of character when put in a strange stable.

What you had thought was a quiet, sensible animal may, if put loose in a strange stable, charge round the box, kick the walls, bang on the door or rear up and try to get its forelegs over the door. If you go into the box you may be knocked over as it charges out, or tries to, or knocked over as it careers wildly round the box. If the top door is shut this may only make matters worse but it may be necessary to do this to stop the horse jumping out. If it is tied up, it may bang, kick and rear up constantly.

Many horses which behave like this when tied up in a strange stable will calm down if allowed to look out over the door, so put the tying up ring and haynet nearer to the door not at the back of the box.

A horse which has always had company may behave like this if it finds itself alone. A horse which has always had the peace and quiet of a lone existence may behave like this in a busy stable with other horses constantly coming and going.

Most horses will calm down in three or four days but if they don't you may have to consider trying different stabling arrangements.

Putting a horse where it can see others and touch noses with its neighbours can have an almost miraculous calming effect.

This is a common problem when a horse goes to new owners and new stables, particularly if the horse has been in its previous home for several years. Some animals will even behave like this when moved out of their regular stable into another one in the same yard.

Some horses which panic in a small box may settle in an open cattle yard.

It can be very disturbing to be led out of a horsebox into a strange place, with nothing familiar – no noises, people, voices, smells or other horses that you know. Put yourself in the horse's place and imagine what it must be like. However, don't despair, your previously quiet, sensible animal will revert to its normal behaviour if you can discover the cause of the problem and put it somewhere that it feels safe and happy.

FRETTING IN A NEW HOME

Not enough thought is given to a horse's mental state. Put yourself in the horse's place. First take a young horse which was born and has spent its first three years in one place where it has become accustomed to the same horses and the same people looking after it and handling it in the same way. The youngster is used to hearing the same tone of voice; the sounds, sights and smells are all comfortingly familiar.

Suddenly it is sent away to be backed or it is sold. Its whole secure world is shattered; there is not a single familiar person, horse, sight, sound or smell anywhere. The calmest of horse will be bewildered, uncertain and insecure. A nervous, highly strung horse will be in a highly traumatised mental state in which it may do things completely out of character.

Do not hit or shout at a horse in this state. You will only make things worse for it and will delay its return to normal behaviour. Find out as much as possible about how it has previously been kept and fed and treat it as much as possible in the same way. Most horses relax and calm down best out at grass so, if possible, turn it out with a quiet, sensible companion. Lead it round the field boundary and show it where the water is. When you bring it into the stable or if you have put it in a stable from the start, make sure there is another horse nearby which it can see and hear. If it is very worried and excited, shutting the top door and closing it in where it cannot see others will make things worse. Put a metal grid over the top door if you have one. If you do not have a grid, fix one or two solid bars above the bottom door so that the horse can see out but cannot jump over or get its head stuck between the bars. Strong staples and baling twine can be used to fix the bars. As the horse calms down more each day, remove the top bar so that it can look out but not jump out, then gradually lower the other bar until it is the same height as the door. When the horse has quite settled, remove the bar. Try to keep the horse in the same stable and have the same people dealing with it until it has settled.

Fretting for a companion

Horses which have been sole companions for some time can be badly affected by the sale or death of their companion. They may box walk, go off their feed or whinny constantly in the stable or when ridden. If they are competition horses this can seriously affect their performance so, if possible, get a third horse as company before or very soon after their old friend leaves.

Fretting in a change of stable in the same home or when travelling to competitions

Some horses are really worried by a change of stable and this can affect their behaviour and performance. If you have a competition horse which is going to have to travel and live away from home for days at a time, move it into different boxes in your own yard and then get it used to spending a night in strange yards before you bring it to peak fitness.

If the horse gets in a really desperate state, consider buying a sheep or goat as a companion which can travel everywhere with it and live in the same stable.

NERVOUS HORSES

Horses, like people, are born with differing temperaments, but the handling of foals and young horses can make a tremendous difference to their opinion of people and the world in general.

A calm, slow-moving, quiet-voiced handler who always behaves in the same predictable way is more likely to have a sensible, relaxed, easy horse. A moody, quick-tempered, unpredictable, noisy handler, tearing about the place and shouting, will produce a nervous, jumpy and perhaps bad-tempered animal.

If you buy a nervous horse which is jumpy and looks at you distrustfully, wondering what you are going to do next and even laying back its ears or turning its hindquarters to you as you approach, it has probably had the latter sort of previous owner.

You have got to convince the horse that you are different. Move slowly and talk frequently, quietly and calmly. Rub its neck, behind the ears (if it will let you) and its forehead; scratch its crest and withers (as other horses do to each other). Let it sniff you all over. Take time to get its confidence. If it lays its ears back at you, ignore it. Don't reprimand it because this act comes from fear not aggression. If it turns its hindquarters towards you when you approach, have a scoop of food to offer it. Move the food about in the scoop and make chewing noises, pretending to eat some yourself. Stand still, sideways on to the horse (this is a submissive attitude). Wait until it turns round and comes to you. If it is a foal or a small pony, squat down low so that you are smaller than it, and turn a little sideways to it. You will not then be so frightening. I do not normally suggest feeding titbits but they are a good way to get a nervous animal to come to you with confidence – 'What present have you got for me this time?' Instead of, 'Oh dear, what are you going to do to me now?'.

If the horse is difficult to get hold of in the stable because of nervousness, leave a headcollar on it with a foot of rope dangling from this so that when the horse comes up to you to eat you can quietly take hold of the rope. Tie the horse up to groom and handle it so that it cannot suddenly dash away because it has just had a bad memory from the past.

Gradually begin to give it a 'police horse' type of training. Place plastic bread bags on your hands and gently rub it all over with them gradually progressing to bigger and noisier plastic bags, an anorak, blankets, rugs. Gradually bring them near its head and between its fore- and hind legs, over its back and right round under its stomach. Never do enough to frighten the horse, just progress very gradually, doing this several times a day. Stop and rub and scratch the horse as a reward and cease to give titbits as soon as it will come up to you in the stable.

Roll a plastic bucket about the stable; drag a plastic bag or rug along the ground. Give the horse experience of more and more things to teach it that it need not be afraid of them. It is necessary to keep a very nervous horse stabled until it has confidence in you, because you would never catch it in a field.

The horse must be lunged or ridden for exercise or could perhaps be led out from another horse. As it progresses, turn it out in a large yard or a small, enclosed area, then a small paddock. Always take titbits or a bucket of food when you go to catch it. Have a tiny feed in its manger every time you bring it in from field to stable, so that there is something to look forward to.

If your horse is very nervous and jumpy when you are on its back, give it the same training from the ground but concentrate on putting things on its back, banging the saddle and waving the saddle flaps. Hold a big plastic sack up in the position a rider would take and move it about, coughing, sneezing, blowing your nose and waving a handkerchief as high as possible above its back. Don't frighten it but try to gain its confidence. Talk to it, rub and scratch its forehead, neck and withers as a reward for accepting your training. Wave whips all round it and stroke it gently all over with one. Get on its back in a stable with a high roof and, very gradually, do these same exercises on its back. It may tense up but you should never do so much that you make it jump. Gradually get it used to your scratching, rubbing, banging of the saddle, making rustly noises with your clothes, blowing your nose, etc.

A horse which is so nervous that it suddenly catches its breath, tenses up and looks back at you as if it is going to explode in terror (and some do) is frightening to ride. You may jump because it has jumped, then it jumps again because you were jumpy. Do not ride a horse like this out in the open; wait until it is calmer.

Some horses have been caught up in something in the past. They might have been tied to a post which has been pulled out of the ground and has banged along the ground, apparently hitting and chasing them. A saddle may have slipped round and flapped underneath them, the stirrups banging their legs. They may have got away when being lunged and the lunge rein pursued them, flapping and catching their legs. A rider may have fallen off and been dragged. A branch may have caught firmly in their tail and, however much they galloped and kicked out at it, they could not dislodge it. Any of these things can so terrify a horse that the memory is with them for years. They are potentially very dangerous and should only be ridden by an expert who can feel the tiniest muscle tension and almost read their very thoughts.

I once bought a pony which was absolutely terrified of the sight of my feet in the stirrups as it looked back at them. It was not a young pony and was not unduly nervous in any other way. I put it in a well-bedded-down loose box, with no buckets, haynets or projecting areas and which had a solid top door to shut. I tied it up, saddled it up and, very securely, tied a large wellington boot in each stirrup iron. I fixed them to the irons, the stirrup leathers and to each other over the top of the saddle and tied the irons together underneath over the girth so that nothing could come undone. I removed the headcollar, hurried out and closed the door. There was soon the most awful commotion which continued, on and off, every few minutes.

I did this every day for a week until the pony had got used to the boots. I then lunged it in a small, enclosed area so that if it panicked I would not lose it. It looked back at the boots, shot forwards once or twice and then settled down. It never completely forgot, however, because, just occasionally, it would still catch its breath and look back at my feet.

You rarely know what has happened in a horse's past but, sadly, few horses spend their entire lives without ever having had a frightening experience.

The calm and relaxed expression in a horse's eye as it looks at you, a low head carriage, ears moving slowly backwards and forwards, tail relaxed, perhaps a leg resting, will all tell you that this horse has never had cause to distrust people. A nervous horse will shoot into a corner as you approach, head high, eyes wide open, ears moving quickly, jerkily, backwards and forwards, perhaps lips twitching, tail swishing, standing square on all four legs, ready to shoot off.

This behaviour warns you that the horse has had a frightening experience in its life and no longer trusts people. Its behaviour is likely to be unpredictable. A sight, sound or smell, normal to you, can trigger some memory from the past and produce violent reactions or even dangerous behaviour from this animal.

The memory will stay for very many years, possibly forever. A very nervous horse should never be bought by a slightly nervous or inexperienced person. A nervous pony should *never* be bought for a child.

2 THE HORSE IN THE FIELD

CATCHING

If your horse is very difficult to catch, you will have no success if you keep it in a field with several other horses. It is essential that it is in a field with, at most, only two others, both of which must be good to catch. In a safe situation you may be able to get your horse to follow loose when you lead the other horse(s) into a yard or pen but this will not improve its 'catchability' in a field. Ask yourself why it is bad to catch. Is it genuinely nervous of you approaching it, of its head being touched or of any movement of your hands, or is it just quick and clever at evading being caught, a trick learnt through years of practice?

If it is really nervous and jumpy when you approach it in the stable, you will definitely not be able to catch it in the field. At first, keep such a horse in a stable. If it is difficult to get hold of even there leave, a headcollar on it and go in to see it as many times as possible during the day, offering it food or hay only when it comes near you for it. Keep very still and allow the horse to

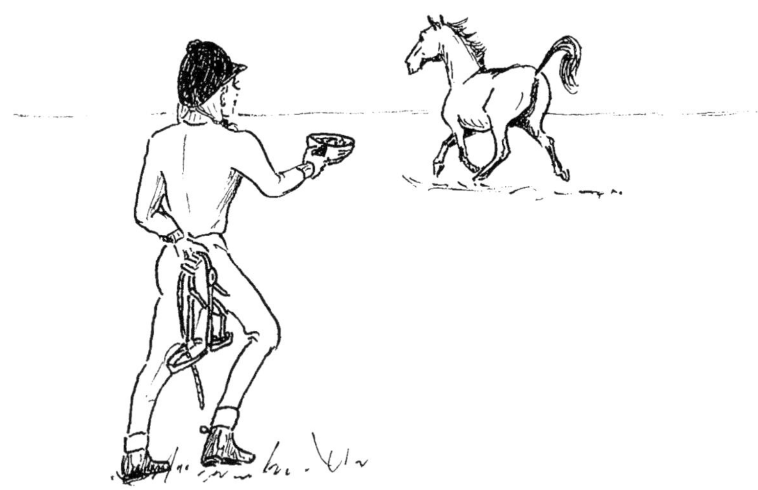

'Catch me if you can!'

19

approach you. Do not look it in the eye. If necessary, squat down low so that you are less frightening. Do not attempt to take hold of it until it will come to you with confidence. Rub and scratch its shoulders and neck, then gently slip your hands through the noseband of the headcollar while still feeding it. Slowly and carefully clip a rope on to the headcollar. If the horse is ridable, exercise it as usual; if not, lead it out or lunge it for exercise. When it will come up to you and let you catch it in the stable, put it in a cow yard or very bare, small paddock, where it will still have to rely on you for its food. Offer it food in a scoop or wide feed bowl because many nervous horses are frightened of putting their heads into a deep bucket. As long as the horse remains easy to catch, continue to put it out into a larger area with only a little grass. It must be kept a bit hungry so that it will continue to come to you for food. Never, ever make a grab at the horse. Wait until it comes to you and is relaxed and confident.

If your horse is just naughty and evasive, you will not be able to catch it unless it really wants the food you have in your scoop, so this horse must also be kept short of grass and a bit hungry. Do not walk directly towards your horse, head on. Do not look it in the eye. Come in from one side and look down and away from the horse but watch it out of the corner of your eye. The second it looks as if it is about to move away, stand still, turn away a little from the horse and make 'rattly' noises with your fingers in the food in the scoop. If you are near enough for it to see what you are doing, pretend to put some food in your mouth and eat it noisily.

If there are one or two other horses in the field, catch them first and get someone to hold them while you feed them within sight and sound of your horse. If it approaches, offer it food but do not attempt to get hold of it. Manoeuvre so that you turn away from the horse and it has to put its head and neck across in front of you to reach the food, then you can put your fingers through the back of the noseband of the headcollar. A few older horses will try to dash off when they feel the pressure on the headcollar but most will give up and allow you to attach the rope. Some horses will not allow you to touch their heads or the headcollar but will allow you to scratch their shoulders and necks. For them, have a rope in your right hand and, as you scratch, slip the rope over the horse's neck and down the other side while the horse is still eating from the scoop in your left hand. When the two ends of the rope are in reach, get hold of them and give a little pull. Many older horses will now give in and stand still while you attach the rope to the headcollar.

The really clever old horse has to be outwitted. I have found that by 'grazing' – pulling grass with my hand in the same rhythm as a grazing horse – while bending down low and totally ignoring the horse, I can make it so curious about what I am doing that it will come up to investigate. I continue to 'graze' until I am beside its foreleg then, still while bending down, I run my hand down its foreleg, say, 'Up' and pick the leg up. I hold it as you would when holding a leg up to restrain a horse, for instance when dressing a wound on

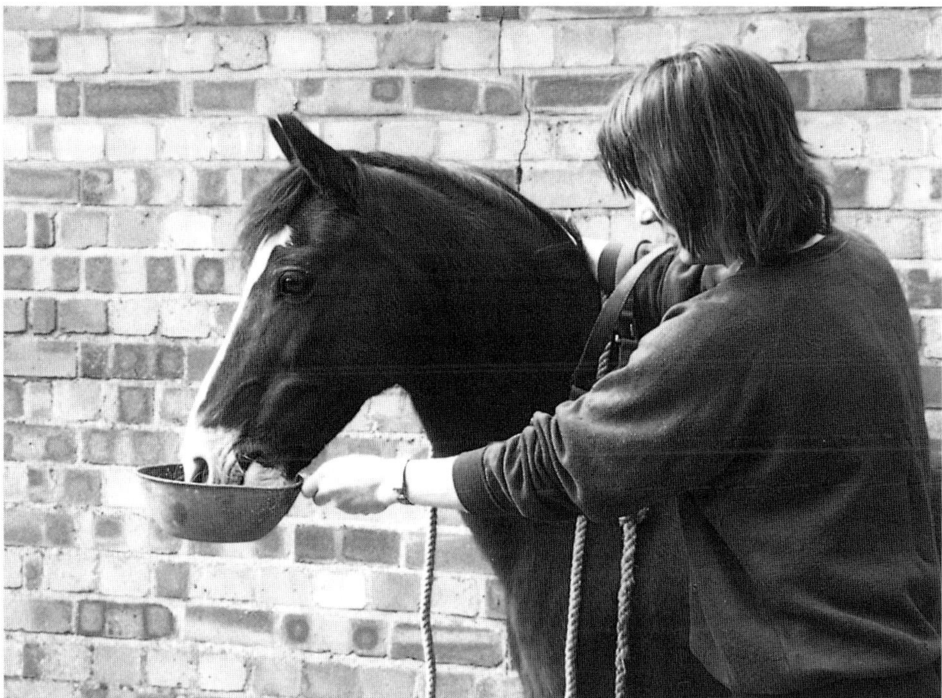

*To catch a pony, encourage it to come well across in front of you before you put the rope
over its neck with your right hand.*

another leg. Horses are often taken by surprise at this treatment when in the
field as they do not associate it with being caught. They *do*, however, associate
it with having to stand still, for example to have their feet picked out every day
in the stable. When the horse is standing quietly, continue to hold the foreleg
up with one hand while attaching the rope to the headcollar with the other
hand.

If, when you are trying to catch it, the horse continually turns its
hindquarters towards you or will not allow you to get near its head, you can
attach a rope 4–6 m (14–20 ft) long to the back of its headcollar and leave this
trailing on the ground. (Do not do this if there are other horses in the field or if
there are bushes or anything else the rope might get caught up on.) Put the
scoop of food on the ground and, while the horse is eating, pick up the end of
the rope. You may need to manoeuvre the scoop of food so that the rope is not
between the horse's legs or you could frighten it when you pick up the rope
(*Do not* attach a long rope to a horse which is inclined to gallop in the field or
it may tread on the rope and fall. Get it used to the sight and feel of the long
rope in the stable.) When you pick up the rope, pull the horse gently towards
you and then reward it with food. You may eventually be able to catch it with
just 1 m (1 yd) of rope attached, in which case it can be out with others.

It may take weeks of patience and equine psychology but you should be able to teach your horse to come to you eventually, although it will probably never come if it is in a field with a large group of pushy horses. Do not take a scoop or bucket of food into a field containing a large group of horses as they are likely to mill around you and may well kick you or each other. If you want to catch one horse from a group, go up to the horse quietly with something in your hand or always call your horse in the same way and try to teach it to come to you for its titbit so that you both avoid being in a group of jealous horses.

If you leave a headcollar on a horse in the field, make sure that the noseband is loose enough for the horse to be able to chew without the headcollar rubbing the two sharp ridges of its lower jaw. A leather headcollar is safer as it will break if the horse gets caught up on something. A nylon headcollar will not break and could be dangerous. A headcollar which is too tight round the nose will soon cause bleeding sores on the sharp ridges of the lower jaw. If your horse constantly rubs its headcollar off over its ears, make a 'throatlash' from a soft strip of material, attach it to the headcollar at the poll and do it up tight enough to prevent the headcollar from coming off over the horse's ears but just loose enough so that it does not restrict its breathing.

If you do succeed in getting a rope round the neck of a horse which is not wearing a headcollar, you are much more likely to be able to hold the horse if you manoeuvre the rope up to a position just behind its ears. Hold the rope with your right hand, pass the free end of the rope round the horse's nose with your left hand and keep hold of it. You have now formed a 'headcollar' and can keep this in place by holding the rope with both hands (see page 327).

Points to remember

- If it has ever been difficult to catch, never try to catch a horse without some food as a reward.
- Never try to corner a horse.
- Never allow small children to be in a field with loose horses.
- Never make a grab at your horse's mane or headcollar.
- Never wrap the rope round your hands as you could get dragged along and trampled.
- Never allow a rope to form small loops round your hand for the same reason.
- Never wrap the rope round your waist. You could get pulled over.
- Never put your fingers or thumbs in the Ds, rings or buckles of a headcollar.
- Never, ever try to hang on to a horse which does not want to be caught by its forelock, mane, nose or with your arms round its neck. It is stronger than you and it will get away. You may hurt your hands or fingers and if you get them entangled in the mane, you may be pulled over and even kicked or trampled.

The dangers of leaving on headcollars

Headcollars can be dangerous. I personally know of the following accidents which have been caused by them.

- A pony scratched its ear with its hind toe while wearing a nylon headcollar. The heel of the hind shoe got caught at eye level on the metal headcollar ring. The pony was caught up this way all night. Its head was very swollen, one eye badly damaged, its back was damaged and it got severe laminitis from stress, never having had it before. It lived, but only just, and recovered only after many months.
- Several foals have died after having got a tiny hind hoof caught up in a headcollar when scratching their heads.
- Numerous horses have got caught up on internal stable fittings.
- Numerous horses have got caught up on stable door catches, bolts and the eyes on the outside of the door on to which the hook for holding a door open fits. Because the horse is hooked up on the outside of the door, if it really panics and goes down the top of the door causes its neck to bend so much that the horse is killed by breaking its neck. This has happened even to knowledgeable people with super stables and expensive horses.
- Horses get caught up on fences or branches in the field.
- Horses get caught up on the taps when an old bath is used as a water trough.

ELECTRIC FENCES

Electric fences are suitable for horses providing that they are introduced to them correctly.

Put the fence up against an existing fence or hedge and approximately 1 m (1 yd) away from it. The sight of the existing fence will slow the horse down so that there is no chance of it galloping through the electric fence or jumping it before it knows what it is. Do not lead a horse up to an electric fence and let it touch it and get a shock while you are holding it. Many horses will then think that *you* have given them the shock. As a result, they may become nervous and difficult to catch.

For years people have used a type of electric fence made of thin, stranded wire and this has been very successful if introduced in the way I have explained, with small strips of plastic tied along it at intervals so that it becomes very visible. If horses gallop through it, however, it can be very dangerous as it can wrap tightly round their legs and cut them badly. If they become entangled in it and the wire is really tight round their legs, it can even stop the circulation. If the horses are not found for several hours, this can be disastrous and may permanently affect the circulation.

The thick plastic tape containing wire threads, which is on the market nowadays, is excellent. Horses can see it and it will not cut them if they do get caught in it. However, I would still recommend introducing it against a permanent fence at first.

Electric fence poles

Metal poles can be dangerous if a horse becomes entangled in the fence. Plastic ones are much safer and come in different heights. Insulated wooden poles are good as long as horses do not learn to rub on them or bite them.

Small plastic insulators can be fixed to an existing post and rails fence to carry electrified wire or tape which will stop horses rubbing on the fence or chewing it.

Dividing horses up

To prevent horses striking out at each other over an existing fence, an electric fence can be set up 1.2 m (4 ft) away from it, which is far enough apart so that the two lots of horses cannot touch noses.

Two electric fences set parallel at 1.2–1.5 m (4–5 ft) apart can be used to divide horses up.

Small paddocks can be formed for horses or ponies whose grazing needs to be rationed. Don't forget to include some form of shelter, hedge, bushes, wall or shed. It is unkind to keep any animal within an electric fence in an open field. Water should always be available.

When a fence has been in place for some time and it is then moved, many horses will hesitate as they approach the line where the fence used to be or may even absolutely refuse to cross the line. They may need to see another horse go first. Be understanding of their overcaution – don't shout at them or hit them.

FIELDS

A field grazed only by horses will soon be ruined because the horses will dung in one part which then grows rank and long and will never, under any circumstances, be eaten down by them. The area dunged on, and therefore inedible, quickly increases until very little grazing is left. The best idea is to get a farmer to put some cattle in. They will soon pull off the long grass. A few sheep kept in with the horses will also keep the long grass down. Alternatively, you can pick up the droppings nearly every day. Spreading the droppings out by harrowing is not much help because horses have a natural instinct to preserve their health by not eating where their droppings lie.

Wire

So many horses are terribly injured by barbed wire that it is far safer not to have it anywhere round your field.

The square-mesh type of pig wire is also dangerous because, in striking out with a foreleg, a horse can get its foot through this. In pulling the foot back out, the thin wire often gets caught under the heel of the front shoe. As the horse continues to pull the wire goes in further under the shoe and is firmly trapped there. The horse is held by one foreleg and may panic and hurt itself. Some horses, on the other hand, will stand patiently waiting for help. If you find a horse in this position (and I have done so on several occasions), you are unlikely to be able to get the wire out from under the shoe, partly because the horse is almost certain to continue to give the odd pull back. The best way to free the horse is to bend the piece of wire up and down just where it disappears under the shoe. This fairly soft wire soon gets hot and will snap if you bend it quickly and far enough. Repeat the action on the other side where the wire goes under the shoe and, when that side snaps, the horse will be free. The broken-off piece of wire will still be under the shoe but it can be removed later. Be aware, however, that a horse trapped in this way can panic, strike out, throw itself down and hurt *you* badly, so be alert all the time that you are trying to help it.

Other fixtures

Wooden fences or hedges are safest. Gates should be strong and sound and, in these dishonest days, fixed so that they cannot be lifted off their hinges, and also padlocked at both ends.

Some form of shelter from the weather, natural or built, is essential. Avoid putting a group of horses in a field where there is a tight corner or narrow passage in which a weak-natured horse can be trapped and kicked or bullied.

A new horse which has always had company may panic totally when put in a strange field alone. It may get in such a state that it will try to jump out over completely impossible places and could end up on a road and cause an accident.

Clean water is essential. Old baths are only suitable if the taps have been removed because headcollars can get caught up on them. (It is best not to turn horses out in headcollars unless they are difficult to catch. If they have to wear headcollars, these should be made of leather which will break in a crisis. Webbing will not break and could cause a tragedy.) Sharp metal rims should be protected by wooden rails. A clean, fast-flowing stream which will not freeze up in winter is ideal.

Mares and geldings are safer if kept in separate fields. If horses are kept where they can sniff at horses in the next field, a dividing fence should never be made from any form of wire as the horses are certain to strike out at each other with their forelegs. (See also Electric Fences, page 23.)

JUMPING OUT OF THE FIELD

Some horses will jump out of a field if left alone. They may be trying to get to other horses which they can see or hear. The grass on the other side of the fence may seem greener or they may just enjoy jumping.

Try to find company for a horse which hates to be alone.

A fairly expensive, but effective, way to keep a horse in when it can jump out anywhere in the field is to put up an electric fence (see page 23) 1–1.5 m (3–5 ft) inside the existing fence.

If there are just one or two places where the horse can jump out, tie poles to the existing fence so that they stick up 50 cm (20 in) or more above the fence. Tie baling twine to the top of the poles, using one to two rows of it according to the size of the gap between the fence and the top row of baling twine. Tie strips of plastic or cloth to the bailing twine so that the horse can see that this place is now (you hope) unjumpable.

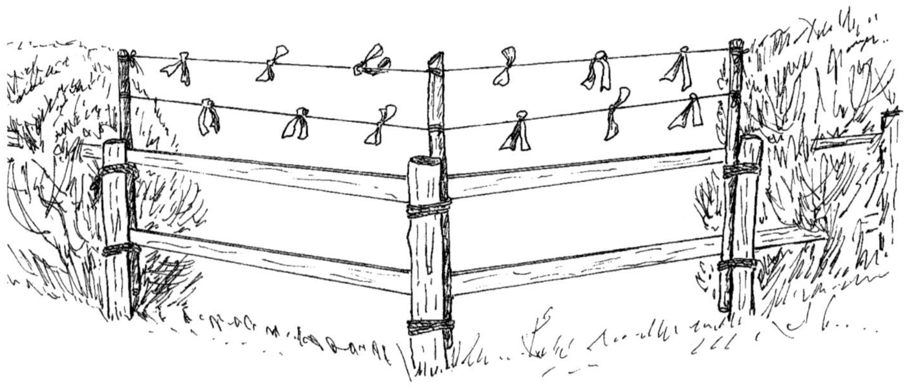

String and plastic strips can be used to prevent a horse from jumping out of a vulnerable place in the field.

TURNING OUT IN BAD WEATHER

If you do not have a New Zealand rug, or for some reason it is impossible to use one, and your horse has to be turned out, spread 225–450 g (8–16 oz) of lard on the horse's back. Brush any mud off first and be sure that the coat is dry. With your fingers, smear the lard over the top of your horse's neck, shoulders, back and hindquarters, always working in the same direction as the hair grows so that the coat lies smoothly.

This application of lard also prevents rain scald, a scabby and sore condition of the skin of the back and especially the hindquarters, which is caused by rain washing the natural grease out of the skin which then cracks and allows dirt and infection to enter.

Shivering in cold weather

It is normal for animals to shiver when turned out in pouring wet conditions. Shivering helps to warm them. Horses and ponies vary enormously. Some do not seem to mind the wet and cold and never shiver, while others, which seem to have just as good, thick coats, shiver and shake when they are even slightly wet or cold.

If the horses have been wet for many hours, bring them in and rub them down if you want to. Lunge them or ride them to warm them up.

TETHERING

In many countries of the world all sorts of horses, even Thoroughbreds, are regularly tethered.

This practice is potentially dangerous when the animal is first tethered as it can panic if the rope gets caught round a hind pastern. The horse backs up because of the pull on its head and its hind leg is then drawn forward toward its head which is being dragged downwards by the pull from its hind leg.

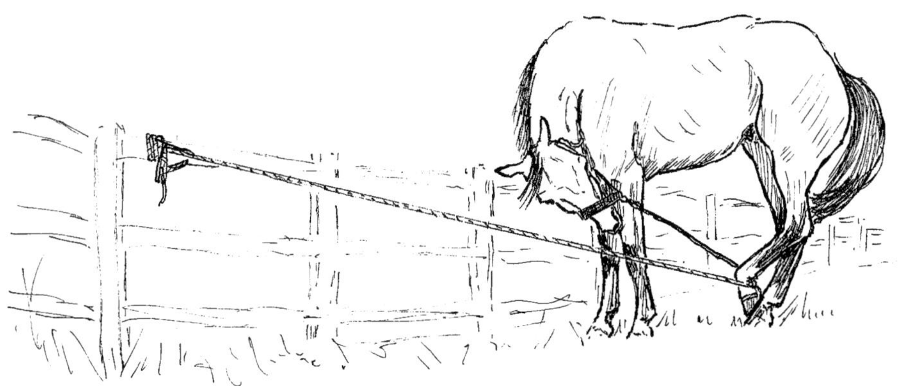

This pony has become hung up because the rope is attached too high.

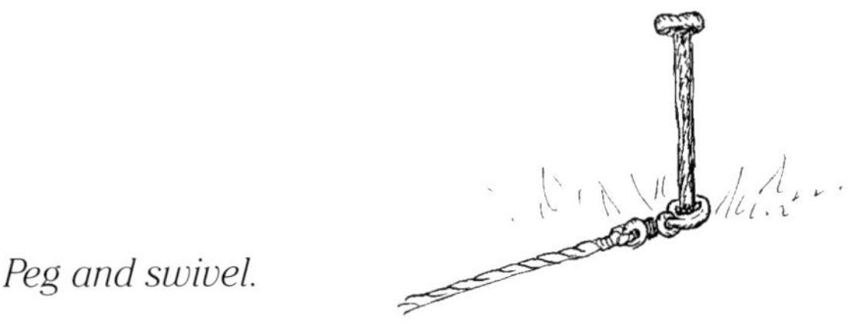

Peg and swivel.

Accustom the horse to the feel of lunge reins or ropes round its hind pasterns. Give a gentle pull so that it gets used to the feel of the pressure there. Keep the lunge rein or rope very low to the ground and slacken it if the horse picks its hind foot up, so that it will learn how to step out of the loop restricting it.

Bandage both hind pasterns with tail bandages to protect them from rope gall if the horse does get tangled and pulls hard. Use a very thick, soft rope, at least 4 cm (1½ in) in diameter, or a thick chain. The weight of this will keep the tether near the ground and the thickness will help to prevent injury to the legs.

There should be two swivels, one near the headcollar and one near the end of the rope or chain. If the animal starts off by being tethered to a post or stake in the middle of an open area, it is more likely to go round and round in circles and get tangled up.

Fix the rope securely to a hedge or fence at ground level so that the horse has only half a circle to move in. Stay with the animal until you are certain that it knows how to pick its feet up to avoid becoming entangled. An intelligent animal learns very quickly. When you first tether an animal, you will know immediately by its reaction whether it has ever been tethered before.

Note the following rules when tethering.

- The tether should be at least three times the length of the animal's body. The longer the tether, the less likely the horse is to get tangled up.
- The tether should always be fixed at ground level to minimise the chances of legs getting caught.
- There should be two swivels.
- No roots, branches, shrubs or thick clumps of weed should be within the tether area as the rope or chain will soon get wrapped round these as the horse circles. It will then be left unable to move or graze and be fixed on a very short length of rope or chain.
- Water buckets, preferably without handles for the tether to get entangled in, should be placed on the outside edge of the tethering area up against the hedge or fence. (They can be tied in place.) Make sure the horse can reach the water but that the tether cannot get around the bucket.
- Stay with an animal that is unused to being tethered.
- Even when it is used to being tethered, check very frequently to see that all is well.
- A horse cannot move about to keep warm when tethered. Even if tied to a hedge there is shelter from only one direction and that may not be where the wind or rain is coming from.
- Do not leave animals tethered at night.
- If more than one animal is tethered, make sure that they are far enough apart not to get tangled up with each other.
- Never tether one animal when there are others loose in the same area as they can get caught in the tether.

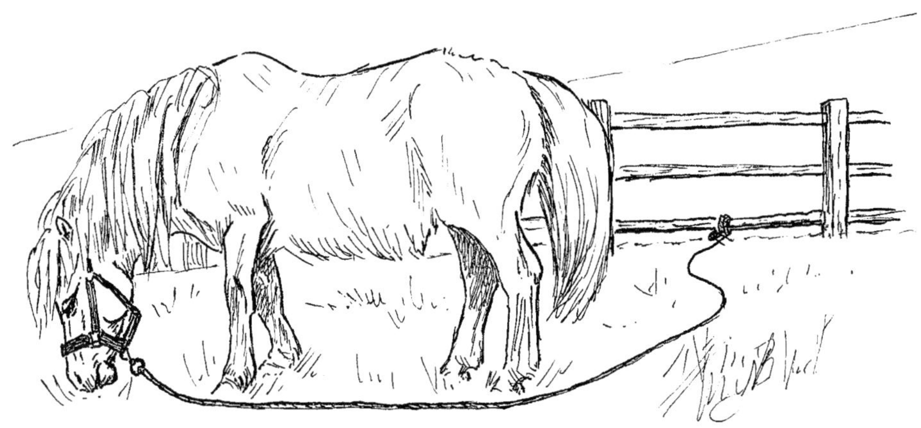

The tether is attached at a low point but is in the centre of the rail – its weakest point. It would be safer tied around the very bottom of the upright post. There should be two swivels – one at each end.

- If tethering in the open so that the horse has a full circle, use a long, strong stake hammered into the ground. It should have a swivel attached to it or a metal ring large enough to move freely round the stake when the tether is attached to it.
- The animal should be moved on to a fresh area of grass every day.
- A tethered animal needs regular exercise as it cannot exercise itself when tethered as it would loose in a field.
- Remember that if an animal is tethered near a public place there is the danger that people may feed it unsuitable foods, try to get on it, tease it or throw things at it. Dogs may chase it round and round.
- In the UK there is a law against 'cruel or illegal tethering'. Any member of the public who thinks, rightly or wrongly, that your horse or pony is in distress, may inform the police or RSPCA.

THE HORSE IN THE STABLE

BEHAVIOURAL PROBLEMS

Lack of exercise

Lack of exercise can cause a horse to be too lively for its rider. It may give cheerful bucks which are not always enjoyed by the rider; it may be stupidly spooky from overfreshness, shooting sideways or whipping round at a tiny bird or an odd-coloured leaf – any excuse to have fun will do. This will most probably start as exuberance but if the horse learns that the rider wobbles, clutches or cannot control it, it will soon learn to be deliberately naughty and, in no time, a bad or even dangerous habit is formed.

If you were kept shut up in a small loose box for 23 out of 24 hours, wouldn't you be overjoyed to get out? You might even leap about and shriek, 'Whoopee!'. Some people only exercise their horses every other day or only at weekends even when they are stabled all the time. You cannot blame any horse for misbehaving under these circumstances. Stabled horses need to be exercised – and not just an hour's wandering about! – but really exercised for at least an hour every day. A rest day is just a day of boredom if the horse is shut in all the time. If you cannot exercise your horse every day, it must be turned out in a field for all or at least half of every day.

You are going to have problems with most horses, especially active young horses, if you cannot give the horse daily exercise or daily freedom in a field. It is far better not to buy a horse unless you can fulfil these conditions.

Being shut in not only makes a horse overfresh, it makes it bored, so an intelligent horse looks for occupation such as chewing the wooden parts of the stable which can lead to crib-biting (see page 33). It may walk round and round the box until this becomes a habit. Have you ever seen caged zoo animals doing this? (See Box Walking, page 31.)

Swinging its head from side to side (see Weaving, page 35) and banging the stable door (see page 31), which will soon give it a big swollen knee, can all start from being shut in a stable too much.

Lack of exercise causes far more problems than too much work!

Banging the stable door

This can be caused by boredom, waiting for a feed, excitement, frustration or lack of company. Try not to leave this horse in the stable for longer than absolutely necessary. Another horse stabled within sight may help. A horse which continually bangs its knees on the stable door may cause them to swell up. Put a bar on the inside of the door, if necessary thickly padded, so that the horse cannot get its chest near enough to the door to bang its knees. Pad the inside of the door panel with something soft, such as straw-filled sacks or a rubber panel, to prevent injury to the knees. Do not use prickly things like gorse which will hurt the horse and may cause an infected cut if a thorn end breaks off in the skin.

Box walking

This is a nervous habit. This horse just cannot rest and settle. Its mind is in turmoil.

The condition can be temporary, for instance if the horse is put in a new stable; if a new horse arrives in the yard; if a companion goes; if there have been strange, exciting noises; if hounds have been hunting nearby; if the horse has been hunting or to a competition. In a few days the horse will probably settle down again but is likely always to be a restless type, taking a mouthful of hay or a mouthful of feed then walking to look out of the door.

A true box walker will tramp round and round the box non-stop, just snatching a mouthful of food or hay in passing. It wears its nerves and body to a frazzle and will not perform to the best of its potential ability for this reason.

Horses with this sort of temperament are best turned out as much as possible with a quiet, steady companion. Often, they will only relax in the field. They will do better if their lives are kept to a regular pattern and timetable.

If the horse is turned out by day with a quiet companion, it should also be kept in the nextdoor stable at night, preferably with only a low division between them so that the companion is always in sight.

If it is impossible to turn the horse out in a field, it should be kept in a large, open yard or in a loose box with a yard in front, somewhere where there is space, a feeling of some freedom and an interesting view to occupy its mind. It may be possible to lead it out to some grass.

Two shorter periods of exercise per day instead of one long one can help to occupy an overactive mind.

A small animal, such as a sheep or a goat, could live with the horse. The advantage of a small companion is that it can live in the same loose box and travel everywhere with the horse more easily.

Feed the horse a little at a time and very often, to occupy its mind. If it will only pick at food during the day, you may find it will eat up during the night, so arrange your feeds accordingly.

Pawing

If a horse is constantly pawing it is either uncomfortable or it wants something.

Discomfort may be caused by colic pains. If the horse is rugged up, it may be too hot or the rugs may be irritating its skin. The roller or surcingle may be too tight. The front of the rug may be too tight and restricting the horse when it tries to eat from the ground. It may have toothache.

The horse may want more food, more water, more exercise or it may resent being stabled and want to get out. It may dislike being alone and want the company of another horse. It may be bored stiff, shut up in a stable for too many hours per day. It may paw because it has seen another horse being taken out of its stable and it wants to go out too.

Some horses will paw when feeding, perhaps in an attempt to get the food down quicker!

If, in pawing, a horse bangs its knee on anything hard, such as a door or manger, it can permanently damage the knee. You must take precautions to prevent this happening (see Banging, page 31). Try to discover and deal with the reason for pawing.

Chewing

Some horses never grow out of the habit of chewing anything within reach.

If your horse chews through halter ropes when tied up, you must use a chain. Use a fairly thick, smooth chain as a thin, sharp one may cut the horse's mouth if it takes hold of it and pulls back.

Catching the reins in its mouth when you are leading it is an infuriating habit in a horse. Be very alert and give the horse a little thump on the lips with your fist as it begins to think of catching the reins. Do this every time so that the horse never gets away with it.

Catching a running martingale in the mouth is a dangerous habit as the martingale can get caught across the mouth, tying the horse's head down. A horse in this position will often panic, run backwards, lose its balance and fall over backwards. If this should happen when you are on a horse, dismount quickly and undo the girth to release the pull on the horse's mouth. You should now be able to get the martingale out of the mouth quite easily.

To prevent this from happening, use a bib martingale which has a solid piece of leather filling in the space between the divided straps carrying the rings.

A gelding grabbing at a martingale could get one of the rings caught round a tush (one of the four extra teeth found between the incisors and molars in male horses). Dismount immediately and undo the girth to release the tension.

Chewing wood in the stable can lead to crib-biting so paint any places the horse is likely to chew with creosote and, if necessary, also dab on some mustard.

Catching the cheeks of a cheeked snaffle or a curb bit in the mouth can sometimes be prevented by using ordinary circular rubber bit guards. If this fails, longer, oval pieces of stiff leather, cut to the shape and size you need, can be used. This habit can be caused by using a bit that is too narrow, so that the cheeks are pressing on the lips.

Chewing at rugs, see Rug Tearing page 105.

Crib-biting

Many horses bite wood, the top of the stable door, the manger or posts and rails in the field. This is not crib-biting. This habit is only so called when the horse bites something with its teeth, arches its neck and actually swallows air, often making a grunting sound. The large amount of air that is taken into the stomach can give the horse a pot-bellied look and can cause indigestion. If the horse is crib-biting in the field, other horses may come up to see what it is doing because they think it is eating something. These horses may also start to bite wood and will eventually also learn to swallow air. Horses which crib-bite are nearly always tense, highly strung, worried individuals, rather like people who bite their nails. Boredom alone does not often cause crib-biting but tension does. Keeping a horse out or turning a horse out every day, working it

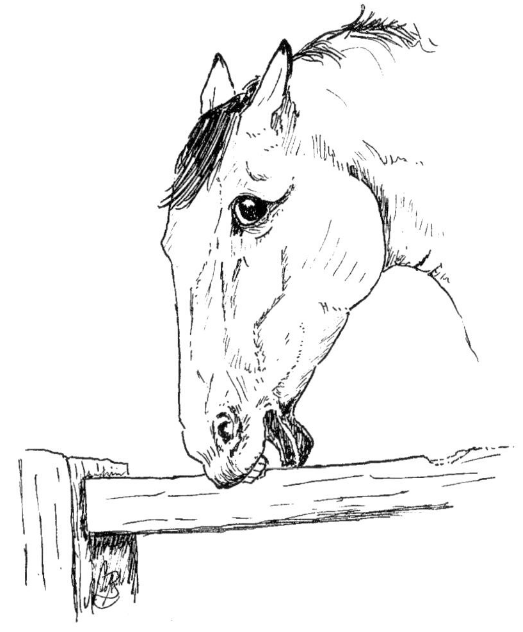

Crib-biting.

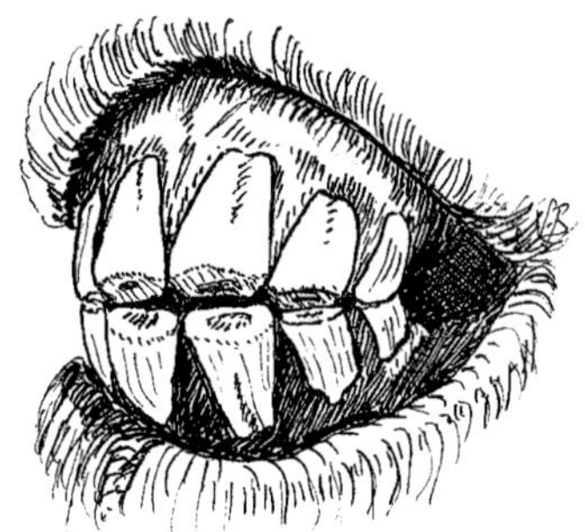

The worn teeth of a crib-biter.

twice a day, trying to keep it relaxed and happy in its work and calm and quiet when you handle it will all help mentally. Putting a cribbing collar on may stop it crib-biting but the tension will now be much more difficult to endure because you have removed the only method the horse had of relieving that tension. It is now likely to become even more screwed up mentally.

Methods of prevention, which can also be used for windsuckers (see page 36), include:

- A collar with a hard U-shaped piece which fits closely round the gullet and prevents air from being swallowed.
- A collar with a shield-shaped piece of hard material with a pointed end which is worn towards the throat so that when the horse arches its neck to swallow air, the sharp part sticks painfully into its throat.
- A collar with a double layer of metal with holes in the inside layer and spikes in the arched outside layer. As the horse arches its neck, so

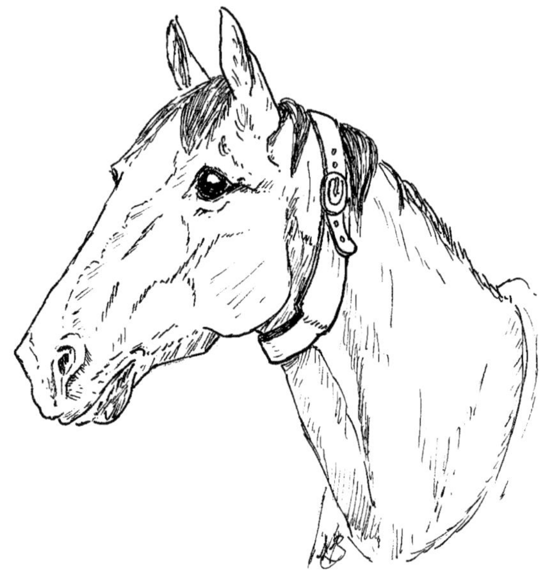

A collar worn to prevent crib-biting or windsucking.

increasing the size of it, to swallow air, the spikes come up through the holes and prick its throat area.

- A flute bit. This is an open-ended tubular bit with holes in so that the horse is unable to form a seal with its lips and therefore cannot swallow air.
- An operation to the muscles of the neck, making it impossible for the horse to arch its neck and swallow air.
- A hole the size of a 5p piece cut above and behind the corner of the mouth so that the horse cannot form a seal and swallow air.
- Electric fencing on every possible surface in the field.
- Electric fencing on every possible surface in the stable.

NB: electric fencing is no use for windsuckers who swallow air without getting hold of anything.

Weaving

Weaving is the name given to the action of constantly swinging the head and neck from side to side, usually over the stable door. Horses weave for a variety of reasons, including boredom, tension, frustration, loneliness, excitement, anticipation and fear.

They rarely weave when turned out in a field, although some will stand at the field gate weaving when they think it is time to come in. Sometimes keeping the horse in an open yard, preferably with company, will stop it weaving. Hanging rounded-edged bricks on string above the stable door so that they hit the horse's head if it weaves has been tried and works with some horses. Narrow, upright bars or V-shaped bars which fit above the stable door can be bought. The horse can still look out but cannot weave. Some horses will, however, then weave in the inside corner of the loose box.

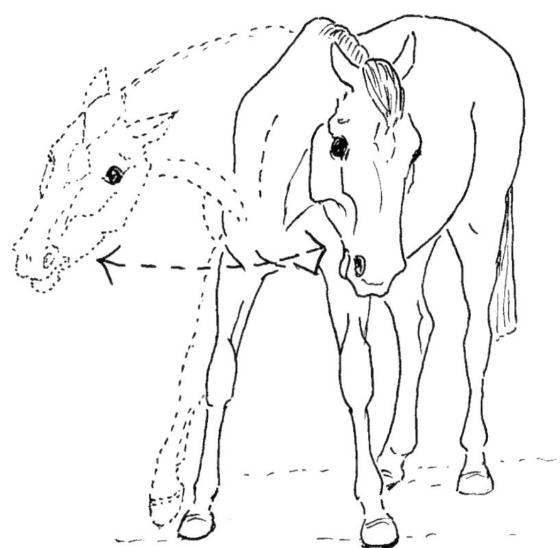

Weaving.

Weaving tires the horse. It can wear its shoes down and the stable floor too. It can also cause damage to the joints in its forelegs.

A change of stable or owner can trigger off weaving, in which case it may cease when the horse has settled, but a long-term weaver is unlikely to be permanently cured.

Some horses which weave will not travel quietly in the normal width of a padded horse box stall because there is no room to weave. They may really throw themselves about here but will then travel quietly, though weaving away, in a double section.

Horses sold in sales which are weavers must be declared as such. A horse can only be returned to a sale with the complaint that it is a weaver if it actually picks up and puts down each foreleg in turn as it weaves. If it stands square on both forelegs and just swings its head and neck from side to side, it is not returnable.

Windsucking

This vice is similar to crib-biting except that the horse swallows air without getting hold of anything with the teeth. (See pages 33 and 34 for causes and preventions.)

Never lying down

Some horses will not lie down in a strange stable.

A horse's main defence is speed in running away from danger, so when it is lying down it is at its most vulnerable.

A horse will only lie down if it feels relaxed and safe. Some horses only feel safe enough to lie down when they are out in the field and will never lie down in a stable.

It is important that horses do lie down as it is the only way that they can rest all their legs at the same time.

A horse may not lie down if it tried this and found the floor slippery so that it had difficulty in getting up again. In this case:

- Put sand or gravel down under a much deeper bed than usual.
- Put down another layer of concrete and mark grooves in it while it is setting.
- With a hammer and chisel, rough up the floor (wear goggles to protect your eyes).

Keeping the horse in a big cow yard instead of a normal-sized loose box will often encourage it to lie down.

Always talk to your horse as you approach the stable so that if it is lying down it will not suddenly leap to its feet in fright when surprised by your silent appearance.

GETTING CAST

Some horses happily roll right over when out in the field but are very careful not to do so in the stable. There they roll on one side, get up and then go down again and roll on the other side. These horses are either naturally cautious or they have been cast when rolling over in the stable and have learnt not to risk doing this again.

Other horses constantly roll right over in the stable, regularly get cast and never learn not to do it. They are a real worry to their owners as they can hurt themselves badly.

An anti-cast roller with a high, hooped metal arch will stop most horses rolling right over. A very agile horse may succeed in rolling over when wearing one, however, in which case, if the horse is now near the wall, the arch can prevent it rolling back again so that it is unable to get to its feet.

The other disadvantage of this type of roller is that unless it is very carefully fitted and well padded, it can give a horse a sore back by inward pressure on each side of the withers.

To help the horse to get up more easily, bedding can be banked up all round against the walls of the box.

Wooden bars can be fixed on all round the walls of the box, to a height of approximately 1 m (3 ft 6 in) from the ground and 30 cm (1 ft) apart. These will give the horse's feet something to push against to help it to get up.

If you find a horse cast, go and get help. It is almost impossible for one person alone to get a horse up. If possible, put a headcollar on the horse.

Get two ropes or lunge lines and form a running loop at one end of each line or rope. Put the loops on the front and hind pasterns of the legs which are nearer to the wall. Pull firmly and strongly on both ropes at once to roll the horse over. As it comes over, let go of both ropes and hold the headcollar rope. When the horse stands up, remove the leg ropes.

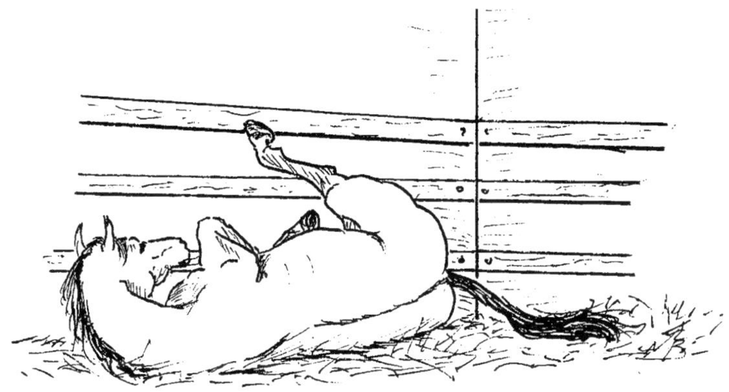

Cast horse using bars to help it get up.

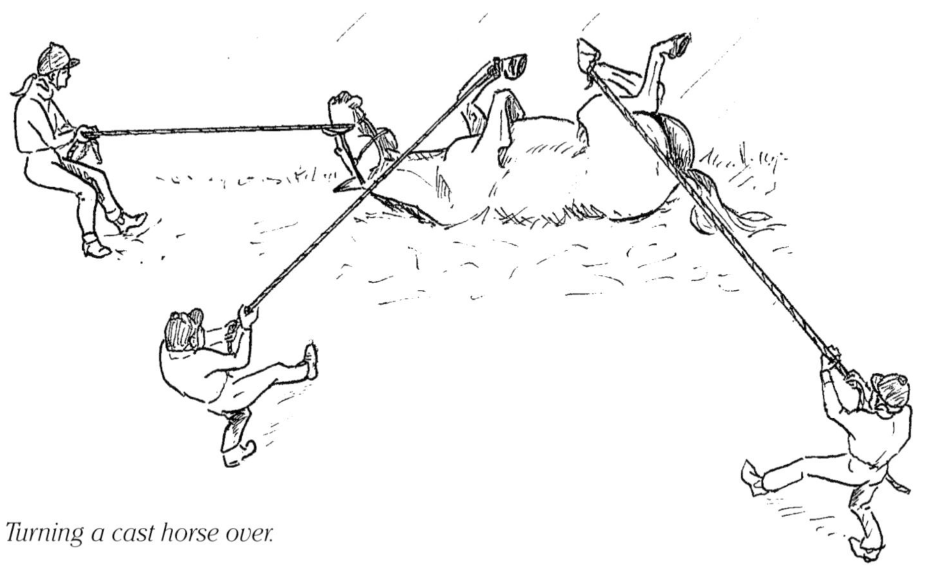

Turning a cast horse over.

A third person to control the horse's head with a headcollar and rope is ideal but if they are not available be aware that the horse's neck and head can be damaged if they are twisted unnaturally when you pull on the leg ropes and as the horse turns over.

If you put the ropes on the legs nearer to you (the ones further away from the wall) you will 'open the horse up' (pull its legs apart) and may hurt it. If you put one rope round both forelegs and the other round both hind legs, the horse will not be able to stand up after you have rolled it over.

The horse may be sweating and shaking with fright when it is on its feet again. It may be in shock. It may be in pain. Examine it for cuts to legs, head or eyes. See if it moves freely round the stable, can turn easily in both directions, move its head and neck in both directions and get its head down to eat off the ground. When you next ride it, see if it feels as comfortable as usual on turns and in all gaits. Listen to its hoof beats. Are they in a regular four-time beat in walk and regular two-time beat in trot? If you have any doubts get a registered equine chiropractor to check your horse's back.

FEEDING PROBLEMS

Overfeeding

Do not overfeed. More problems are caused by this than almost anything. An overfed horse, jumping out of its skin, is going to learn bad habits, do silly things and frighten its rider (who will then probably overshorten the reins and hang on to the horse, making it hot up or nap).

A new horse, or a horse that has just been brought into work after a rest, wants just as much good hay as it can eat and a double handful of horse or pony nuts twice a day. If it is turned out to grass during the day, this will help to keep it sensible. If the horse or pony is very fat or gets laminitis, ration the amount of grass and hay it gets but do not leave it with nothing to eat for more than four or five hours. Instead, offer clean wheat straw which has little food value but provides bulk so that there is still something in the horse's gut. In the horse's normal way of life the gut is never empty and if it is allowed to be so for long periods, the animal may develop a twisted gut which is nearly always fatal.

Increase the amount of feed you give the horse gradually and feed according to its body condition, age and temperament, the work it is going to do and your own riding ability.

Really fussy feeders need extra thought and care. Could the problem be sharp teeth? (See Quidding, page 44.)

The overweight horse

An overweight horse is putting extra strain on its legs, feet, muscles, tendons, ligaments and heart.

Its feed or grazing must be rationed and it must be worked in walk for gradually increasing periods of time.

It may develop:

- laminitis (see page 144);
- girth galls (see page 128);
- scalded back (see page 127).

Its legs are likely to swell and it may get windgalls (puffiness above the fetlock joints). A very fat horse is going to need at least eight weeks of slow, steady work and may take twelve weeks or more to be fit for fast, hard work.

The overweight horse will be shorter-striding than normal because the bulges of fat will restrict the movement of its shoulders. It will waddle along and may be so fat that it is difficult to keep the saddle in place and it may slip to one side.

As it gets slimmer, the same saddle may no longer fit the horse. If you have bought a very fat horse you may be pleasantly surprised to find that, when slim and fit, the horse is a far better ride than you expected. Don't do too much too soon, however, or you may do permanent damage.

If you only use your horse for half the year and it is your practice to turn it out in the field for six months, take precautions to see that it does not get too fat. Some horses just blow up like balloons on grass. This is bad for them and it takes ages to get them fit again.

Possible plans of action include:

- Turn the horse out in a small paddock.
- Turn it out for a few hours each day.
- Ration its grazing with an electric fence (see page 23).
- Keep it in a big yard and give it a ration of hay.

- Turn it out on rough, poor, hilly land where it will have to search for grass and walk up- and downhill as it does so.
- Arrange for someone to ride it regularly three or four times a week.

Your horse will have a longer working life and stay sounder if you do not let it get too fat.

The thin horse

Is the food kept in clean bins where no mice, rats, hens, dogs or cats can get in? Was the food clean and sweet smelling when you bought it? Is the manger/feed bin very clean? Is the hay clean, sweet smelling and a greenish-yellow colour – not dusty or mouldy even in part of the bale?

Some horses will not eat because of their excitable temperament (see Box Walking, page 31). Others just do not seem to be interested in eating so you have to tempt them. Give very small feeds, very often, add grated carrot, grass chopped up small and well mixed in, grated apple (grated because many horses are clever enough to pick out the bigger pieces and still leave the feed), black treacle, herbs, garlic, etc. You have to find out what appeals to your horse.

If your horse eats well but loses weight, or is thin and does not put on weight, take a sample of droppings to your vet and get a worm count done. Even if you have always wormed the horse regularly, this extra check up is still necessary. If worms are not the problem, get the vet to do a blood test to see if the horse is anaemic.

The field-kept horse

Normally there is very little food value in grass by September in the UK so you may need to start feeding hay or giving a hard feed as early as this if your horse is losing weight.

Patches of long, lush, green grass surrounded by areas of grass eaten right down to the ground do not mean that your horse still has plenty of grass to eat. The long green patches are where horses have dunged and they will starve before they will eat this grass.

If your horse lives out, some of its food will be used up in keeping it warm so a sheltered field, and a New Zealand rug if the horse is well bred and therefore fine-coated, or partly clipped, will help to keep condition on it.

Hay

Meadow hay is made from permanent pasture and is softer and finer than seed hay. It contains a large variety of natural grasses and herbs and, for this reason, many animals prefer it.

Seed hay is sown as a crop and can be a one-year, two-year or three-year ley.

(A ley is the length of time the field will be kept in grass before being ploughed and cultivated to grow cereals.) By the second year some natural grasses will be present and in the third year more still.

Horses working hard or fast, such as racehorses, are usually fed seed hay because it should be higher in protein and less dusty than meadow hay.

The most important points to note about hay are:

- When it was cut. Hay needs to be cut early in the year so that the seeds are still in the grasses, because they contain protein.
- It will be more palatable and higher in protein if it has had no rain on it between cutting, baling and getting it under cover.
- The hay should feel loose and move easily within the bale. Very heavy bales containing hard, immovable hay may have been damp. Sometimes this is from rain, sometimes because they have been baled too quickly while the grass was green and full of sap. The centre of the bale may be caked hard, blackish in colour and quite inedible or there may be patches of white mould which will seriously damage a horse's lungs.
- When you push your hand deep into a bale and pull out a small sample of hay, it should be a greenish colour (meadow hay) or lighter yellowish colour (seed hay) and look bright and shiny. It should smell sweet and clean and there should be no dust.

Haynets

Many haynets, particularly those put out in fields, hang dangerously low when empty. Many animals will paw at an empty net in the vain hope of getting more hay out of it. In so doing, they may get a foot stuck in it and injure themselves.

In a stable, tie the haynet up as high as possible, passing the string through the very bottom of the net before pulling it up again as tight and high as possible. When empty, it will then hang in a U-shaped loop well clear of the ground.

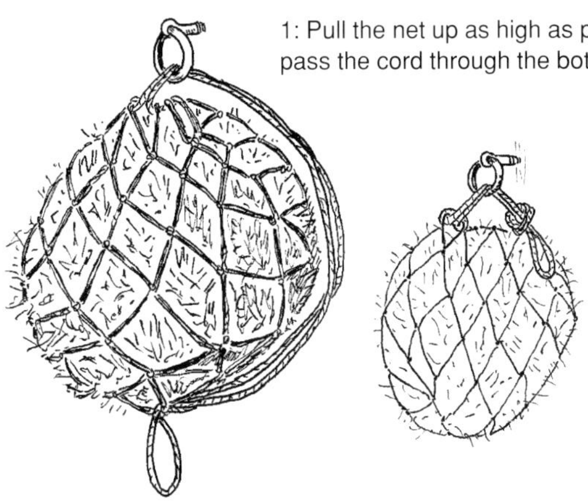

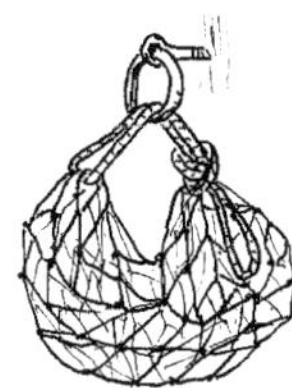

Tying up a haynet.

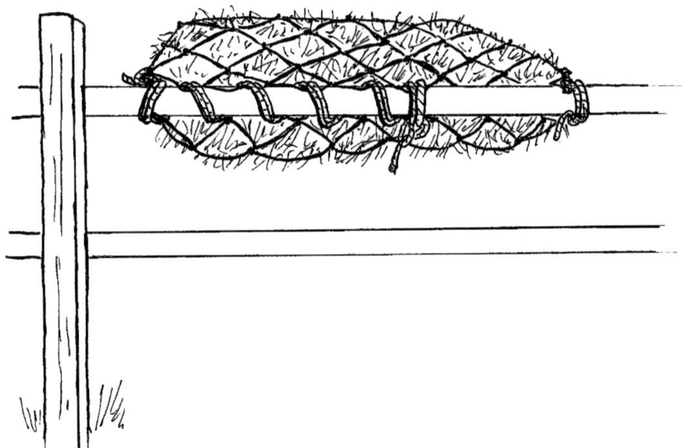

A hay net 'laced' to the top tail of a fence so that it will not hang down dangerously when empty.

In a field it is often very difficult to find anywhere high enough to tie a haynet, so it is often tied to the top rail of a wooden fence. It looks high enough when full but it will be very near the ground when empty. To make it safer, tie the top end of the net as high as possible on the fence using its own string. Attach a second piece of string to the bottom of the net and pull this end up as high as possible, using the remainder of the string to 'lace' the middle of the net on to the top rail before tying the string safely. Tied in this way the net cannot sag on to the ground when empty.

Perhaps there is a tree branch well out of reach to which you would like to tie your haynet. Get a stone or a fairly heavy, small piece of wood and attach a long, lightweight piece of string to it. Throw this weight up and over the branch and then use the light string to pull a heavier piece of rope over the branch. You can then tie your haynet to the rope at a safe height.

If several horses are given hay in nets in the same field, the nets should be tied well apart. There should always be one or two more nets than there are horses so that the weaker characters will get their share of food.

Making a haynet

Haynets are very easy to make if you have a large supply of baling twine or have kept the twine you cut off your bales of hay or straw. (Hint: cut beside the knot.)

Take 20–24 full-length pieces of twine (less for a smaller net but always an even number). Arrange all the knots together, level, at the top and make one enormous single knot with them all. Pull each string very tight individually. Thread a piece of string through below the knot so that you have eleven or twelve pieces on each side of it and use this string to tie them up approximately at eye level. Take one pair of the pieces of twine and knot them

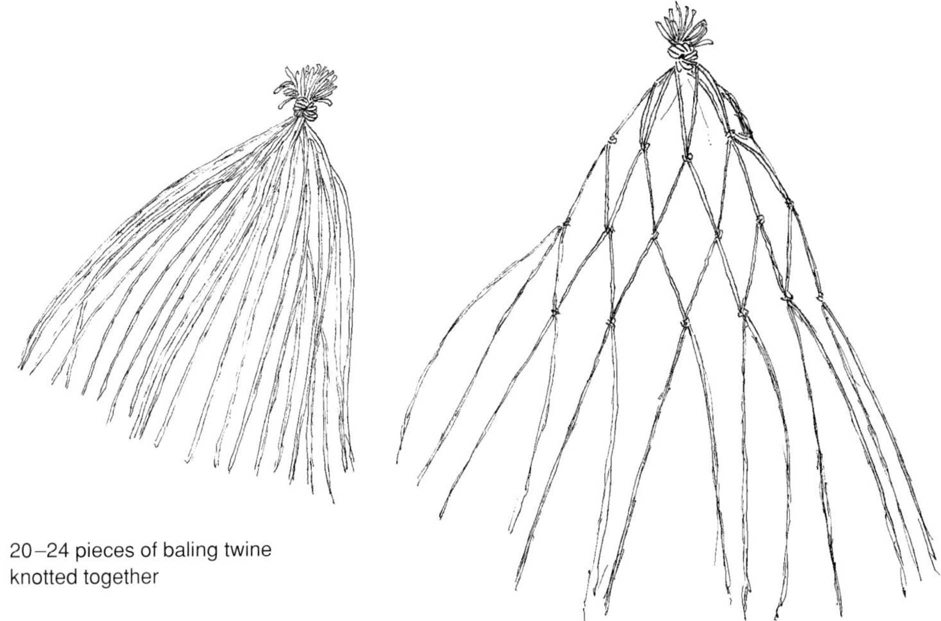

20–24 pieces of baling twine
knotted together

Knot pairs together to form 'diamonds'. To finish off, trim the
ends level and thread cord through

Making a haynet.

together with a single knot 10–12.5 cm (4–5 in) below your large central knot.
Continue knotting pairs all the way round, keeping the knots at the same level,
until you have a circle of eleven or twelve knots. Now (being careful to keep
the circle open and not join any pieces across it) take one string from one
knot and one from the knot next to it and knot this pair together 10–12.5 cm
(4–5 in) below the top layer. You will see that you have now formed a
diamond shape. Continue in this way, row after row, keeping the 'diamonds'
the same size and the rows of knots neat and level. Tighten each knot after you
have made it.

When you have made the last possible row of knots (leaving about 10 cm or
4 in of unused twine beyond them), tighten these last knots extra strongly and
trim off all the ends to a level 10 cm (4 in).

To make the cord to thread through, take three lengths of baling twine. At
least one should be of a different colour to the net, if possible, so that it will be
easy to find the cord when you are filling the net. Knot one end and plait the
three strings, putting another knot at the bottom end. Thread your plait in and
out through the top diamonds of your haynet and knot the two ends securely
together.

Warning: if you simply pull the loops of baling twine off your bales of hay or
straw without cutting them open and then leave them lying about the field or

stable, a horse could get one hind and one front foot caught in the same loop, with disastrous consequences.

Quidding

If a horse chews its hay two or three times then starts to spit partly chewed wodges out, suspect that it may have sharp teeth. The discomfort is more obvious when a horse is eating hay than when eating hard feed but the same pattern of spitting out partly chewed food may also be seen then. Ask a vet, or a reputable horse dentist, to check the horse's teeth and rasp any sharp edges off.

Because the horse's upper jaw is wider than its lower jaw and it chews with a sideways motion, the outside edge of the teeth in the upper jaw do not rub against anything to wear them down. They can become razor sharp and will cut the insides of the horse's cheeks when it tries to chew.

The same applies to the inside edges of the teeth in the bottom jaw, which can make the tongue sore if they are sharp. The top teeth, however, cause trouble far more often. All horses' teeth should be checked once a year, even youngsters'.

Throwing food out of the manger

This habit wastes a lot of food. Two large, rounded stones placed in the manger may help.

A manger with an inward-curved lip all round it, or one with a bar set across it a few inches in from each end may be used.

Droppings

All horses' droppings vary in consistency according to what they are eating. If you look at the droppings of eight horses all fed in the same way, their consistency will vary enormously too. Learn to recognise the normal state of your horse's droppings, then you will notice if there is a problem.

Scouring

Looser, more runny droppings can be caused by wet grass, a move on to richer grass, excitement, a chill, new hay, a lot of sugar beet or too much protein. If caused by excitement or wet grass, for instance after heavy rain, the condition should clear up on its own in 24 hours or so. If the cause is a field with very rich grass, beware of the horse developing laminitis (see page 144). If the scouring continues for more than 48 hours, ration the grazing hours in that field and feed some hay or clean straw to provide more solid bulk.

If the horse is stabled and fed sugar beet or carrots, cut them out of the diet and see if that helps. Feed less protein and more hay and offer clean straw. If the horse continues to scour badly, call the vet.

Constipation

Firmer, harder droppings than usual can be caused by the horse not drinking enough water, being fed food which absorbs a lot of moisture, such as a complete feed or horse and pony nuts or by a change from being out at grass all the time to being stabled all the time.

Make sure the horse's water bucket or trough is really clean. Refill the bucket several times a day and clean out the bucket daily. Many horses prefer to drink from a trough in the field and will hardly touch water in a bucket in the stable. A constipated horse must be encouraged to drink, so lead your horse out to a clean trough or stream and see if it will drink there. If it does so, continue to offer it water there at least twice a day.

Feed soaked sugar beet regularly every day and also carrots. Give the horse a bran mash. Put 1.4 kg (3 lb) bran in a bucket and pour on boiling water until it is all moist but not sloppy. Cover it with a clean sack or piece of blanket and leave it to steam for two to three hours. Feed when just warm. If necessary, continue to give a bran mash three times a week. If you have been feeding horse and pony nuts or any other form of nut, either change to an equivalent coarse mix or soak the nuts for twelve hours so that they will absorb a lot of moisture before the horse eats them instead of soaking up moisture once inside the horse.

Know the number of droppings your horse usually does overnight when stabled and notice if there are fewer than usual. No droppings may mean a stoppage which could be very serious, so notice as soon as there is a real difference in the number of droppings or their consistency and do something about it.

You can tell how a new horse has been kept and fed by the state of its droppings. The droppings of horses eating mainly grass are dark green, soft and of very fine texture. Fully stabled horses' droppings are firmer, yellowish-brown and much coarser in texture, the actual stalks of hay often being visible. Undigested cereals can sometimes also be seen in the droppings. If sharp teeth are making it painful for the horse to chew, this could cause a problem (see Quidding, page 44).

Feeding too much protein (more than the horse can digest) often produces yellow droppings with a foul smell.

A stabled horse's droppings should be moist and some should break when they fall. Some horses constantly produce dry droppings, which is a worry to their owners.

Hard, dry droppings can become impacted inside the horse, so try to improve the situation naturally. Perhaps the horse is not drinking very much. Here again, the quantity each animal drinks varies enormously and bears little relation to body size. To encourage the horse to drink more, make sure that all water containers are clean and regularly refilled with fresh water. Immerse the hay in water before feeding it or pour a bucket of water over it. It is surprising how much moisture hay will absorb.

Turn the horse out on to good, edible grass every day. Feed sugar beet pulp at every feed and add extra water to it. Feed carrots or swedes.

These natural methods should improve the state of your horse's droppings. If you are at all worried or there is a sudden change, call the vet.

BAD MANNERS

Biting

There are several reasons for a horse biting you.
- Fear: the horse associates people with something frightening or painful and it is trying to make you keep your distance.
- Tension: biting is a quick, often unthinking reaction to something or someone different.
- Greed: the horse has constantly been fed titbits and is annoyed because you have not got any for it this time.
- Aggression: the horse is a bully and wants to put you in your place. It has found that people are frightened and will retreat if it lays its ears back and snaps at them.
- You are grooming tickly places or tightening the girth without due care and thought.

If fear, tension or aggression is the problem with your horse, take a scoop containing a handful of nuts or coarse mix when you go into the stable so that a fearful or tense horse will gain confidence in you and an aggressive horse will be pleased to see you. As soon as the problem has been overcome, gradually cease to offer the food.

If greed is the problem, never feed titbits (unless it is essential, as when catching the horse in the field). Leave a headcollar on the horse. When you go into the stable try to get hold of the headcollar and immediately rub and scratch the horse's forehead, behind its ears or along its withers and crest – wherever your horse shows that it enjoys this attention. (Do note, however, the dangers of leaving headcollars on in the stable, page 23.)

It is always safer to tie a horse up when working in a stable or grooming. This is especially true with a horse which bites or kicks.

Kicking in the stable

This habit involves two main groups – the aggressive horse and the timid horse.
1 The aggressive or bossy horse wants to put you in your place and show that it is in charge. If it is eating, it wants to keep you away from its food. If you have just fed it and are walking out of the stable past it, it may kick out to

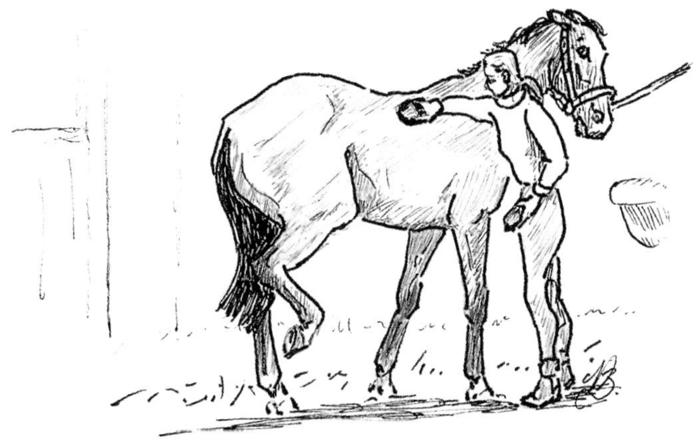

If a horse tries to kick when being groomed, tie it up short and stand close to its shoulder.

make sure you go away quickly and do not return to take some of its food.

If you show you are frightened of a horse of this type, it will get worse and may well start to bully you, chase you out of the stable or try to corner you. Feed it near the door or have a removable manger to fix on the door. Feed it and go away.

When dealing with the horse in the stable, you will have to try to overcome your fear, which is easier said than done! Horses know by the way you approach them whether you are frightened or not. They fully understand body language in other horses and in people. It will be necessary to convince the horse that you are not frightened of it by looking it in the eye and moving towards it with confidence, with shoulders squared towards it, not creeping in sideways in a submissive attitude. Talk to it firmly – don't shriek at it (this is a sign of nervousness). Tie it up when you go into the stable.

A horse which is aggressive and bossy with one person may show no signs of such behaviour when a person of a stronger character approaches it showing no signs of nervousness. If you are frightened of your horse in the stable, it will know that you are and may well also take advantage of you when you ride it.

2 The nervous horse may have been badly treated in the past and may shoot into a corner, literally shaking with fright, if you approach it in the stable. It may put its head into a corner as far away from you as possible and turn its hindquarters towards you, moving them from one side to the other to prevent you from getting to its head. Some young horses which have not been handled much will also behave in this way. They are unsure of what is going to happen next and their heels are their defence.

Horses which have been badly treated will do everything they can to prevent you from getting near to them because they think you are going to hit, hurt or frighten them.

Spend as much time as you can in a corner of the stable near the door, squatting down low with your shoulders sideways on to the horse. This is a submissive attitude and the horse may begin to think that you are not going to hurt it. Do not look this horse in the eye. Talk quietly and constantly and place a scoop of coarse mix near enough to the horse to tempt it to investigate. Do not move if the horse comes towards it or eats it. Repeat these actions every time you go into the stable and gradually see if the horse will allow you to touch it and scratch it. Gradually and carefully, scratch and rub towards its neck and head. Always take some favourite titbit for it until it comes to you with confidence, then cut down on the titbits and reward it with a scratch or rub only. Never give titbits for no special reason as horses get pushy and may even nip when they find you have nothing for them.

Cow kicking

This is the name given to the kind of kick which comes forward at you; for instance when you are grooming a ticklish horse's tummy and the kick is aimed at your head. Horses will also kick forward at the clippers if they are ticklish around their tummy, elbows or near their stifle so, if using electric clippers with a lead attached to the mains, great care must be taken to ensure that a cow-kicking horse does not get a foot over the cable and tug the clippers out of your hand when being clipped. The type of clipper which works from a 12-volt battery strapped to your waist and has a short lead, working like a coiled spring, is safest for clipping a kicking horse. Many difficult horses are far quieter when clipped with this lower-voltage type of clipper.

Cow kicking at you is far more dangerous because the horse brings its hind leg forward under its tummy, swings it out sideways then forcefully backwards. It deliberately aims at you and gets you on the backward swing which is very powerful. To groom a horse that cow kicks, tie it up and have a second rope on the headcollar on the side D-ring nearer to you. If you are on the near (left) side of the horse, pull its head towards you with the rope in your left hand. Stand close to the horse's left shoulder, facing its tail, and reach forward to work with your right hand. With horses which are very tickly to groom, it may be necessary to use your hand to get dry mud and sweat off or to wash the horse instead of using a brush in the normal way. Very few clipped horse will allow you to use a dandy brush on their tummies or inside their hind legs. This must be uncomfortable on sensitive areas, so respect their wishes and use something softer instead of having a fight with the horse which may turn it into a bad-tempered kicker when being groomed.

Kicking at other horses in the field

Aggressive horses

These horses are aggressive and bossy and want to make other horses frightened of them. They kick to show power over others.

In the field an aggressive horse may lay its ears back and veer sideways, trying to head off a horse about to overtake it, then quickly swing its hindquarters across and kick out. This horse may charge towards others with its ears back and, sometimes, mouth open, then whip round and kick at them. The aggressive horse will also back up to another horse, sometimes quite fast, then lash out at it. It may try to get another horse into a corner so that it can attack it.

If your horse is aggressive when turned out in the field, this could be caused by jealousy between horses of different sexes. If possible, keep mares and geldings in separate fields and divided from each other by a safe fence. Horses may strike out at each other and get a leg over a barbed wire fence with disastrous results. Ideally, a sound post and rail fence or a thick hedge is best but an electric fence will also make horses keep their distance.

If you have to mix the sexes, try not to put two geldings in with one mare or they might fight over her. If you put one new horse in with two horses which have been turned out together and are friends, one or both may attack the newcomer. Put the new horse out alone with one of them, then swop them round and put it out alone with the other before putting all three together. If you know a horse is aggressive in the field, it is better to have its hind shoes taken off before putting new horses out with it.

An aggressive horse will often attack other horses when hay is put in the field so you must either remove this horse, if possible, and feed it separately or put out several more piles of hay or haynets than there are horses in the field and space them far apart.

When you go into the field to catch one of the horses, the aggressive horse will come to you first and try to keep the others away. It may be necessary to catch it and remove it from the field, or tie it up, before you catch the others.

Do not take children into a field with loose horses, whether aggresive or not.

Kicking when ridden

When riding an aggressive horse you must discipline it. When your horse tries to kick another, your instincts are to move it away by turning its head away from the other horse. This, in fact, moves its hindquarters towards the other horse, putting them in the ideal kicking position, so do not do this. Be very quick to realise what your horse is thinking of doing. Ears back, head slightly raised, tension in the back are all signs of thoughts of kicking out. As soon as you begin to feel or see any of these signs, use the rein and your leg nearer to the other horse to move your horse's hindquarters away from it so that it cannot kick it. Moving your horse's head towards the other horse helps to move its quarters away. Use a cross voice and a strong leg to correct the horse. If your horse starts to move its quarters towards the other horse, hit it really hard very quickly so that it knows why you are hitting it. However, do not hit

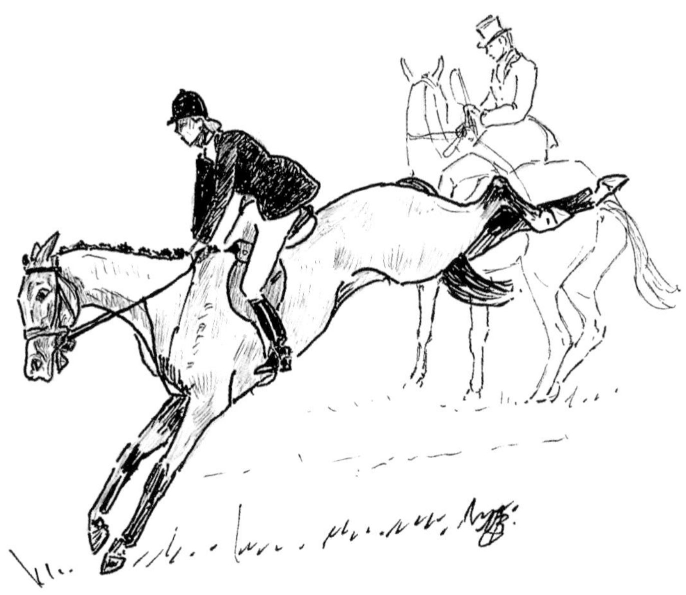

Kicking out at another horse.

your horse if there are other horses close enough to be hurt if your horse should kick out when you hit it.

When being ridden, an aggressive horse may suddenly veer across to head off a horse which is about to overtake it, then swing its quarters across and lash out at it. Watch your horse's ears and head carriage and feel for any tension in its back. As another horse approaches from behind to overtake you, increase the feel on the rein nearer to that horse to bend your horse's neck towards the horse and increase the use of your leg on that side to prevent your horse from kicking. Steady the horse with the rein further away from the other horse to prevent it from veering across.

A red ribbon on a horse's tail warns other riders that the horse kicks but does not give you the right to go into crowds of horses and just hope that others will keep their distance. A person riding a kicker should consider the safety of others and keep to the back or well to the outside of a group of riders.

Timid horses which kick

These horses are normally nervous of others, young or lacking in self-confidence. They kick defensively and often move away from other horses as they do so. It is often a 'keep your distance' warning kick, not a vicious lash out.

A horse that is nervous of others may kick out as another horse gallops past it or as others crowd round it when a group of horses is coming up to be caught from the field. This horse may not get its fair share of hay in the field so be prepared to feed it separately.

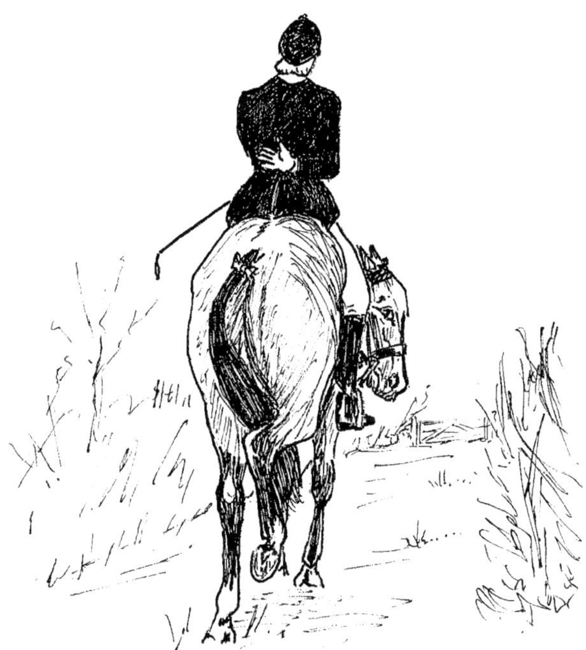

A warning to other riders coming up behind – 'Keep your distance; this horse may kick!'

When ridden, the nervous horse may kick out when crowded in a gateway, so if you are riding such a horse, put one hand in the small of your back, palm outwards. This will warn the people coming up behind that your horse may kick if crowded. If you are riding a young horse, put a green ribbon on its tail to warn people to give it extra room and not gallop past close to it. Horses galloping past too close to a young horse, probably showering it with mud as they do so, can make a young or nervous horse kick in fright. This type of horse is always ready to shoot backwards or veer sideways if other horses show aggression or if it is in a situation where it thinks they might do so.

Do not hit a young or nervous horse for kicking out in fright to protect itself. If you do, it will then have two things to be frightened of, the other horse and you hitting it. Try to ride at the back or out to one side of a group of horses until your horse gains confidence.

If you are able to watch a group of horses in a field you will learn to recognise and differentiate between aggressive and timid behaviour.

Refusing to enter a stable

It is no good pulling on a horse's head when it refuses to go into a stable. It will only put its head up even higher to show you that it can't possibly get through that doorway without hitting its head, or else it will run back.

People are very often taken by surprise when this happens and have no assistant handy, no extra rope and no whip. Sometimes a growl and a really good thump in the ribs with your right hand, while keeping the horse straight (but not pulling on its head) with your left hand, may work.

Sometimes turning the horse round and backing it in works. This is especially true if no one has ever tried to do this before. The horse is taken by surprise and has not yet learnt how to resist this method.

Always give the horse a small feed of something especially nice in its manger when it does go in. This is better than giving it a titbit from your hand because it will then associate the stable, not you, with something pleasant to look forward to and go in willingly.

If a horse consistently refuses to enter a stable, an assistant or the rope or crupper methods mentioned on page 185 can be used.

Not standing still

Teach your horse to stand still in the stable with a headcollar on. Use the same word in the same tone: 'Whoa' or 'Stand'. One word only is best. Stand in front, but slightly to one side, of the horse. Put one hand on its nose, level with the noseband, and the other on the point of its nearer shoulder. Apply pressure on both places as you say, 'Whoa/Stand'. If the horse resents the hand on its nose, put it on the back of the headcollar noseband.

If the horse is really bargy, ask it to stand as it approaches the side of the box. Do not try to teach a horse to stand if it is tense or excited because of other noises or happenings in the yard. If you are to succeed, all must be calm.

If the horse takes even one step forward, push it back, if necessary tapping your toe on the coronet of the offending foreleg. If the horse is willing to stand still for several seconds, keep it there then ask it to 'Walk on' again, being consistent in your use of the same words and tone of voice. If your horse is very impatient, expect it to stand for only one or two seconds at first. Repeat the lesson five or six times several times a day, gradually increasing the length of time that you expect the horse to stand still. Repeat the lesson outside in hand with the horse wearing a headcollar and a bridle. This will give you more control and, if the horse does not respond to the headcollar and your fist on its shoulder, you can then put your hand on the reins and move the bit in its mouth.

Standing still is a very important lesson and one day your safety, or the horse's, may depend on its obedience to this command. It is much better to teach the horse to stand still in hand first. If you wait to teach an impetuous horse to stand still when you are on its back, its natural reaction will be to do little lifts of both forelegs: 'If you won't let me go forward, I feel I must go somewhere so I will go up'. You will then be giving your horse its first lesson in rearing as a resistance, something you never want it to do.

Mounting a horse that will not stand still

Face the horse towards a fence or wall and get on as quickly as possible. Get someone to hold its noseband (not reins or bit) while you mount in the normal way. If the horse is really stroppy and tries to go up if asked to stand still for a second, get someone to lead it forward and someone else to give you a leg up as the horse is walking. Hopefully, the horse will gradually calm down with regular work and then you can ask for more discipline when you mount. (See also page 206.)

Difficult to trot up in hand

Have an assistant to encourage the horse to go forward so that its shoulder is level with yours at all times.

Use your voice to ask for trot and run with your horse, getting the assistant to flick a whip if necessary. Use your voice and slow down yourself to steady the horse to walk.

If you have no assistant, a long whip held behind you in your left hand can be used on the horse's quarters to encourage it forwards. In practice, knowing that you are carrying a long whip and that you will use it if they don't trot, many horses shy away from you by swinging their hindquarters out of reach. Some will end up facing you and may even run back because of the whip. Be very careful as this method can make a horse more difficult to lead.

Another method is to have a rope or rein going from the girth on the off side round the horse's hindquarters above its hocks. Both stirrups should be down and tied together over the girth and under the stomach. The rope is then threaded through the nearside stirrup iron and so to your hand. When the horse does not keep up level with you or trot when asked, give a tweak on the rope, which the horse will feel round its hindquarters and should respond to.

NB: accustom the horse to the feel of a rope round its hindquarters in the stable before you lead it outside.

Sometimes fitting a crupper and tweaking the crupper just behind the saddle works. Again, accustom the horse to the crupper in the stable first.

Your horse must move straight when trotted out in hand. It will not do this if you pull its head round towards you, so learn to adjust the reins and hold them so that you can use them to keep the horse's head straight. Holding the reins in your right hand so that the left rein enters your hand under your index finger and the right rein under your little finger, so that they cross in your palm, is one way of controlling a horse and keeping its head straight.

If you are trotting up a young horse in a headcollar or bitless show bridle, use a length of chain (made for this purpose) with two clips which attach to each side of the noseband and have a central ring to attach the lead rein to. This will help to keep the horse straighter than just a lead rope attached to the back D-ring of the noseband.

The same type of chain can be used to clip on to the bit rings of a show bridle so that you have only a single rein instead of a pair of reins as on an ordinary bridle.

The white rope halters used on some breeds when showing in hand do cause problems by pulling round on to the horse's offside eye because the lead rope starts from the near side of the noseband loop.

The pattern known as a Yorkshire halter, where the lead rope comes from the centre back of the noseband, is preferable. The disadvantage is that unlike an ordinary rope halter, the size of the noseband is fixed and cannot be adjusted.

Showing

Trot the horse directly at the judge and continue trotting in the same straight line as you pass him or her, when they will step aside and then step forward again to be directly behind you to see if your horse moves straight.

Rearing when led

A horse may rear when being led for several reasons.
- If it is being led in a bit which is hurting it or if it is very young and unused to a bit, it may rear.
- There may be a sore place on its nose or in its mouth which hurts when pressure is put on it.
- It may not want to leave other horses or to leave the stable yard.
- It may be frightened of the person leading it or of something it has seen or heard and be trying to get away from it.

First try to figure out the cause of the rearing. If it is caused by pain, try to make the horse more comfortable, perhaps by using a lunge cavesson or padded headcollar.

If the horse does not want to leave others, you will need a bridle (if it is old enough to wear one) with a lunge rein attached, or a lunge cavesson with a lunge rein. You will need an assistant behind the horse to encourage it to go forward with a lunge whip if necessary. You may need three people, one on each side of the horse holding lunge reins to keep the horse facing the way you want it to go, and one behind it. Do not try to drag it forward. This will only make it fight and it is stronger than you. Use the lunge lines to keep it straight or to straighten it if it tries to turn round but do try to have 'allowing' hands so that the horse feels that it *can* go forward. Be ready to lift your hands really high to prevent the horse from getting a foreleg over the rein if it strikes out at it.

If the horse is genuinely frightened, lead a quiet, older horse in front, then alongside, then, when the nervous horse has become used to the places you pass, try to lead it in front of the older horse. Finally, lead it alone.

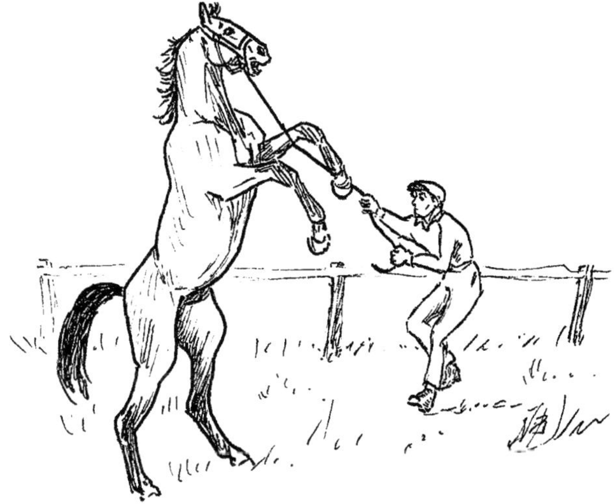

The wrong way to hold a rearing horse. The man has crouched down and his hand is low, allowing the horse to get a leg over the rope. The man should be wearing a hard hat and gloves.

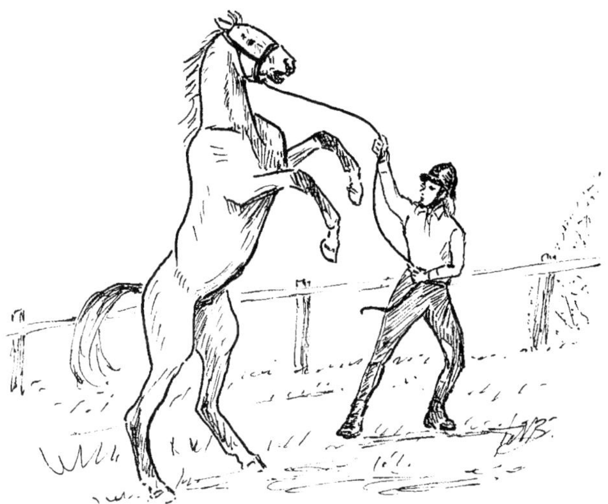

The right way to hold a rearing horse. Stand up very tall and raise the hand holding the rope as high as possible to prevent the horse from getting a leg over the rope. Do not pull. Wear a hard hat and gloves.

A standing martingale attached to the noseband of a bridle and to the girth or a roller may help. A rope running from the back 'D' of the headcollar, between the forelegs and to a roller can help to control a horse which rears in hand. For safety, a tail bandage can be used as a neck strap going over the rope so that there is no danger of the horse getting a leg over the rope if it puts its head right down. If you fit the martingale or rope too tightly (literally tying the horse's head down), it may run back, lose its balance and fall over backwards because it will be unable to use its head and neck freely to regain its balance. While such a fall backwards may frighten it and stop it rearing again, it could also injure its spine and do permanent damage.

When leading difficult horses, always wear gloves. When leading difficult horses, young horses or horses inclined to rear, always wear a hard hat as well. Use only experienced assistants who are neither nervous nor bad tempered.

Running backwards when led

Horses which run backwards when you try to lead them forward are difficult to deal with without an assistant to drive the horse forward from behind the very second it begins to think about running back.

Some horses will respond to a person leading them who is carrying a long whip in their left hand. The leader must be level with the horse's girth so that, when the horse hesitates, the leader can use the whip behind their back and apply it round the horse's hindquarters to drive it forward.

Many persistent offenders anticipate their leaders' actions, however. As the leader makes a move to use the whip as described above, such a horse will shoot violently backwards or sideways because this method has been tried on them before and they know all about it.

When leading a difficult horse, always wear gloves so that you will not get a rope burn if the horse pulls away.

All horses are different; some lead better in a bridle than in a head collar, and vice versa.

- If you are leading in a headcollar, use either a very long lead rope or a lunge line. Pass the spare end over the horse's withers to the off (right) side and round its hindquarters just above the hocks and back to your right hand. Use your left hand about a foot from the headcollar to ask the horse to go forward and, with your right hand, tweak the rope passing round the horse's hindquarters to encourage it forward. There must not be any backwards pull on the headcollar.
- Have two ropes, one of which should be an ordinary lead rope attached to the headcollar to lead the horse forward with your left hand (if you are using a bridle, use the reins for this). With the other rope, make a loop running from your right hand over the horse's withers, round its quarters just above its hocks and back to your right hand. Tweak on the rope to encourage the horse forward. If you find that the back rope is inclined to slip down too low, attach an extra piece which passes over the hindquarters and keeps the back loop in position.

These two methods can also be used when a horse refuses to go into a stable or when it is reluctant to load (see pages 51 and 184).

Taking off when led

Horses which are inclined to get ahead of you and trot off, possibly when being led out to the field in a headcollar, can be controlled by attaching a chain over the nose, wrapping a rope round the nose or putting the rope through the mouth. Remember that the nose and mouth are *sensitive* areas!

You will have more control using a bridle when leading.

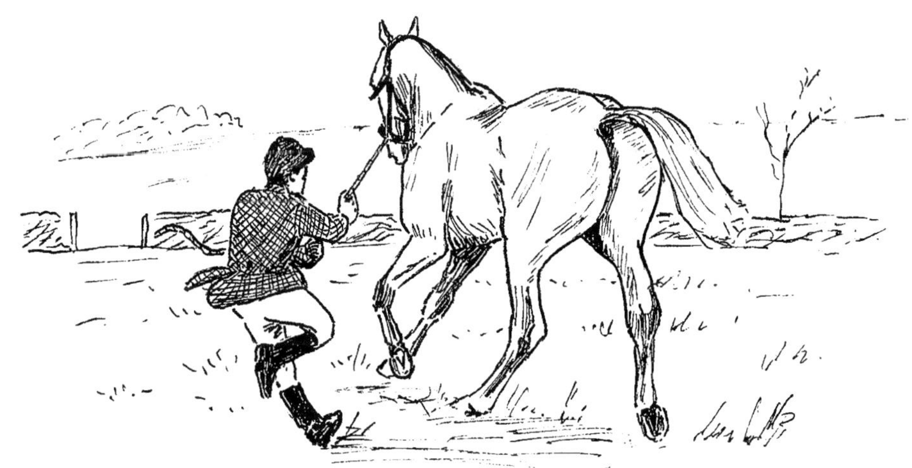

Taking off when led.

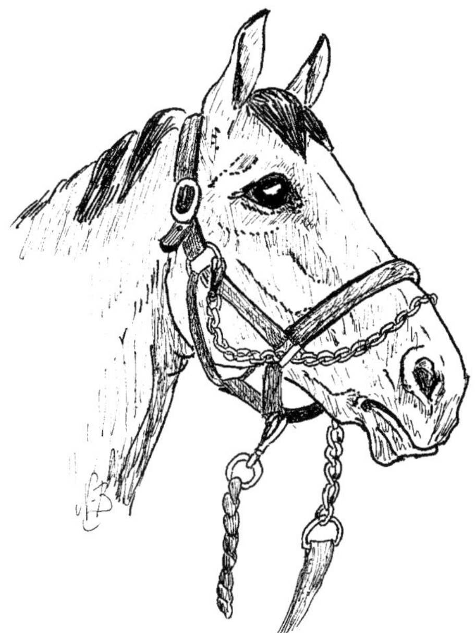

A chain over the nose can give extra control over a horse which misbehaves when led. Use a chain with large, flat links.

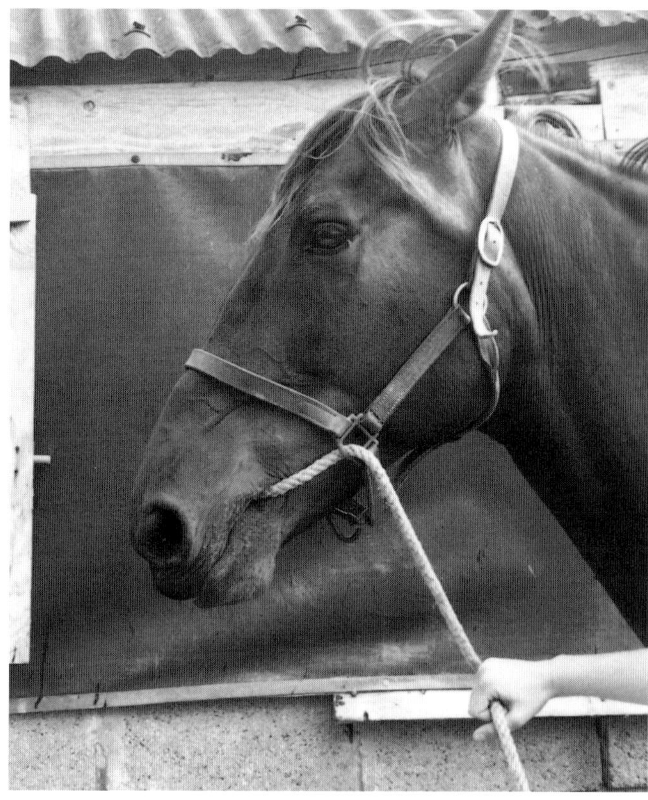

Extra control can be achieved by putting the headcollar rope through the mouth.

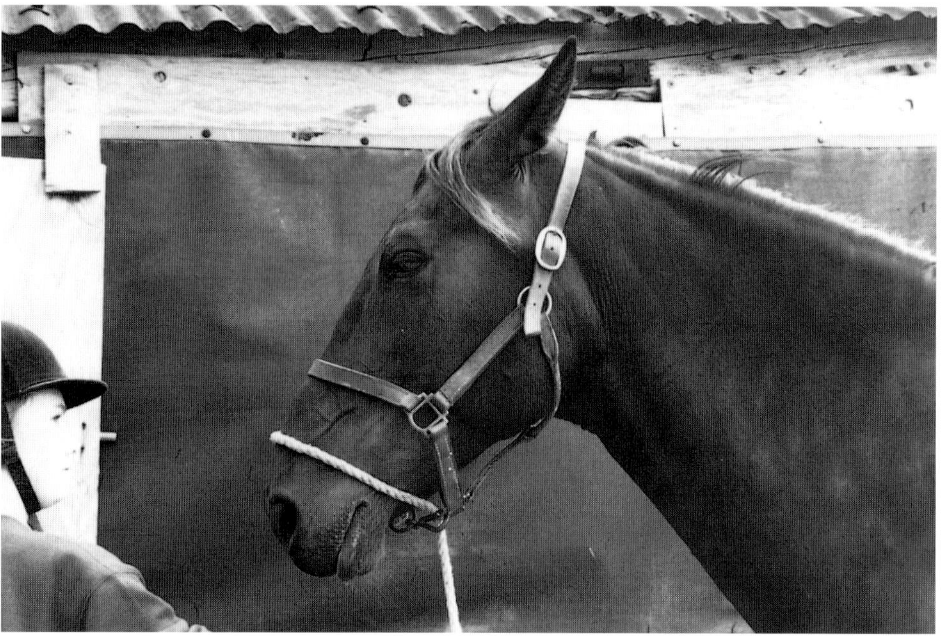

Extra control can be achieved by putting the headcollar rope round the nose well clear of the nostrils.

Crushing against a wall

Some horses will quite deliberately try to crush you against a wall to prevent you doing something that they do not want you to do. This is a painful and dangerous habit. You must make it equally painful for the horse by using something strong, hard and deeper than your own body to place next to you between the wall and the horse. A metal bucket with the sharp lower rim towards the horse and the open end against the wall works quite well. Be careful not to hold the bucket by the handle or your fingers will get trapped! A piece of wood with a blunt end against the wall and a sharper end towards the horse should also make it think.

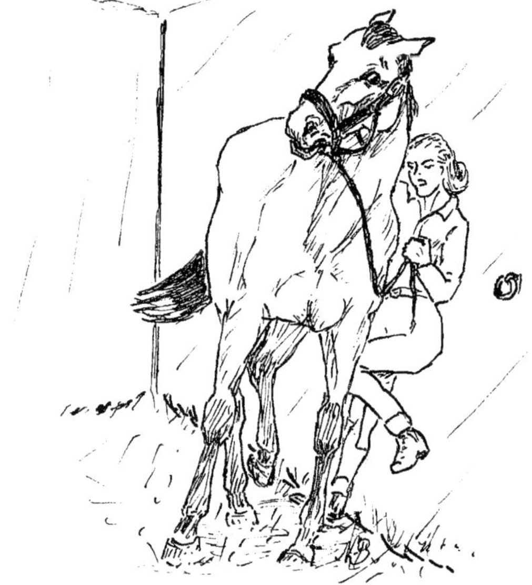

Crushing the handler against the stable wall.

Most horses with this habit try to crush you with their shoulders, sides or hindquarters when they are tied up, so a second rope in your hand can be used to pull the horse's head towards you while you jab it hard with something fairly sharp (but not sharp enough to wound it!) to make it move away from you. Bringing its head towards you has the effect of making its hindquarters move away from you.

ESCAPING

Escaping from the stable

Horses and ponies which barge out of the stable as soon as you start to open the door are very dangerous as they can knock over a child or even an adult and trample on them. To break this habit, fix a bar or a length of strong chain

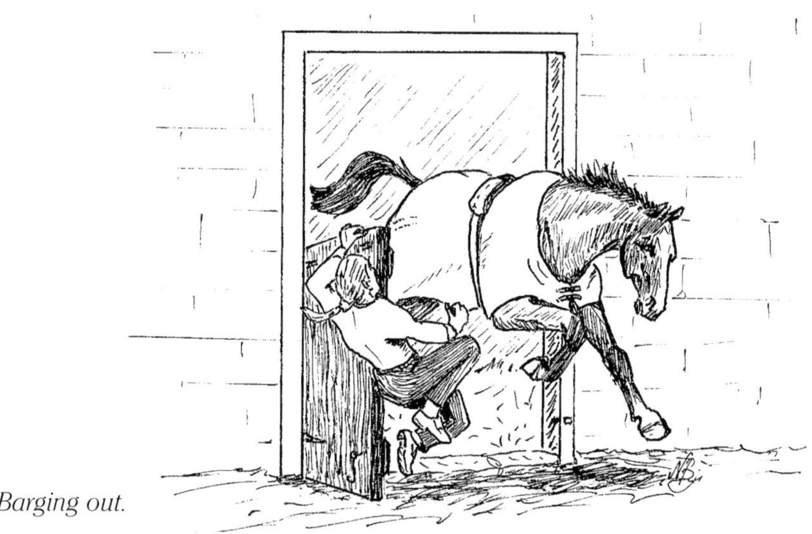

Barging out.

across the inside of the stable doorway, just high enough to prevent the animal from getting under it. You yourself can get in and out by ducking under the chain or bar. For reasons of safety, you should still tie the horse up when you are grooming it or mucking out.

Discipline the horse by making it back away from the doorway when you enter the stable under the chain or bar. When you wish to lead the horse out of the stable, make it halt at the doorway and wait until you ask it to walk on out.

Escaping from the field gate

It is sometimes very difficult to get just one horse out of a field when several horses are in a group near the gate. One or more of them can easily barge out as you lead your horse out, and if the field leads on to a road a bad accident could occur.

Create a pen just inside the field gateway with two strong posts and three poles. Lead your horse into the pen and close the entrance pole before opening the gate. This pen will also help to prevent the gateway from becoming poached and can also be used for feeding a shy horse or tempting in a horse which is difficult to catch.

Escaping when tied up

Some horses are experts at undoing knots and will untie their ropes and escape however correctly you have tied them. The answer to this is to have a very long rope, pass it through the baling twine loop or ring you normally tie your horse to, then tie the knot well out of the horse's reach.

Other horses are experts at removing their headcollars by rubbing them off over one ear. To prevent this, attach a loop of leather to the top of the

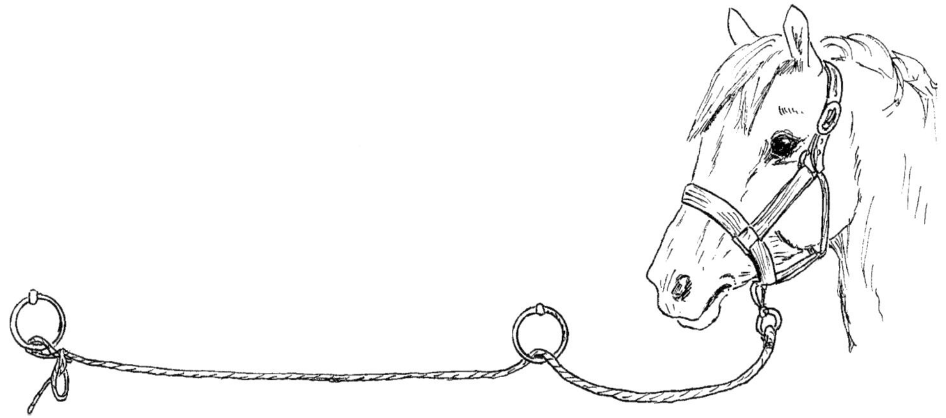

How to tie up a pony which can untie knots.

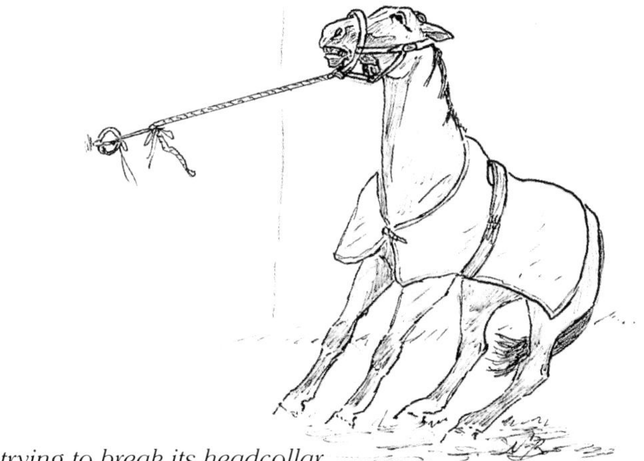

A horse trying to break its headcollar.

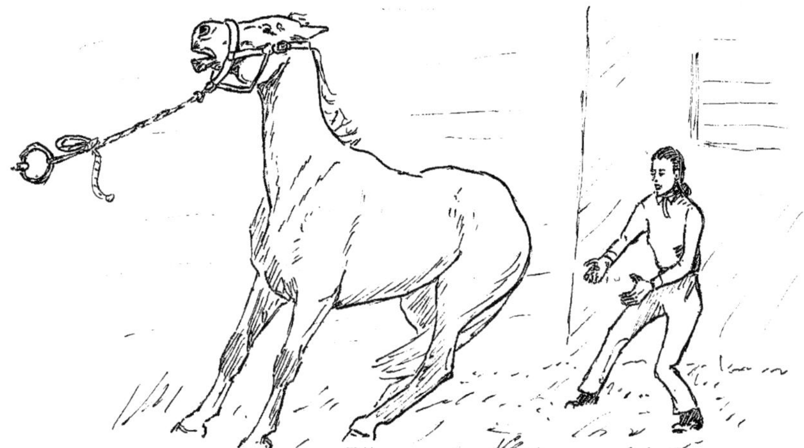

When a horse pulls back, don't go to its head, go behind it and 'shoo' it forward to take the pull off the headcollar.

headpiece of the headcollar and, through this, thread a leather strap to form a throatlash. Do this up tight enough to prevent the headcollar from coming off over the horse's ears but loose enough not to restrict its breathing.

If your horse runs back when tied up and breaks ropes and headcollars, use two really strong ropes and two really strong headcollars. Try to tie the horse up so that when it runs back its hindquarters will contact something solid. To do this, it may be necessary to cross tie the horse. Everything you use must be virtually unbreakable but do have a sharp knife ready to cut the horse loose if it goes down. When the horse starts to run back and pulls on the rope, chase it forward vigorously from behind each time it does so.

TYING UP

Horses which have learnt to run back in order to break the headcollar or rope and get loose can sometimes be cured with the help of a motor car tyre.

One side of a small tyre, such as a Mini tyre, can be securely and closely roped to a ring or, preferably, a strong, upright post. The horse is tied to the opposite side of the tyre using an extremely strong rope and headcollar. When the horse pulls back it does not meet a dead pull because the tyre stretches. The tyre also pulls the horse forward again as it regains shape. The horse should be encouraged forward from behind. It is not so easy to break a headcollar or rope when there is no dead pull. A strong horse may pull the tyre out almost straight but it will not be able to break the tyre.

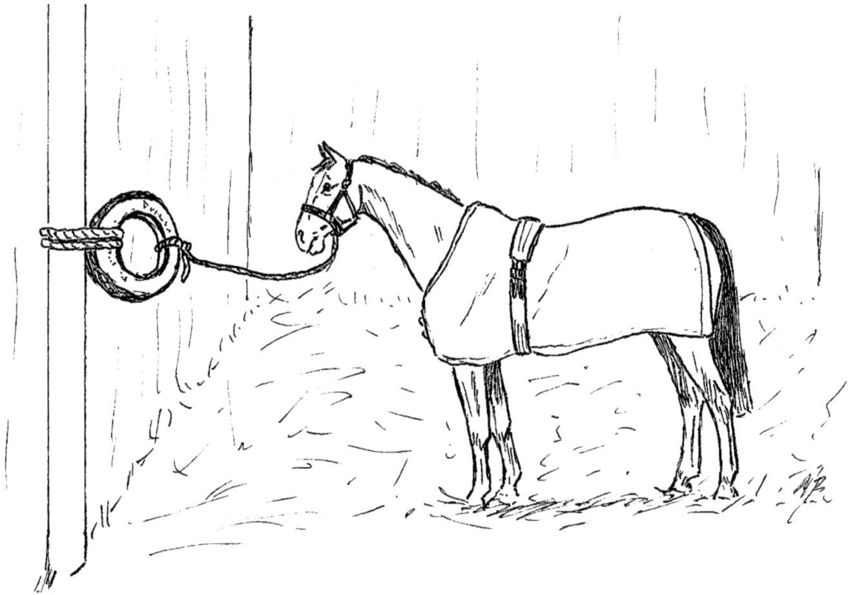

A horse tied to a car tyre which will give when the horse pulls back so that the headcollar will not be broken.

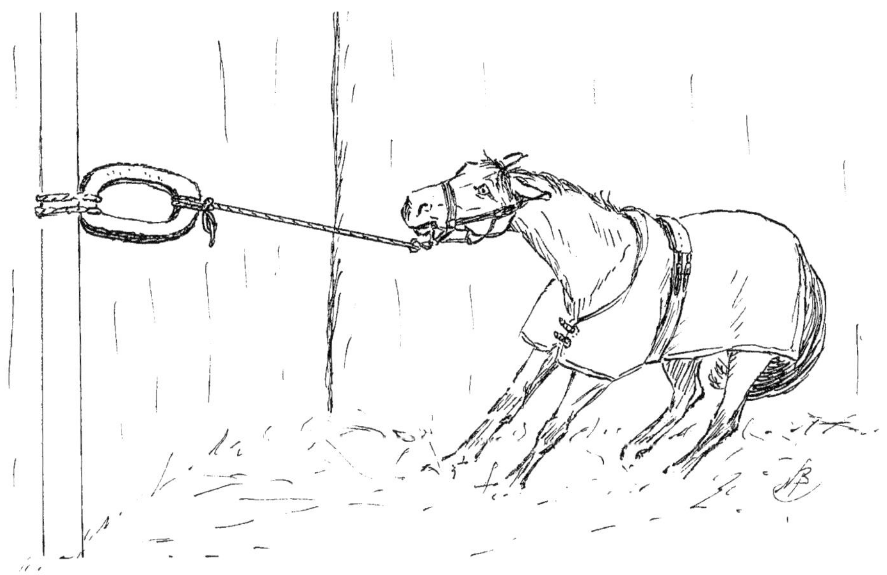

The tyre has stretched but the horse has not been able to break anything or get loose.

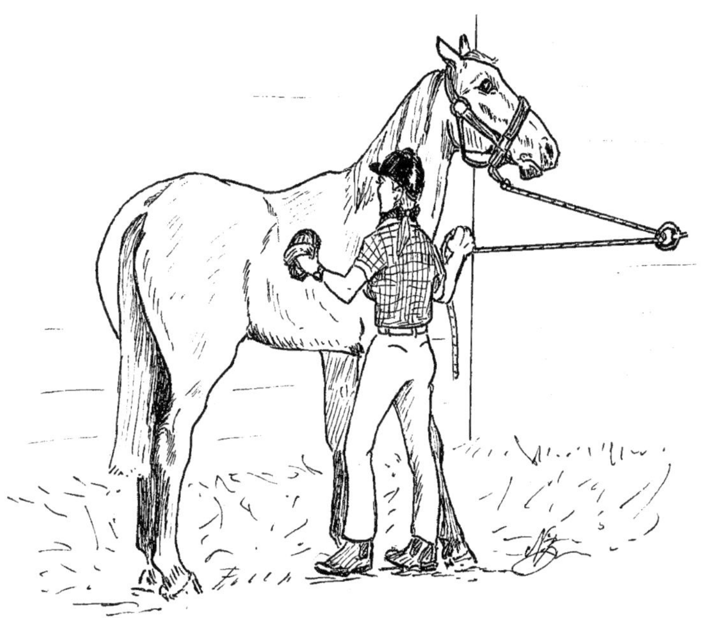

How to control a horse which runs back when being groomed.

If your horse constantly runs back when being groomed, do not tie it up but put it on a long lead rope and simply thread this through the tying up ring. You can then hold on to the end of this lead rope and give and take on it, at the same time talking firmly but not angrily to the horse and praising it when it does not resist and stands still. Make sure your grooming methods are not too rough!

Pulling back when tied up – the sack halter

Horses which pull back and try to break their headcollars can be taught to accept being tied up by using a folded sack with a headcollar.

Fold a strong hessian or nylon sack in half lengthways. Cut holes at each end far enough in so that they will not tear. Put a strong headcollar on the horse then put the sack halter in place just behind the horse's ears, pass a very strong rope through the holes and secure it firmly. Pass the end of the rope through the D in the back of the headcollar noseband and tie the horse up securely. The pressure will now come on a wider area of the horse's neck. The rope through the back of the headcollar noseband keeps the horse's head straight, so that it will not feel that it is choking, as it might if it turned sideways. The rope to the sack must be short enough for the pull to be taken by the sack not the headcollar.

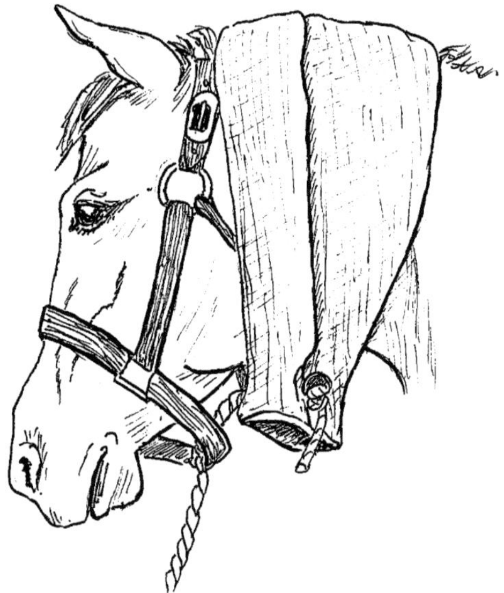

Sack halter for horse which runs back when tied up.

STABLE DOORS

Stable doors must be low enough for a horse to be able to look out in comfort when standing with a normal relaxed neck and head position.

If the horse has to stand with raised head and neck to see over the stable door, you are encouraging it to develop a ewe neck and hollow back.

Little ponies are often kept in loose boxes with normal horse-sized doors. These are so high that the pony cannot see out at all. How would you like to be shut up within four walls with nothing to do and nothing to look at?

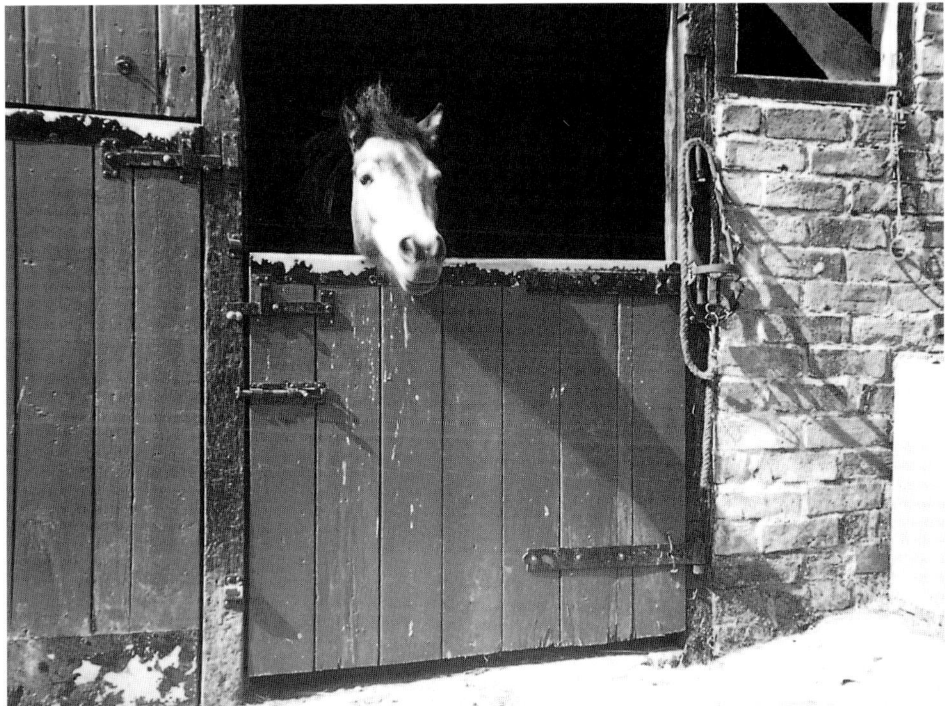

Little ponies should be able to see out. The stable door may need to be lowered. Note the normal height of the stable door on the left.

There are several ways to rectify this problem.
- Lower the stable door.
- Replace the higher door with a lower one.
- Fix two slip rails inside the existing door which can then be left open by day. (Put some stops on the slip rails because clever ponies will soon learn how to slide them sideways and escape.)
- Fix a hurdle inside the doorway.

LITTLE PONIES THAT ARE DIFFICULT TO HANDLE

Young little ponies will sometimes rear up and snatch their feet away from you when you attempt to handle their forelegs.

Tie them up really short at their own eye level. Use two headcollars and ropes if necessary to make sure that they cannot get loose. Against a solid wall or smooth solid wooden barrier is an ideal place. They cannot rear when tied like this so you are more likely to be able to keep hold of the foreleg. (See the method of holding up a foreleg when the other foreleg has been injured and needs dressing, page 154.)

Some little ponies really do fight and, for your own safety and theirs, they need to learn that they must allow you to handle their legs and feet. Do not get rough with them. Be gentle but firm. Hold the foreleg for a short time and only let it go when the pony is *not* struggling. Talk to the pony, rub and scratch it. Try to convince it that you are not going to hurt it, then pick a foreleg up again for a short time. You will need to do this every day, if possible two or three times a day until the pony accepts that it can't win this battle and that when it is tied up really short you are in charge. Some ponies will give in almost immediately after just one struggle – others may take a few days.

HANDLING NEW FOALS

Do not 'play' with a foal, letting it chase you, push you around, nip you or try to kick you as it would when playing with another foal. If you do, it will continue to do this as it grows into a big strong horse which will not be so funny. From the start the foal must respect you but not be frightened of you.

For your own and the foal's safety, having control of it is essential so, in the first few days of its life, put a foal slip on it and teach it to be tied up.

To put a foal slip on the first time will certainly take two, and perhaps three people. One person holds the mare in a corner of the box. The foal is manoeuvred into a position between the mare and the wall. One person stands close to its quarters and rubs and scratches them to prevent the foal from running back. Whoever is nearest to its head gently puts the foal slip on and quickly does it up. They must not pull hard on the rope or the foal is likely to throw itself over backwards and may get hurt. 'Play' the foal as you would a big fish, giving and taking a little until the foal settles. Allow it to remain close to the mare where it feels safe.

To tie the foal up for the first time, tie the mare up first. For the foal, use a long rope and thread this through a ring at the foal's eye level or higher. Keep hold of the end of the rope and stand behind the foal in such a position that if it runs back you can encourage it to go forward with a hand on its hindquarters. You are teaching it that if the rope pulls on its head it can relieve that pressure by stepping forwards.

When the foal has learnt this lesson, tie it up with something it cannot break but still stand in a position to encourage it forwards from behind. In case it panics and goes down, have a knife ready to cut the rope and free it if necessary. Tie it up for five minutes every day, even twice a day. The lesson of accepting being tied up and not attempting to run back and break loose is one of the most important lessons of a young horse's life, both for its own safety and for yours. Leaving this lesson until the young horse is big and strong is the cause of many problems later in life. Stay with the foal while it is tied up. Always tie the mare up also.

Leading a foal

Use a lungeing rein and wear gloves. At first allow the foal to follow the mare, again 'playing' it like a big fish, giving and taking a little. As it begins to accept your control, discipline it a little more. Ask it to stand still and not move when the mare stands still. Never try to pull the foal along; always encourage it forward from behind and, at this stage, let it follow the mare.

At the next stage it must learn to go in front of the mare. Again, do not try to pull the foal forward as it will only pull back against you.

With your left hand, hold the lunge rein about 30 cm (1 ft) from the headcollar as you stand on the near (left) side of the foal. With your right hand, pass the lunge line over the foal's neck to the off (right) side, round its hindquarters just above the hocks and back to your right hand. (Obviously, you must have handled the foal well first and got it used to the feel of first your hands and then a rope round its hindquarters when it was in the stable.) Your left hand gently encourages the foal by leading it forward. Your right hand gives little tugs which it feels round its hindquarters just above its hocks to encourage it to go forwards.

4 PLAITING, PULLING AND CLIPPING

PULLING A MANE

Many horses object to having their manes pulled and find the process really painful. It seems to be less painful immediately after exercise when the horse is warm and the pores are open.

Tie the horse up short, or cross tie it short, to limit its movement. Start near the withers or at the centre of the neck because most horses protest more when you are working nearer their heads. Take a very few of the longest hairs, six to eight, hold them firmly in one hand and, with the other, run the comb right up to the roots. Twist the six to eight hairs round the comb and give a quick pull. Use a narrow, short-toothed metal or plastic comb that is blunt between the teeth so that it will not cut the hairs. For the effect to last, the hairs must come out at the roots. Be prepared to take as long as ten days to finish the job, doing just a little each day, if you want the horse to learn to accept mane pulling. You can also offer food to distract the horse.

Some horses throw themselves about frantically and will try to squash you against the stable wall, trample you or strike out at you. Possible ways of coping with this include:

- Find an old-fashioned stall or a cow yard with a strong high manger in which you can stand. Tie the horse up short and work from within the manger.
- Put the horse in a trailer or horse box with divisions in it and work over the division.
- Use thinning scissors. (The problem is that the short ends stick out as they grow and give a bristly appearance to the mane.)
- Only use a twitch if every other method fails.
- It really is absolute torture for some horses and in such cases I have clipped the underside of the mane to a level just below the top of the neck. I have graded the width of my clip so that an equal bulk of mane is left unclipped all along the neck. Of course, it has to be clipped regularly but it looks neat and tidy and is easy to plait. The length of hair can be regulated with scissors. Many people will condemn this but in my opinion it is better than torturing an otherwise kind, obliging animal.

Pulling a Tail

You never know until you start whether an animal is going to object to its tail being pulled or rather enjoys it. Some horses which absolutely hate their manes being pulled don't mind when their tails are done and vice versa.

Tie the horse up. If necessary have an assistant to feed the horse grass, nuts, coarse mix – anything to distract it. Stop as soon as a quiet horse gets really fidgety. Do a little each day.

Remember:
- If the horse is warm after exercise the pores will be open and the hairs will come out more easily.
- You are in a very vulnerable position, so stand to one side, not directly behind the horse.
- Take out just a few hairs, say, four to ten at a time.
- Just because it stands like a rock do not abuse your horse and pull great bunches out.
- Do a little each day so that the horse's tail does not become sore and painful.
- Once you have pulled a tail you will have to go on pulling it. Even when it looks good and you have got it just right, you will need to keep on pulling a few hairs each week to maintain its appearance. You will also need to bandage it regularly to keep it looking nice. If you don't want to let yourself in for all this work perhaps you would prefer to leave the tail unpulled and plait it on special occasions. (See page 71.)

Possible ways of coping with a difficult horse include:
- Get someone to hold up a foreleg.
- Work round the end of a stall or division.
- Put straw bales behind the horse to protect you.
- Work over the ramp of a trailer with the horse inside.
- Work over or round the division in a horsebox. (Be warned: the horse may come to associate tail pulling with loading and become difficult to load.)
- Use thinning scissors. The result can look quite reasonable but it is difficult to maintain the good appearance and the hair tends to grow into a coarse bush.
- Only use a twitch as a last resort.

Plaiting a mane using elastic bands

The mane must be pulled short (see page 68), combed through and damped thoroughly. The mane should lie on the off (right) side. There should be an odd number of plaits down the neck. Use small elastic bands, the same colour as your horse's mane, sold for this purpose. Start near the ears.

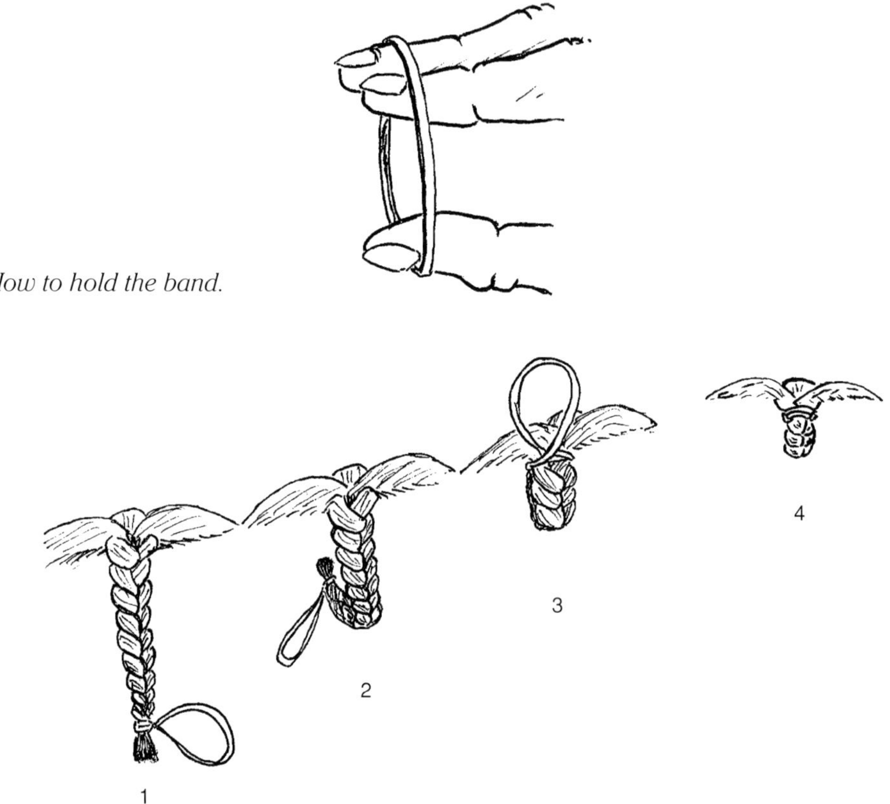

How to hold the band.

Plaiting with elastic bands.

1 Make a parting with a comb and divide off a 5–7.5 cm, (2–3 in) wide bunch of hair.
2 Have an elastic band ready round the index or second finger of your right hand (and several spare ones in your mouth!).
3 Divide the bunch of hair into three equal parts and plait to the end using your thumbs to push the hair smoothly and firmly into place.
4 Hold the plaited tip firmly and wind it round the end of the plait. Hold this end firmly.
5 Push your thumb inside the elastic band together with two fingers and open the band out wide. Wrap it twice round the tip of your plait, stretching the band as much as possible and leaving half of it spare in your hand.
6 Twist the spare part once and double your plait under so that the tip is underneath, close to the top of the horse's neck.
7 Bring the spare part of the band round the plaited loop and up to the top of the plait.
8 Twist it once and put it round the whole plait, again close to the top.
9 Push the finished plait gently up and in, close to the neck.

Plaiting a forelock

This method can be used either when sewing plaits or when using elastic bands.

1 Comb and dampen the forelock.

2 Take a small bunch of hair from the centre back of the forelock and divide it into three strands. Plait it to the tip.

3 Divide the rest of the forelock hair into three equal bunches so that your plait is included to make the centre strand equal in size to the outside ones.

4 Plait normally as for the mane.

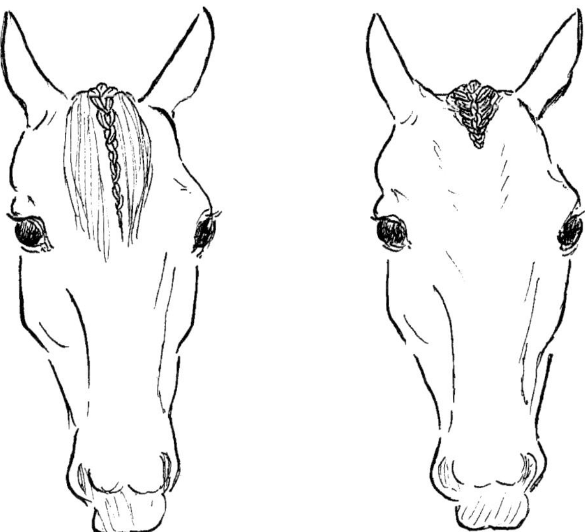

Neat method of plaiting a forelock.

Plaiting a tail

A tail which has been pulled or partly pulled cannot be plaited. The hair at the top of the tail must be quite long.

When plaiting a tail you are in a very vulnerable position because, to do it accurately and neatly, you must stand directly behind the horse.

1 Brush the tail out well and damp it.

2 Take a few strands of hair from the left and right sides, as near the top of the tail as possible. Take a third small group of hairs from the centre top of the tail and plait the three strands over each other once, using your thumbs to push the hair smoothly and firmly inwards.

3 Hold the plait firm with one hand. Use the other to collect a few more hairs from one side and towards the back of the tail and bring them in to join one of the three strands of hair from the other side of the tail.

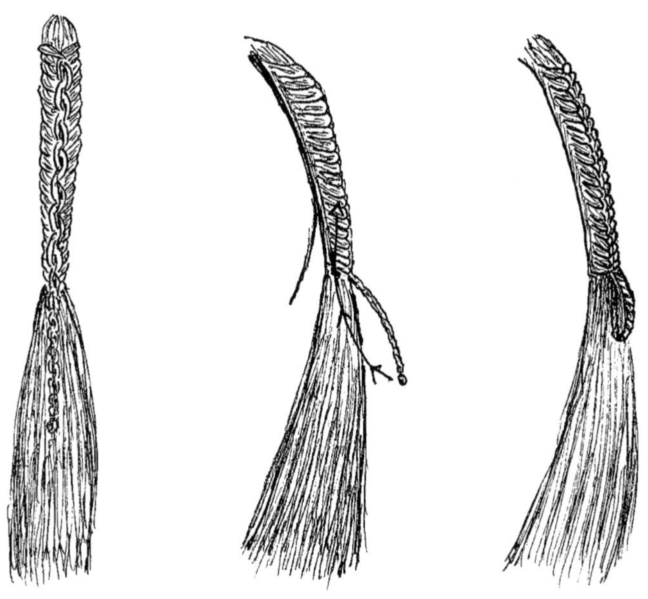

Tail plaiting under.

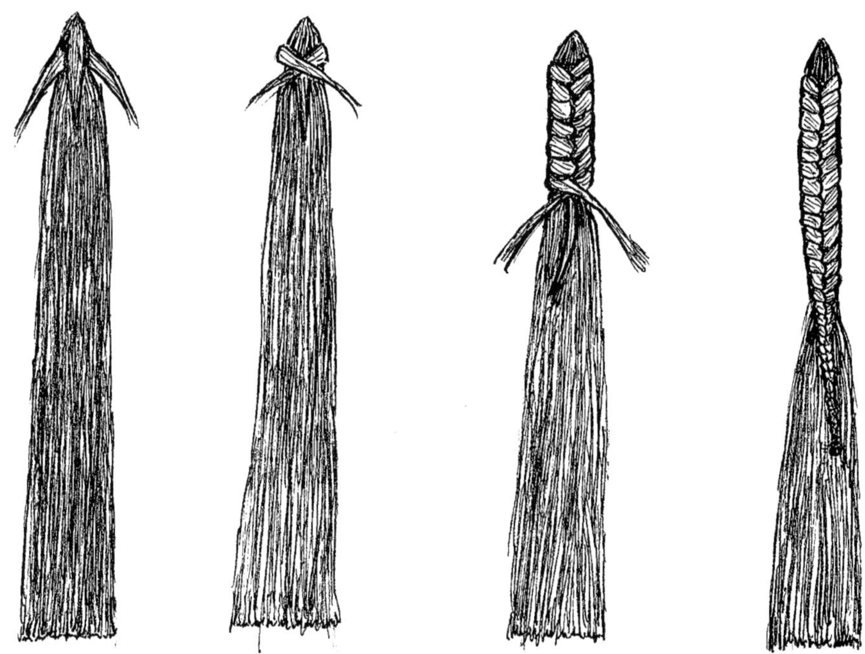

Tail plaiting over.

4 Always use your thumbs to smooth and push the strands into place, each time keeping up the tension (but without *dragging* and making the horse uncomfortable). Continue down, taking a few strands from each side until you get to the end of the dock.

5 Make the strands you have been plaiting into a long pigtail. Wrap the small loose ends round the tips and secure them with an elastic band or thread.

6 Bend the plait under to form a loop and push the tip of the elastic band (or sew it if you prefer) up inside the bottom of your plaited tail far enough to leave a loop of about 10–15 cm (4–6 in) long protruding.

7 Close the loop flat and sew it closed. Sew the tip in place and sew the last few strands of your plaited tail and the first few strands at the top where you started.

Bandage the tail if you are going to travel the horse. Plait the whole of the free part of the tail and bandage that to keep it clean. When removing the tail bandage over your plait remember to unwrap it, not just pull it straight down as you would normally do, or you will untidy the plait.

By following this method you will plait *over and over* to form a very flat, plaited surface down the centre of the tail.

If you plait *under and under* you will create a raised ridge down the centre of the tail. It looks great but is quite tricky to do.

Whichever method you use, it takes endless practice to produce a neat job which will stay in all day. Do not do it the night before. The horse is almost certain to rub its tail. Allow yourself plenty of time in the morning.

Clipping

Horses are very sensitive to electricity and horses which are really bad to clip may, unknown to anyone, have had electric shocks. The type of clipper which runs from a rechargeable 12-volt battery slung round the waist has changed the behaviour of many horses – they don't get shocks; they can be clipped anywhere; there are no long leads to get tangled up in.

Clipping procedure for difficult horses:

1 Let the horse which is bad to clip stand near quiet horses while they are being clipped. Do this as often as possible for as long as possible.

2 Run the clippers every time the horse feeds.

3 Let the clippers run outside, then inside the horse's own stable. Rub the clippers gently over the horse when *not running*.

4 Turn the clippers on when well away from the horse. Let the horse feel the vibration of the running clippers *through* your hand.

5 If you can't get near the horse in the stable with the clippers, try in the stall of a trailer or, better still (because the vehicle is more stable), in the stall of a horse box.

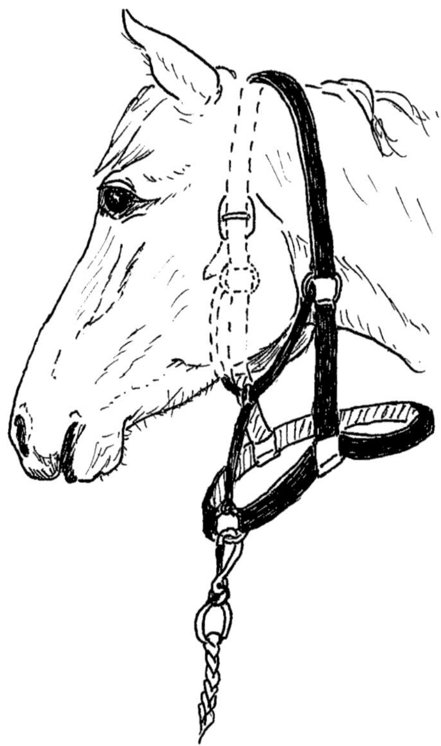

Reverse the headcollar when clipping the head.

Battery-operated clippers can go anywhere. Once you have these clippers touching the horse and gently moving on its body, without attempting to clip, the horse may calm down as these clippers are quieter and vibrate less than other clippers.

Endless time, patience, and calmness and sympathy are more successful than getting cross and short tempered.

Some horses can only be clipped with a twitch on their nose (see page 156); some have to be doped by a vet before they can be clipped. Avoid the latter if possible.

Start clipping the area the horse objects to least – probably the shoulder – and clip the same amount from each side before proceeding further so that, if you have to stop, the horse still looks fairly presentable. If possible, have someone the horse knows and trusts at its head. Let them distract it with feed, carrots or grass.

Some horses dislike having their heads or legs clipped, probably because of the vibration. You could leave the legs as in a hunter clip. You could leave a bridle line on the face. You could try quieter dog clippers on the head.

5 SADDLERY

HALTERS

When using a rope halter, always tie a knot to secure the rope after it has passed round the horse's chin and through the circular eye. Do it in such a way that the knot fixes the size of the noseband and it cannot tighten if the horse pulls back. Without this safety knot the noseband will tighten in a vice-like grip if the horse pulls back and then it will panic, pull back even more and may go down on the ground.

If horses in halters are tied up without such a safety knot when travelling in the back of a lorry, bad accidents can occur without anyone realising what has happened.

Because in this type of halter the pull on the rope is all from one side, the halter can be pulled on to the horse's eye and this can make it panic. A throatlash made from baling twine or cord can help to stop this happening.

A Yorkshire halter, made of hemp, with the rope permanently fixed at the centre back, is preferable. It comes with a cord throatlash. It is not adjustable but comes in different sizes.

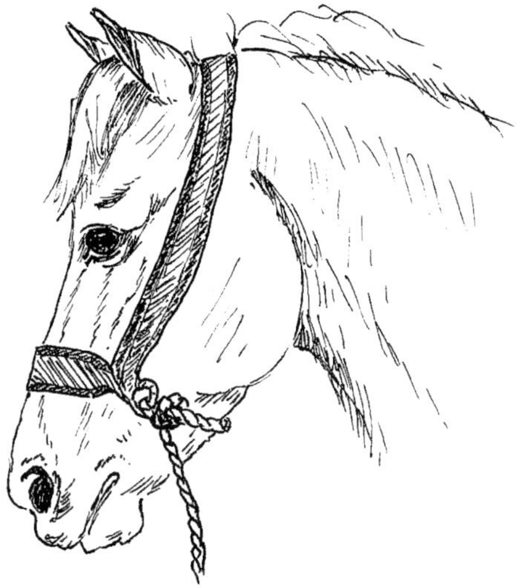

A hemp halter knotted so that it will not tighten around the pony's nose if it pulls back when tied up.

75

BITTING

General points

- A fussy, excitable horse usually goes better in a milder bit or even in a bitless bridle.
- Some horses have very thick tongues and are happier with a thinner bit or a double-jointed bit.
- Many big Thoroughbred horses have very narrow jaws and would be far more comfortable in pony-sized bits.
- It is usually easier to turn a horse and guide it accurately in a jointed bit than in a straight-bar bit.
- A severe bit with curb chain can make a horse hot, fussy and a tearaway.
- Many horses refuse to jump because of the severe bit in their mouths (and the heavy hands of the ignorant rider on their backs).
- The height of the bit in the mouth can change the horse's reaction to it.
- A jointed bit allows more freedom for the tongue and a double-jointed bit even more so.
- A Dr Bristol bit has a flat, sharp-edged plate forming its two joints. Put on one way up (the correct way) the plate lies flat on the horse's tongue. Put on the wrong way up the plate digs into the horse's tongue and is severe. Few people realise this and it is often pot luck which way up it is put in the bridle.
- A French snaffle (double joint with a soft figure of eight forming its two joints) is accepted by most horses.

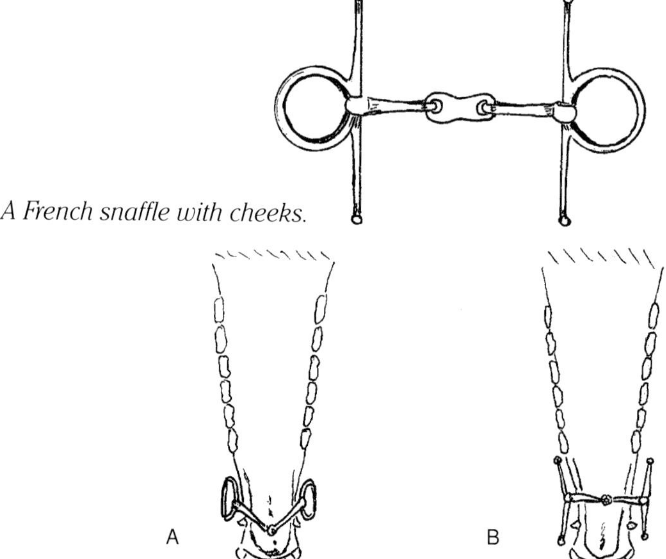

A French snaffle with cheeks.

A: The jointed ring snaffle sits much lower in the mouth than the cheek snaffle used with keepers in B.

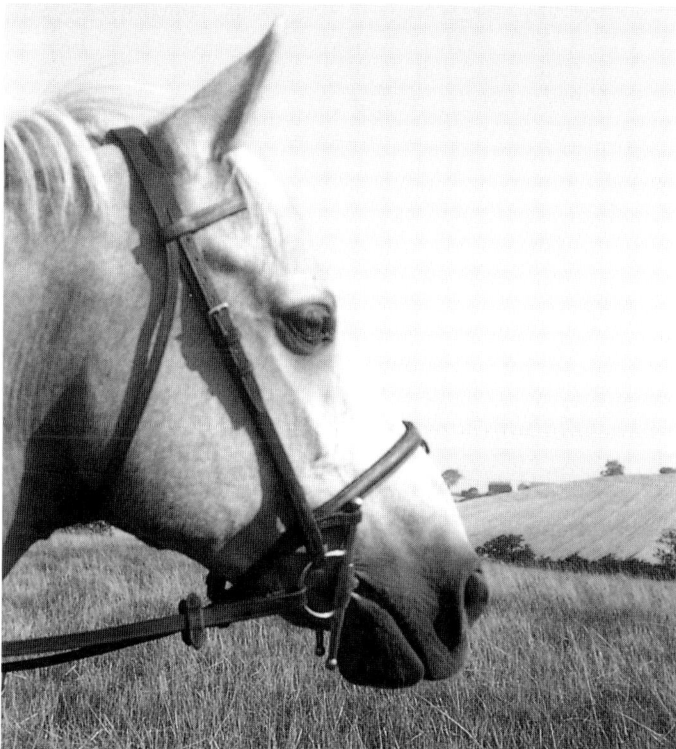

A cheek snaffle held in place by keepers.

- A jointed bit with cheeks hangs much higher in the mouth than a jointed bit with rings. The cheeked bit should be held in place by loops of leather, called keepers, attached to the cheekpieces of the bridle.
- Being higher in the mouth, a bit with cheeks puts pressure on a different part of the bars of the mouth. A horse may go quite differently in this bit.
- A cheek bit (in conjunction with a drop noseband) makes it more difficult for a horse to get its tongue over the bit.
- A single-jointed ring snaffle which is too wide for the horse's mouth hangs very low on the tongue.
- A single-jointed cheek snaffle which is too wide for the horse's mouth causes the joint to press up into the roof of the horse's mouth when the reins are used. The horse will probably open its mouth to avoid the discomfort. Check the fit of the bit before putting on a drop noseband.
- The hands that hold the reins make more difference than the bit in the horse's mouth.
- Curb bits are *not* stronger brakes.
- A double bridle is not severe in itself. A experienced rider has the choice of riding just on the bradoon (snaffle) rein or using a varying combination of bradoon and curb.

- When used with a curb chain, a Pelham with leather loops joining the two rings and one rein attached always gives some curb action. Its severity is controlled by the tightness of the curb chain.
- A Pelham used with two reins and a curb chain gives the rider the choice of using the curb action (bottom rein) or no curb action (top rein) as they like.
- A gag pulls upwards in the horse's mouth and tends to raise the head. It may be used for a strong horse which leans on your hands or dives its head down. It is not suitable for a horse with a high head carriage and a hollow back. It should be used with a second, normal rein so that the rider can use the gag action when necessary but not always. Because of the upward action it is not easy to turn and guide a horse accurately in a gag with only one rein. A second rein attached in the normal way is an asset in turning and in giving accurate control and also means that the gag action need only be used when required.
- A hollow-backed horse with its head in the air will not improve its outline and way of going in a severe bit.
- Sharp teeth cause many problems of head carriage, control and bit acceptance. Have your horse's teeth checked at least once a year.
- A rider sitting behind the movement can cause a horse to go hollow backed with head high.

DRY MOUTH

A horse with a dry mouth tends to have a less-sensitive, less-responsive mouth.

Some people use a breaking bit with keys to encourage the horse to move its tongue and salivate. I have found, however, that horses may learn to play with the keys and will then continue to play and fiddle with any bit put in their mouths.

Possible methods of alleviating this include:

- Using a French snaffle with cheeks. The cheeks lift the bit so that the mouthpiece hangs higher in the mouth. The central, small, figure-of-eight-shaped French link means that there are two joints in the bit, allowing the horse more freedom of its tongue.
- Using a bit with a copper mouthpiece or copper insertions as this metal encourages a horse to salivate.
- Tie a small, double-ended piece of string 4–5 cm (1½–2 in) long to the centre joint of the bit. Put honey, syrup or treacle on it. The taste and position of the string will encourage the horse to salivate.
- Tie a Polo mint to the central joint of the bit.
- Put the bradoon bit and bradoon headpiece of a double bridle on with your normal snaffle bit. Have the reins attached only to your snaffle bit in the normal way.

If your horse responds successfully to any of these methods, gradually use them less and less often so that you do not come to rely on them.

NOSEBANDS

Cavesson noseband

If fitted too low, a cavesson noseband can cause problems such as head tossing and cut and bleeding corners of the lips. When the rider uses the reins the bit is lifted up in the horse's mouth and the corners of the lips are pinched between the bit and the noseband .

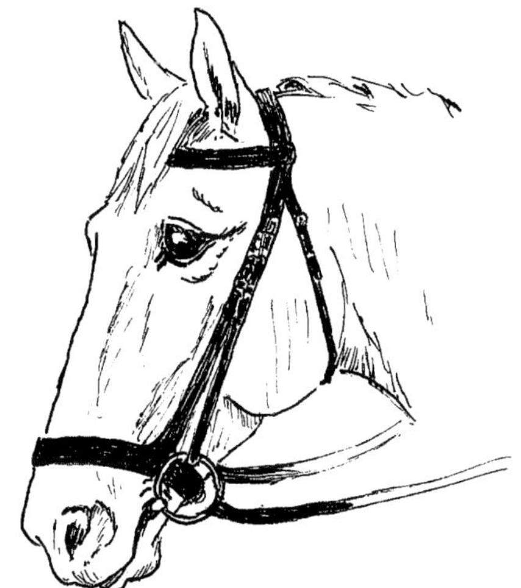

This cavesson noseband is too low.

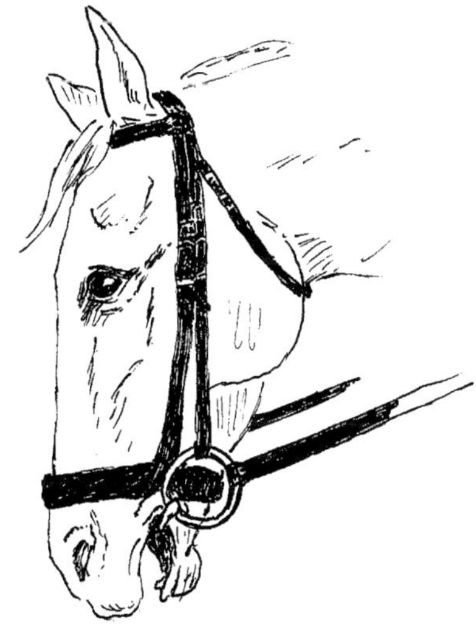

The corners of the lips are being pinched between the noseband and the bit when the rider feels on the reins. The resulting damage is often thought to be caused by the bit.

This problem is much commoner than people realise because when they put the bridle on there is a clear space between the bit and noseband. It is only when a strongish contact is taken on the reins that the trouble occurs, so the rider does not see it happen. It can, however, be seen by an experienced person observing from the ground.

If the horse throws its head about when the lips are pinched, the rider usually thinks that the bit in its mouth, or perhaps sharp teeth, is causing the problem. If the corners of the lips are cut and bleeding, they think something sharp on the bit is the cause.

Having seen horses bleeding from this cause, I have had great difficulty in convincing riders of the true reason unless I can persuade them to dismount and use the reins while on their feet, watching the way the pinching occurs.

Some people use a drop noseband as an ordinary cavesson worn *above* the bit. Because the backstrap drops down it is almost certain to cause pinched lips.

The correct fitting of a cavesson's height is two fingers' width below the horse's projecting cheek bones. To be safe, feel on the reins from the ground to make certain that your horse's lip cannot be pinched.

Drop noseband

The drop section of this noseband must not be used fitted above the bit as the horse's lips will be pinched between the bit and the back strap of the noseband when the reins are used.

Correct fitting will ensure that the front of the noseband is high enough to rest on the bony part of the nose.

This noseband is not meant to be done up like a girth, so tight that the horse's jaws are really fixed and clamped. Would you go quietly and happily if your jaws were immovably fixed? There must be aching and discomfort unless a slight movement of the jaws is allowed.

To accept the bit and be soft in your hand when ridden, the horse must relax its lower jaw. With its mouth clamped shut by a very tight drop noseband, it cannot do this.

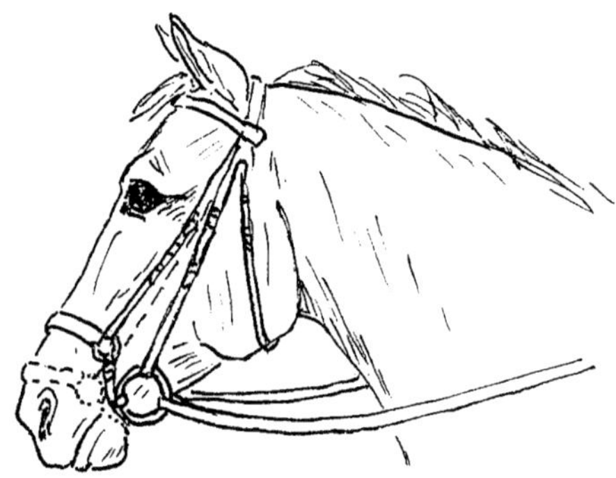

A drop noseband correctly fitted. The dotted line shows the too-low position that is all too often seen. In this position the noseband can be irritating and also make it difficult for the horse to breathe.

Grakle noseband

This figure-of-eight, crossed noseband must be fitted so that it crosses well up on the bony part of the nose. Make sure that the top strap of the Grakle does not rub the horse's projecting cheek bone. The lower strap goes below the bit as in a drop noseband.

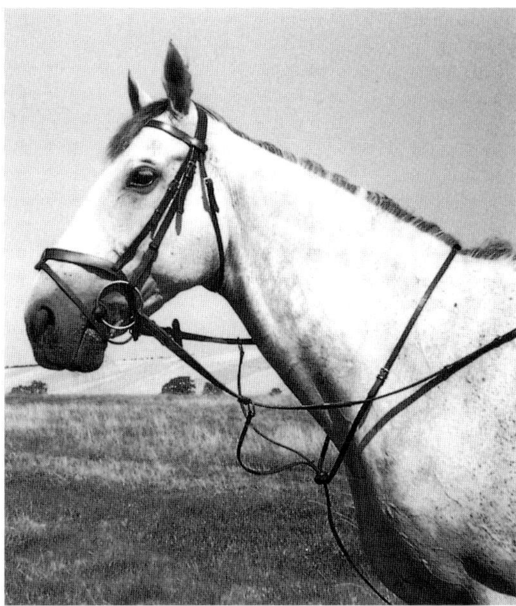

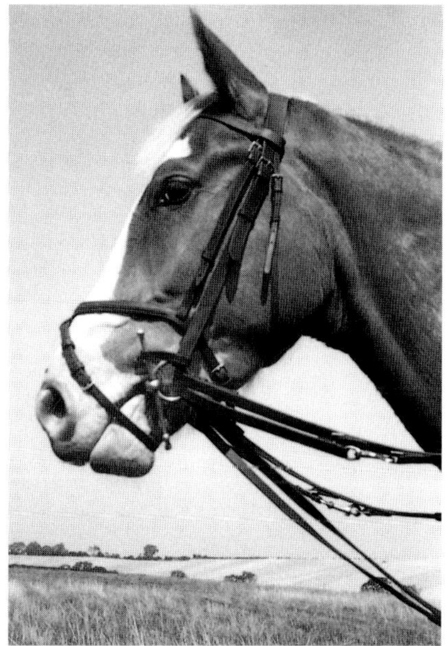

A Flash noseband correctly adjusted.

A sagging cavesson noseband allowing the Flash noseband to hang too low.

Flash noseband

The extra strap of the Flash noseband must be attached to a thick, strong cavesson noseband to keep it up at the correct level. A soft, limp cavesson noseband allows the Flash strap to hang too low.

Rubber rings

Rubber rings or 'biscuits' can be used to prevent the rings of a loose-ring bit from pinching the horse's lips.

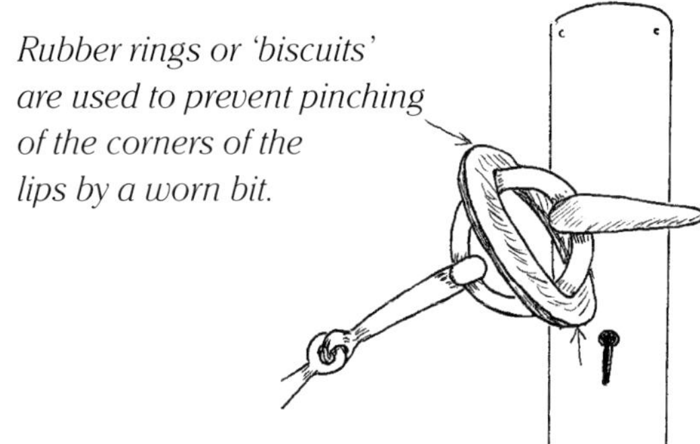

Rubber rings or 'biscuits' are used to prevent pinching of the corners of the lips by a worn bit.

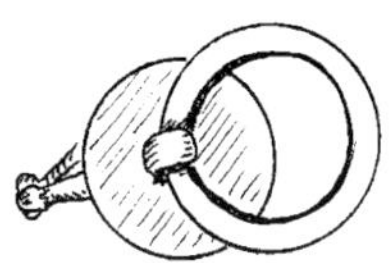

To get the rubber ring on, place it just over one end of the bit ring then hook the bit ring over a door handle and then use both hands to pull the rubber ring over the bit ring.

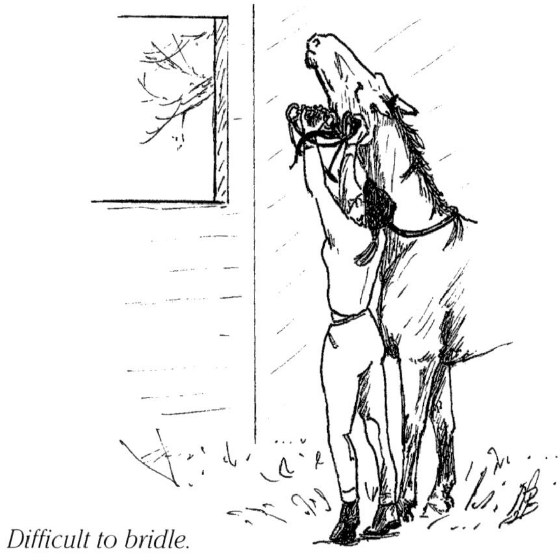

Difficult to bridle.

DIFFICULT TO BRIDLE

Some horses do not mind the bridle going on over their ears but absolutely refuse to let the bit come anywhere near their mouths. They clamp their teeth shut, toss or shake their heads violently or, in the case of tall horses, put their noses as high as possible in the air so that they are out of your reach.

They may run backwards or charge forward or sideways very suddenly and can knock you over as they do so.

Young horses being bridled for the first few times and not understanding what you are trying to do may be mildly evasive but if they have been properly handled previously, they are not likely to react in a violent manner. Great care and patience are needed when first bridling a young horse as a nervous, inexperienced handler or a rough, impatient one can soon cause problems.

A straight bar bit is easier to control and guide with your hand than a jointed one. A rubber or nylon bit is less likely to upset the horse (or hit you in the face) than a metal one.

Fear of the bit

If it is only the bit that the horse objects to, the following remedies may be tried.

- Have the horse's teeth checked carefully (it may also strongly object to this).
- Put it in a small, low-ceilinged stable. (Yes, it may bang its head but it may learn not to do it again.)
- Back it into a corner and, if it will accept it, cross tie it.

- Tie one side of the bit to a headcollar where it will remain fairly close to the mouth so that you have only one side to manoeuvre.
- Lay the bit (attached to bridle or headcollar) across your hand and cover it with your horse's favourite nuts or carrots. (Something lumpy so that it has to open its mouth wide enough to get it in.)
- Halve and hollow out a carrot, insert the bit in the hollow and tie the carrot halves together. Lay the bit in the carrot across your hand and offer it to the horse. (The bit should be attached to bridle or headcollar on both sides.)

Sensitive ears

A horse which is very frightened of its ears being touched may not even allow you to pass the reins over its head. Use reins which have a buckled centre joint and undo the buckle to put the reins round the horse's neck. Make a browband from soft leather or braid with a loop at one end only. Make a popper or Velcro fastening for the open-ended loop at the other end. Undo the nearside cheekpiece of the bridle and the cheekpiece of the noseband. Pass the headpiece of the bridle over the horse's head from the off side and hold it with your right hand. With your left hand put the bit in the horse's mouth. Do up the bridle and noseband cheekpieces. Do up the open loop of the browband on the near side.

Some horses will not allow you to put the bridle on over their ears but will allow you to take it off in the normal way. If there is also a problem taking the bridle off, however, undo all parts of the bridle as you did when putting it on.

If your horse puts its head up so high that you cannot reach to bridle it, try standing on a box or bale of straw. If you have a building with a smooth, fairly low roof, put the horse in there to bridle it. Have a titbit to encourage the horse to lower its head and always give it something when the bridle is successfully on. It will then associate the process with something pleasant. Check its mouth, teeth and lips for sore places and check the bit for sharp or worn places in case one of these is the cause.

Running back and throwing the head up when taking the bridle off

This is usually caused by someone snatching the bridle off too quickly and roughly. The bit has caught painfully on the horse's teeth so it now runs back and throws its head up in anticipation of the pain. Back the horse into a corner so that it cannot run back. Put one hand on its nose, well above the nostrils, to steady it, and slowly ease the bridle off. Never take any bridle off without using one hand on the nose to prevent the horse from throwing its head up. This applies to all horses and all bridles and is a practice which helps to prevent this problem occurring in the first place. If a horse has this problem, do not try to take its bridle off out in the field.

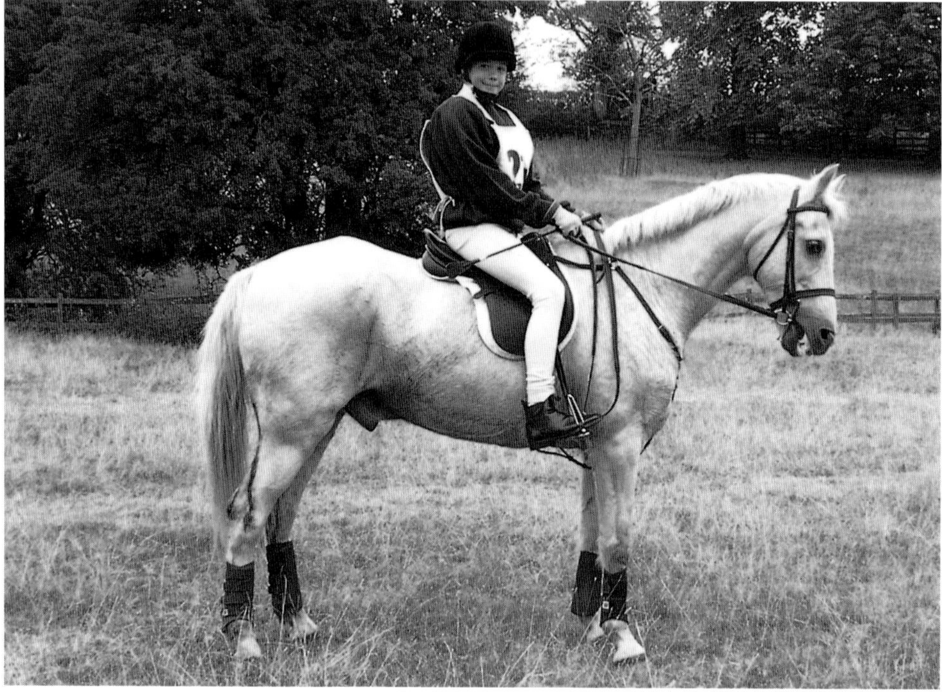

Loops of rein hanging dangerously low can get caught round the rider's toe.

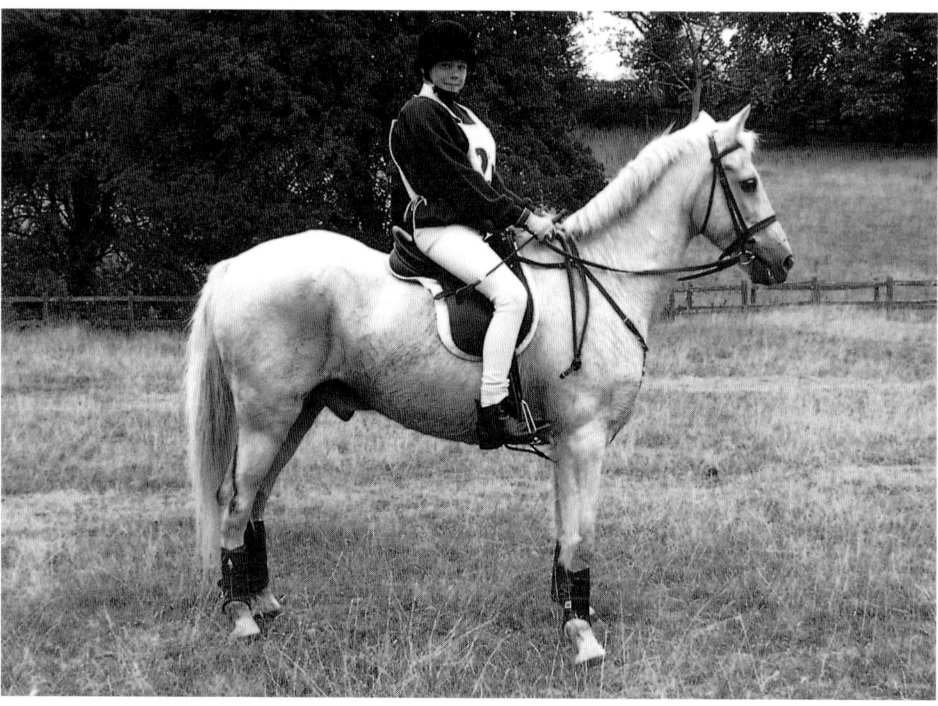

Put a knot in the end to make the reins safe.

REINS

Reins which are a safe length when you are riding on the flat may become dangerous when you shorten your stirrups to jump.

When riding yourself or when you are responsible for others, especially children, always check that the loop of the reins does not hang down so low that it can get caught round the rider's toe. It may appear safe at first but remember that when they shorten their reins to sit in a forward position the loop will hang lower.

If a loop of rein is caught on a rider's toe, it can be difficult to guide and control the horse. If the loop of rein goes right over the rider's foot and round their ankle, it could hold the rider's foot in the stirrup if they fell off. They would then be dragged along the ground with their foot fixed in the stirrup by the reins. This has actually happened so do be aware of the potential danger and put a knot in the end of long reins.

If your reins are wet and slippery, you cannot control your horse properly and this can be very frightening. Dismount and, if possible, get someone to hold your horse while you put a knot in each rein, positioned so that the knot comes just in front of your thumb and index finger when you are holding the reins. These knots will then prevent the reins being pulled through your hands, as will elastic bands (see page 323). When riding normally, the knot should lie in front of your hand on the reins, i.e. between your hand and the horse's mouth. Only when you shorten your reins to gain more control should you place your hand between the knot and the horse's mouth.

Rubber reins
These give you a good grip in wet or sweaty conditions but I think they tend to make riders heavy handed. They are thick and bulky to hold and the rider tends to take a firm hold of them. The rough surface can rub the hair off on each side of the horse's neck.

Plaited reins
These are difficult to clean but less likely to slip than plain reins.

Laced reins
These give a better grip and are easier to clean.

Continental reins
These do not slip and their notches of leather are helpful. Check carefully that they have not frayed where they are attached to the leather fitting near the bit or where they run through the rings of a running martingale if you use one.

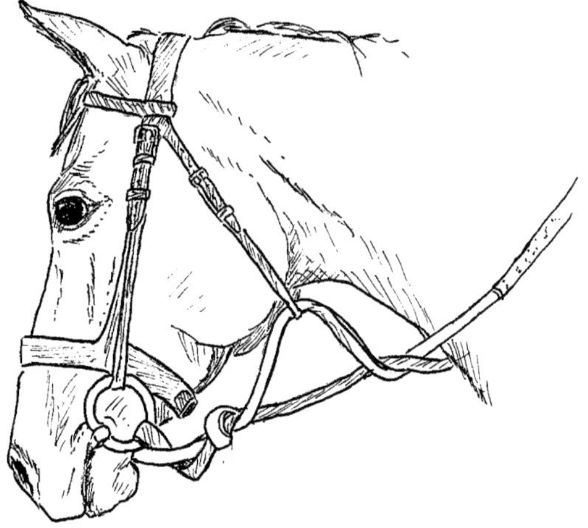

Making reins safe.

Making reins safe

There are several occasions when it is necessary to make the reins safe.
- When the horse is tied up in the stable with a bridle on under its headcollar.
- When it is travelling in a horse box or trailer with a bridle on.
- When it is being lunged prior to being ridden.
- When you are riding and leading a horse with double reins.

If the horse has a saddle on, your can put the reins behind and under both the run-up stirrup irons and leathers. If you twist the reins once, one over the other, at the withers before putting them behind the irons and leathers, they really do stay in place.

Looping the reins round the horse's neck is not a safe idea because if the horse puts its head down or shakes its head when low, the loops come off over its ears. The same is true if a horse bucks on the lunge when the reins are looped over its head.

The safest way is to place the reins on the horse's neck with the buckle at the withers so that they are of equal length. Undo the throatlash then pick up both reins just below the throatlash and twist one over and over the other until they are quite tight and the loop of rein round the neck is now a snug fit. Put the throatlash strap through one loop of rein only and do it up again. This method keeps the reins well up and out of harm's way and they will not come undone.

Making stirrup irons safe

When lungeing or riding and leading, you need to keep the stirrups up. Run the iron up to the top of the leather in the normal way, then bring the loop of

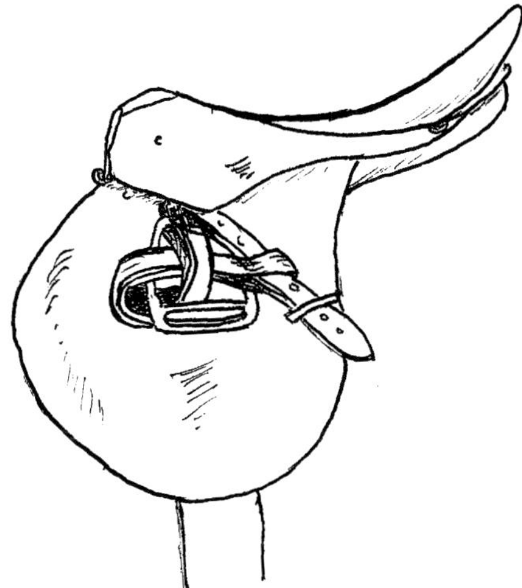

Making stirrup irons safe.

the stirrup leather forward from behind the iron and pass it over the side of the iron and through it from outside to inside so that there is now a small loop sticking out behind the iron. Thread the pointed end of the stirrup leather through the loop to hold everything in place. With safety irons which have elastic on one side, wrap the stirrup leather round the solid side of the iron and pass the pointed end through the loop.

Running reins

Running reins have their place in reschooling but only in the hands of an expert.

If they are attached to the girth straps on each side of the saddle and then go through the bit and back to the rider's hands, they ask the horse to arch its neck but they also ask it to take a shorter step. They inhibit the action of the shoulders and the horse soon ceases to 'swing along'. It can also learn to come up and back towards the rider with its head.

When attached to the girth between the forelegs, then through the bit to the rider's hand, running reins give the horse more freedom of its shoulders and are therefore less likely to shorten the stride. In this position the horse is more encouraged to lengthen the top of its neck and lower its head.

The disadvantage of attaching the reins to the girth between the forelegs is that if the horse stumbles, lowers its head suddenly or bucks, the loops of the running rein can drop right down below its knees.

A safer way of attaching running reins is to use a breast plate, or a strap with a ring, coming from the girth between the forelegs to a martingale neckstrap. Attach the running reins at the bottom of the neckstrap level. There is then no danger of the horse getting a leg over the running reins.

Always use running reins in conjunction with a normal rein. It is so very easy to hold the running reins too tight and short in your hands or to get one rein shorter than the other that I feel they can do much more harm than good except when used by an expert with sympathetic hands. Never jump or lunge over jumps in running reins.

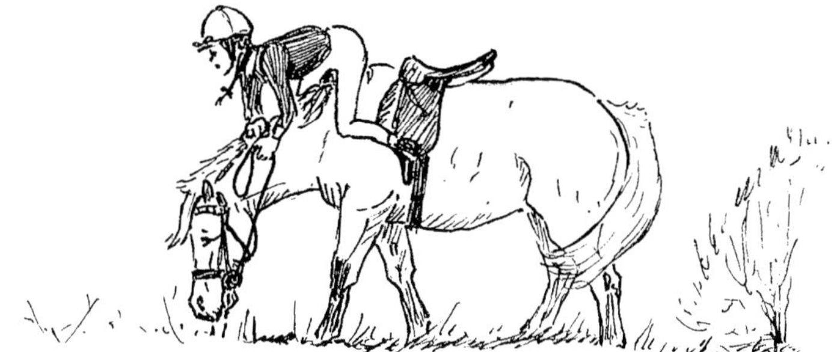

A sight often seen in the summer with a pony that is not wearing grass reins.

Grass reins or side reins

Grass reins or side reins are often used on small ponies which constantly dive their heads down to eat. Three methods of fitting these reins are commonly used.

1 When the reins are attached to the bit, crossed and knotted on the crest (so that they cannot open up and separate) and attached to the Ds on each side of the front of the saddle, they do not need to be tight. The pony has quite a lot of freedom but is just unable to reach the grass because of the knot on its crest.
NB: *do not jump* with reins attached in this way.

2 The reins can be attached to the bit and directly back to the saddle Ds on the same side, as side reins sometimes are when lungeing. Fitted too tightly, however, they can shorten the pony's stride and make it reluctant to go forward. When the pony is asked to turn, the side rein on the opposite side can also act on the bit. I have found methods 1 or 3 more successful as they control the grass eating yet give the pony more freedom of other movement.
NB: *do not jump* in side reins like this.

3 This method needs two lengths of strong blind cord or something similar. Attach each piece of cord to the bit, follow the line of the bridle cheekpiece and thread the cords through the loop of the brow band. Take them along the neck to the highest point of the crest where the two pieces are knotted together. Separate the two ends and attach them to the Ds on each side of the front of the saddle. Adjust the length so that the pony can only just not reach the ground to eat grass. To make for easy attachment, leave them permanently attached to the bridle and attach two strong dog lead clips to the ends which go on the saddle Ds.
NB: this type of rein *can be used when jumping*

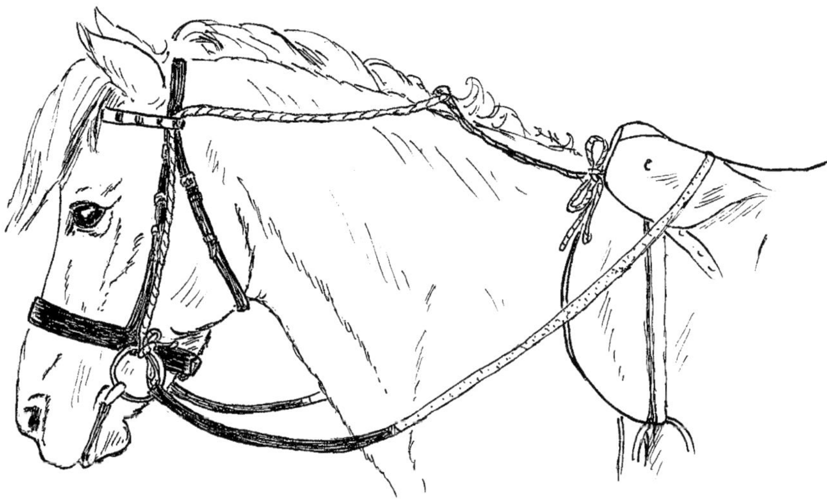

This method of attaching grass reins prevents the pony from reaching the ground but still allows it to stretch its neck out so it can jump. Get an experienced person to check the fitting of grass reins before jumping in them.

DOUBLE BRIDLE

Just because you are going to a show do not suddenly put on a double bridle and expect a horse to go well in it.

A double bridle consists of a normal bridle, the cheekpieces of which carry the curb bit, and a bradoon headpiece which consists of one cheekpiece and a long leather strap which goes from the bradoon bit on the near side up over the head through the loops of the browband and under the normal headpiece to do up on the off side of the horse's head. It does up on the off side to avoid having more than three buckles (cheekpiece, noseband and throatlash) done up on the near side.

If the horse is going happily and correctly at all gaits in a snaffle, you can introduce a double bridle. Hold it up against the horse's head to get a rough idea of size and then adjust it as necessary, leaving all the keepers undone so that the fit can be quickly altered. Put the bridle on. As you put the two bits into the horse's mouth, place the bradoon bit over and on top of the curb bit. If you do not do this the bradoon bit will be lying behind the curb bit although, as soon as the bit is in its mouth the horse will probably use its tongue anyway to lift the bradoon bit and put the joint of it above the curb bit. Adjust the height of the bradoon as you would a snaffle bit. Make sure it is wide enough to be comfortable but not so wide that the joint hangs too low. It must fit into the corners of the mouth without dragging. Don't just look from the outside; gently open the horse's mouth and see how the bit is sitting. Next, adjust the height of the curb bit so that it is resting just below and touching the

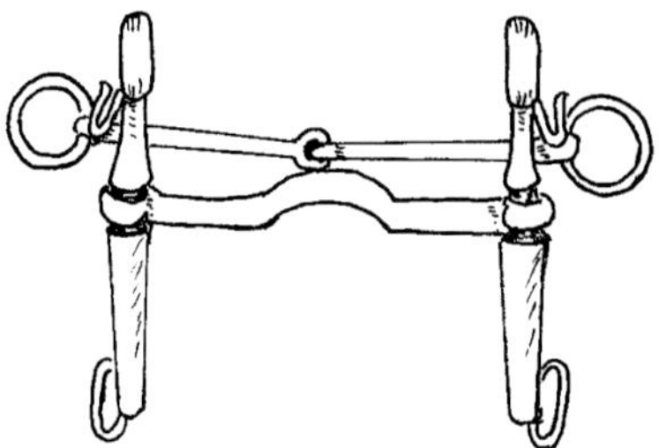

When you put a double bridle on, the horse lifts the bradoon bit with its tongue . . .

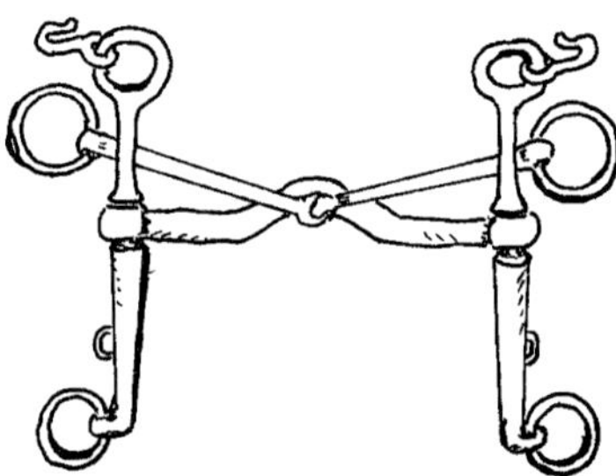

. . . and puts it over the top of the curb bit. This is how the two bits sit at rest in the horse's mouth.

bradoon. Make sure the curb bit is wide enough so that the cheeks do not press on the outside of the horse's lips.

Attach the top of the first link of the curb chain to the offside curb hook so that the central loose ring – the fly link – is hanging from the bottom of the chain when the chain is twisted clockwise until lying flat and smooth. Attach the top of the last link of the curb chain to the hook on the nearside. Take the *bottom* of the link which fits correctly and attach that also to the nearside hook. The curb chain is fitted on to the correct link if the curb chain comes into action against the horse's chin when the cheekpiece of the bit is at an angle of 45 degrees to perpendicular. The lip strap goes from the D in the cheeks of the curb bit and passes through the fly link in the curb chain to keep it in place.

Hack the horse about quietly on a loose rein until it is used to the feel of the two bits. Use the bradoon rein as the guiding and controlling rein, held outside your little finger or in the position in which you normally hold the snaffle rein.

The curb rein is used to ask the horse to flex at the poll and relax its lower jaw so it must be used delicately. The curb rein should never be tighter than the bradoon rein. The curb should be held with one or two fingers between it and the bradoon rein. When looked at from the side the reins appear to cross as they pass from the bits to your hands.

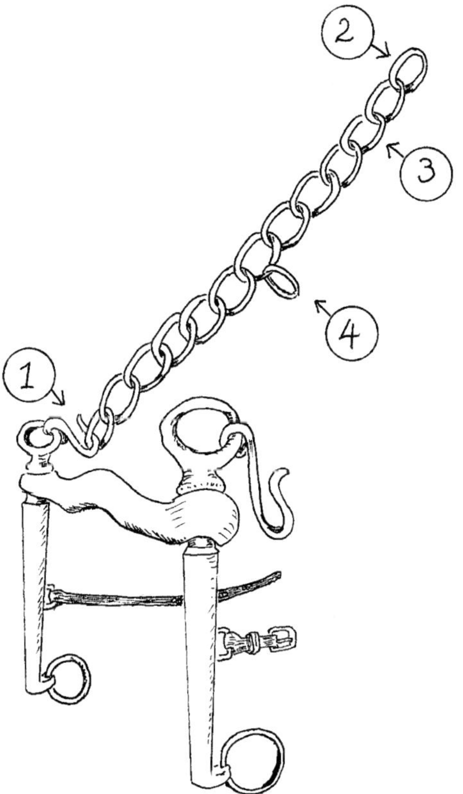

The correct way to do up a curb chain.
1: Put the top of the first link on the offside hook. Twist the chain clockwise until it lies
    smooth.
2: Put the top of the end link on the nearside hook.
3: Put the bottom of the next link that fits on the nearside hook. The curb chain should
    come into action when the cheek of the curb bit is at 45 degrees to normal.
4: Thread the lip strap through the fly link and do it up.

A horse can be badly upset by a rider who is incapable of controlling the exact tension on the different reins, so practise for some time with the two reins on a snaffle bit and only progress to riding in a double bridle when you are absolutely certain that you will not get in a muddle.

Do not put a double bridle on for a Working Hunter class unless you are absolutely certain that you will not pull the horse's mouth by mistake nor get too much tension on one or both curb reins at any time. Do not jump a horse in a double bridle unless you are absolutely certain that it will jump as round and boldly as it does in a snaffle.

To avoid accidentally using too much curb rein or getting one curb rein shorter than the other, you can adjust the right reins so that the bradoon rein

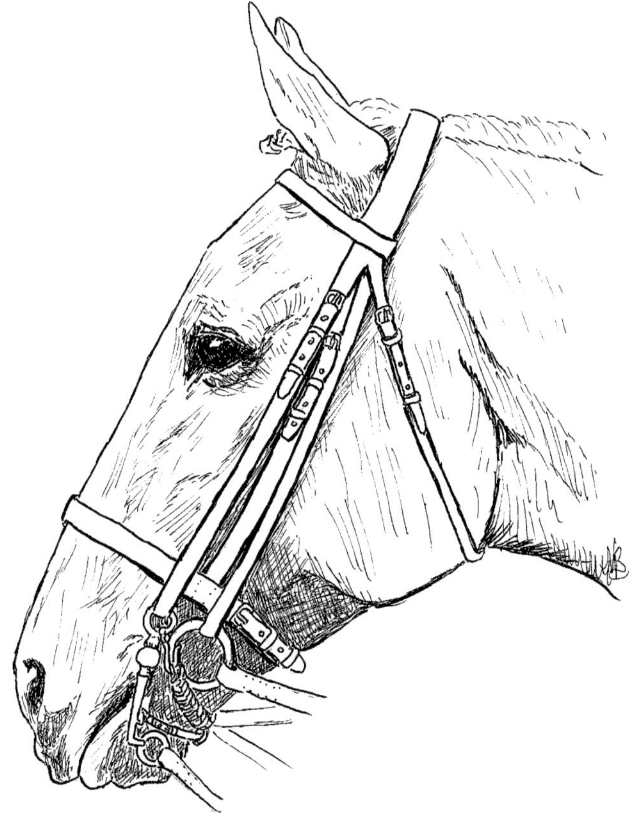

A double bridle correctly fitted.

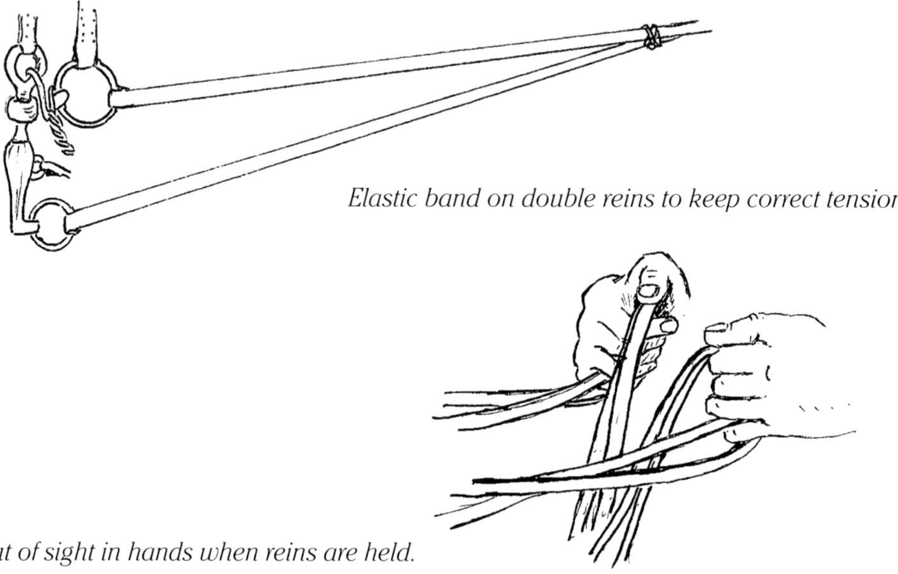

Elastic band on double reins to keep correct tension.

Out of sight in hands when reins are held.

tension and the curb rein tension in your right hand is just as you want it then hold the two reins on the left side in the exact same spot and wind an elastic band tightly round both of the left reins. Do the same on the right side, making sure that the two elastic bands are the same distance from the horse's mouth. Hold the reins in the normal way, adjusting the elastic bands so that they are hidden inside your hands when your reins are at a comfortable length. (This method is ideal for small children in the show ring.)

If the horse does become overbent you must be able to keep the contact on the bradoon rein and ease off the curb rein. You must learn to use the reins independently and make minute adjustments to suit each individual horse or the varying behaviour of your horse in different situations.

GIRTHS

Many horses, especially mares, will nip or even cow kick (kick forward under their tummies) when being girthed up. Tie them up and do the girth up very slowly and gradually.

Some horses will suddenly throw themselves on the floor when being girthed up. A girth with an elastic insert may be a help as there is no rigid, restricting tightness. In some cases a nylon fur or sheepskin sleeve over the full length of the girth may help.

These two methods may also help the sort of horse which suddenly catches its breath and bucks at the girth. If they have not been ridden for some time, there are horses which will behave as if they have never had a girth on before,

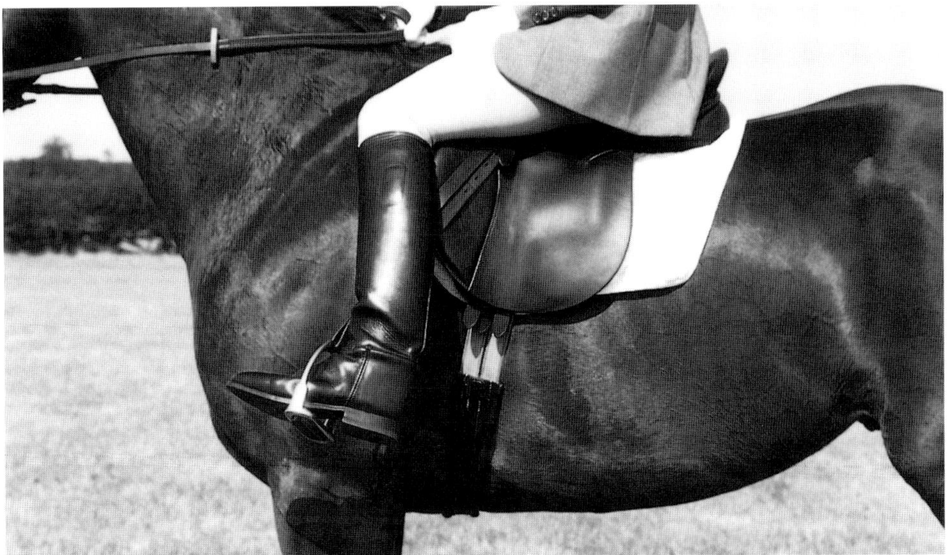

A girth with an elastic insert.

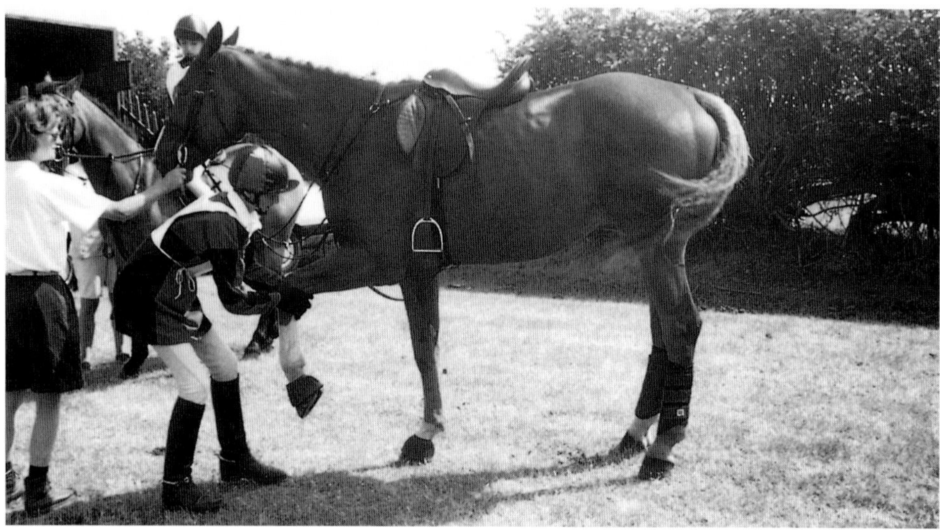

Pulling a foreleg forward so that there are no wrinkles under the girth.

catching their breath and humping their backs in the stable and really bucking at first when ridden. Put the saddle on several minutes before you want to ride. Use a numnah and a furry sleeve on the girth or a girth with an elastic insert. Tighten the girth very smoothly and gradually. Lunge the horse before you ride it or at least circle it in both directions before you mount.

Some horses react very strangely to pressure on a nerve just behind the elbow. Any girth which creates extra pressure here can cause problems. For instance, a nylon girth is joined and held together in several places by string sections. If one of these string sections happens to be situated directly over the nerve and presses on it, it can cause problems. The horse may throw itself down in the stable or it may, after being ridden for a few minutes, suddenly give way on one foreleg and drop as if it had put its foot in a deep hole. It is as if the pressure on that nerve has paralysed the foreleg. Changing to a smooth, soft girth usually completely cures the problem.

When you have done the girth up and are preparing to mount, take each foreleg in turn and pull it forward to make sure there are no wrinkles of skin under the girth.

Tightness of girths

A horse with a high wither which will help to hold the saddle in place does not need to be girthed up very tightly.

If an animal is almost circular, with no wither to speak of, it is necessary to tighten the girth gradually and to check the girth several times when you are riding and always before jumping. When mounting such a horse it may be necessary to have someone to lean on the stirrup on the off side to prevent the saddle from slipping round, or to mount from a mounting block. A piece of wash leather that has been dampened and wrung out, put on flat under the front of the saddle, may help to stabilise it.

OILING SADDLERY

New saddlery

Oil or Hydrolan will soften new saddlery quicker than saddle soap. They will also help to prevent any saddlery drying out hard and stiff after you have been riding in the rain.

Apply whichever you choose liberally on both sides of bridles, martingales and stirrup leathers but apply it only sparingly on the seat of a saddle and on the tops of the saddle flaps as your clothes will come into contact with these areas.

Bend every single inch of your tack in one direction, apply more oil or Hydrolan and then bend every single inch in the other direction. The leather will drink in whatever you apply and you just repeat the process until it is really soft and will take no more. The saddle flaps can be rolled in one direction really tightly, then rolled in the other direction. It may take an hour to do a saddle or a bridle thoroughly but the effect lasts for weeks and the tack can be cleaned normally after the first major application. If it does dry out hard or stiff after rain, give it one more thorough go and repeat the bending because it is this that makes the leather absorb whatever you choose to apply.

Old saddlery

Old saddlery which is dry and hard needs very gentle treatment. Soak it overnight, either by immersing it in oil or by wrapping very oily rags round it. Do not try to bend it or it will crack. After it has absorbed as much oil as it possibly can, try a slight bend, very gently. Work it about very carefully until you have got it soft and supple. If you hear cracking or see cracks appear as you bend the leather, stop immediately and soak it for longer.

Do not use old dry leather which has cracks. It will snap very easily and so is dangerous.

SADDLES SLIPPING

Saddle slipping forward

This problem is commonest with fat little ponies with large tummies and narrow shoulders. The saddle moves forward until the rider feels they are perched precariously over the pony's withers. If the pony then dives its head down to eat, the saddle slides up its neck, the girth descends to the back of its

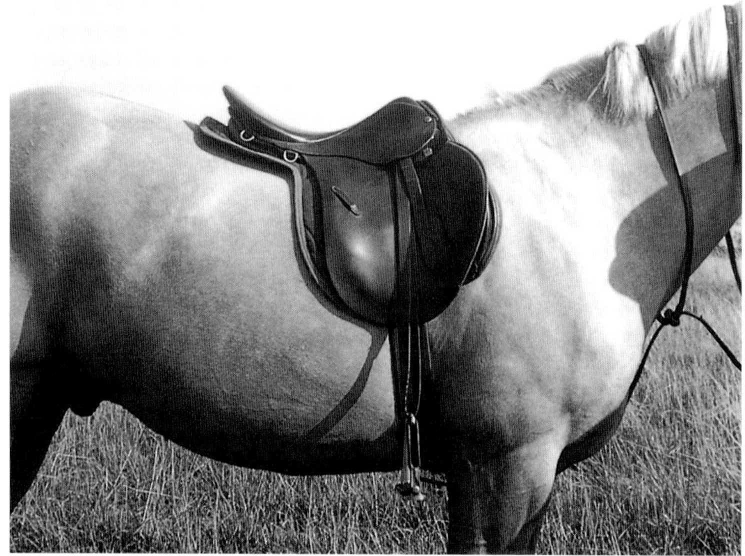

A well-fitting saddle.

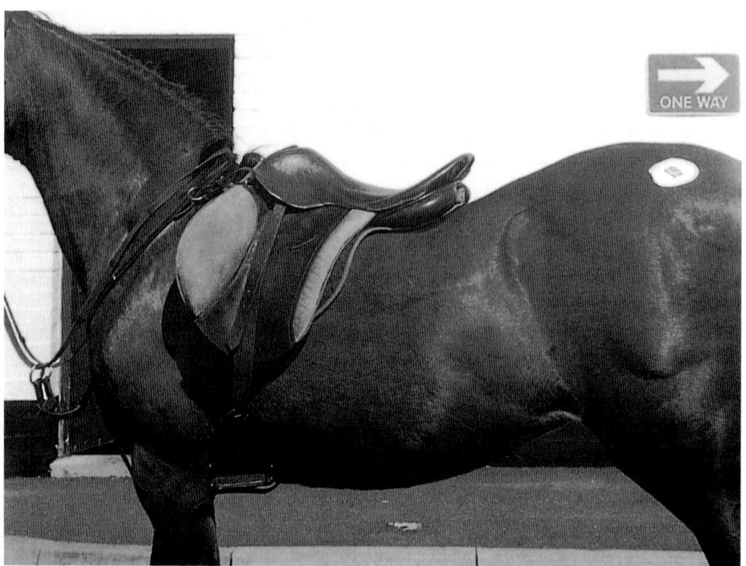

This saddle is cocked up in front and does not fit the horse. It will make the rider slip to the rear of the saddle and sit with their legs stuck forward.

knees and the rider shoots off over the pony's ears. Going downhill on such a pony can be dangerous as the saddle moves further and further forward.

Exactly the same problem can occur with horses which have a narrow, straight shoulder but they usually also have some wither to help to stabilise the saddle.

More stuffing in the front of the saddle (which I have heard being recommended) is certainly *not* the answer because if you raise the front of the saddle the rider sitting in it will push it forward even more. The extra padding will also encourage the saddle to go forward.

One possible solution is a crupper attached to the back of the saddle and passing round the root of the tail. This will stop the saddle slipping forward and is suitable for donkeys and little ponies with very small riders. The disadvantages are that this is ugly; it can be uncomfortable for the animal and some really dislike it and will not accept it; the animals cannot round their backs freely when jumping.

If the front of the saddle slides forward, have your saddle checked to see that it is a good fit. A normal saddle has either two or three girth straps on each side. The front ones are attached to the saddle and each other by one piece of webbing, the second (or second and third together) are attached to the saddle and each other by another piece of webbing. This is a safety factor so that if one breaks the other still holds. It is, of course, necessary to have a girth with two buckles at each end, or a pair of girths, and to attach one buckle to the front girth strap and one to the second or third strap on each side.

Point straps

These are extra girth straps which can be attached to the point pocket (the small leather pocket at the front of the saddle in which the point of the saddle tree sits). You will now have either three or four girth straps on each side of your saddle. Attach your girth to your new point strap and either the second or third girth strap. If the back of the saddle cocks up above the pony's back when the girth is attached to the second strap, move it on to the third strap. Point straps have the effect of anchoring the front of the saddle down and really do work. They can also be used very effectively in the show ring on both horses and ponies as they make the saddle sit further back and so give the impression that the animal has a much better shoulder.

Because attaching the girth to a point strap creates a lot of pressure on small areas of the back, check carefully for any discomfort. Notice if there is sweat

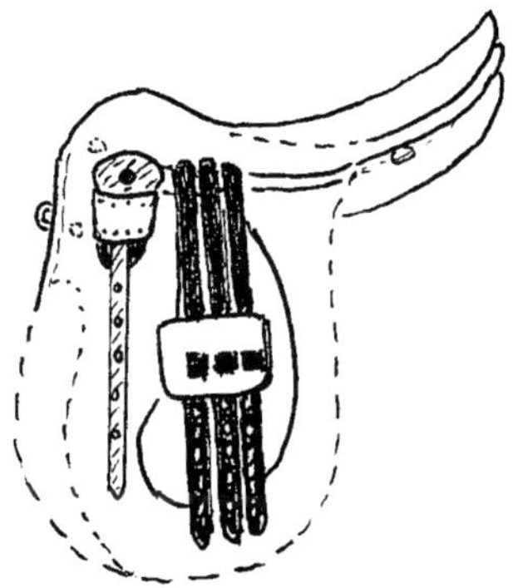

A point strap.

only in this area, notice any swelling or discomfort when handling or grooming this area. If, as you lean forward to dismount, the animal throws its head up or lays its ears back, or both, these are sure signs of discomfort. As you rise up from the saddle in trot or sit forward with your seat out of the saddle in canter, you are putting more weight on the animal's back under the point of the tree and under the stirrup bars. Ears back or head up when you are in these positions can also be signs of discomfort.

Saddle slipping back

This problem is caused by the horse's conformation. Look at the lower line of your horse's body from just behind the elbows, where the girth should lie, back to the flanks and hind legs. If there is the slightest uphill slope towards the hind legs, the girth will slip back and the saddle will then also move back.

During the summer, when they are fat, some horses will keep the girth, and therefore the saddle, in place with no problem as the bulge of their tummy outwards and downwards holds the girth firmly. If they lose weight during the winter or when fit and working hard, however, their shape will change and the girth will slide back, followed by the saddle. I am emphasising the fact that it is the girth going back which mostly causes the problem because if the movement of the girth is only slight it can be prevented simply by putting on a martingale. As this is attached to the girth it will prevent a *slight* tendancy to slip back. If the horse really does slope up sharply just behind the elbows, its whole body will be narrower to the rear and girth and saddle could move dangerously far back very quickly when going uphill or when jumping. This conformation is known as herring gutted because it resembles the rapidly narrowing shape of that fish.

Breast plate

For a horse with this confirmation, a leather breast plate can be used. This is attached to the girth between the forelegs and has two small straps attached to its neck strap, one on each side of the withers. These straps attach to Ds on the saddle just in front of the stirrup bars. Adjust the breast plate so that it does not feel tight but so that it will prevent the girth from moving back from the elbow more than 7–10 cm (3–4 in). A breast plate of this type usually has a ring on the neck strap to which a running martingale attachment can be fixed. Adjust the two small straps so that there is some room for movement of the shoulders.

Breast girth

This is normally made of webbing but can be made of folded leather. It is attached to the girth straps on each side of the saddle and is kept in place by a narrow, adjustable strap passing over the neck just in front of the withers.

If fitted too low, it can press on the shoulders and limit their freedom of action. If fitted too high, it can press on the windpipe. There is no attachment to the girth between the forelegs so a breast girth works by keeping the saddle forward.

Both breast girths and breast plates can be seen in use in racing and show jumping. Breast plates are more common where the horse is to be ridden for a long period of time, as in the hunting field.

If the problem is desperate, a breast girth will hold the saddle forward more effectively. Use it with a martingale which will help to keep the girth in place.

HEADCOLLARS

If a headcollar is to be left on in the field it must be carefully adjusted so that the noseband is loose enough for the horse to chew without having the sharp edges of its lower jaw rubbed. If the noseband itself does not adjust, the height of the noseband governs how tightly or loosely it fits. There may be only one buckle to do it up by or one at each side. Put the headcollar on and make sure that there is plenty of room for the sharp edges of the lower jaw by putting your fingers over them while the horse is chewing. Constantly check for signs of the headcollar rubbing on:

- the lower jaw
- the frontal nosebone
- the bulgy bone near the eye
- the top of the head

If it does rub anywhere, a piece of sheepskin-like fabric stitched right round the area can help. NB: if you have a foal or very young horse, check constantly and be prepared to put on a bigger headcollar because their heads grow very quickly.

Check the field for any dangerous places on which a headcollar could get hitched up if the horse rubs. Nylon headcollars do not break and so can be dangerous if a horse gets caught up. Leather is safer because it will break. See also page 22.

Getting a headcollar off

Some horses are experts at removing their headcollars – a quick rub behind the ear and a hitch from a suitable aid such as a gate, fence post or tree, and the headcollar is on the ground. An extra strap can be attached to the two rings that lie just below eye level, and used like an extra throatlash.

Two or three loops can be fitted on to and behind the headcollar headpiece and an extra strap can be threaded through them to do up fairly tightly as an extra throatlash. Both methods involving the extra strap must be adjusted just tight enough to prevent the horse from removing the headcollar but not so tight as to affect its breathing.

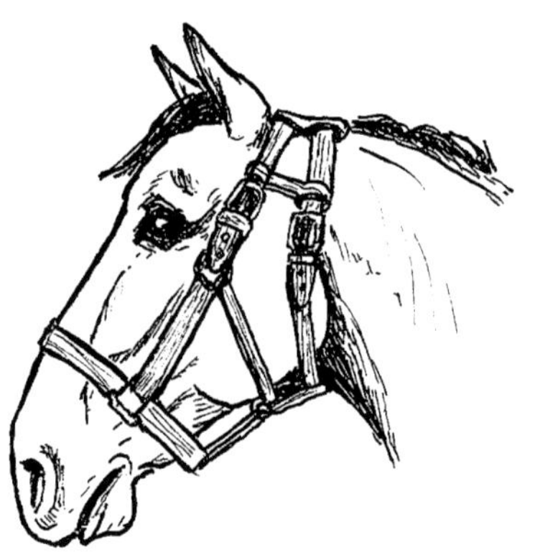

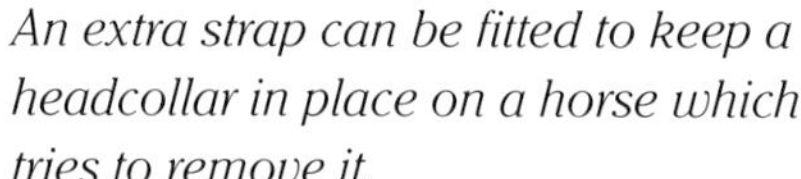

An extra strap can be fitted to keep a headcollar in place on a horse which tries to remove it.

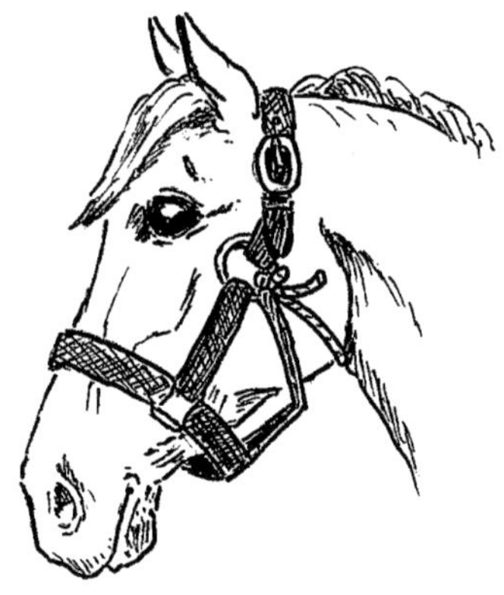

An extra throatlash can be made out of string.

Warning: when scratching their heads with a hind toe, foals have been known to get their hoof stuck in the headcollar. If they are unable to remove their foot they can badly injure or even kill themselves. This may seem unlikely, or even impossible, but I do know a pony which, when wearing a nylon headcollar with narrow metal rings, managed to scratch its head with a hind foot and get the too-long heel of its hind shoe caught in the headcollar ring. It was caught up all night and was severely injured.

MARTINGALES

Running martingale

A running martingale should be fitted so that when it is attached to the girth the martingale rings reach up into the horse's gullet when its head is at a normal height. There should be a rubber stop to keep the martingale in place where it passes through the loop of the neck strap. Reins with buckles or stud billets should have leather or rubber stops on them between these fittings and the martingale rings so that there is no possibility of the martingale getting caught up and jerking the horse's head sideways.

A running martingale should only come into action if the horse puts its head up. It is a help when riding an unruly horse because it prevents it from raising its head beyond the point of control. It does not prevent the horse from stretching its neck out and down so it does not restrict its freedom when jumping. The neck strap is handy to hold on to in an emergency, to save pulling the horse's mouth.

If the martingale is fitted too tightly there will be a downward and slightly backward pull on the reins and so on the horse's mouth. This will shorten the

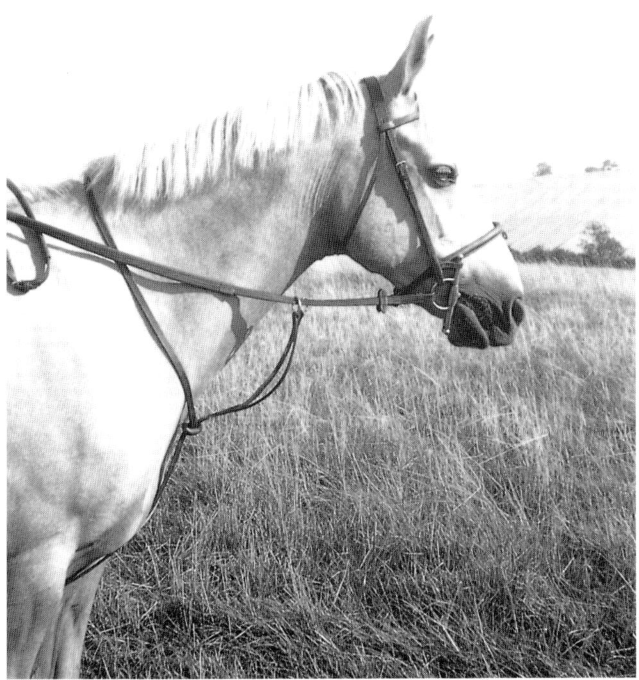

A correctly adjusted running martingale.

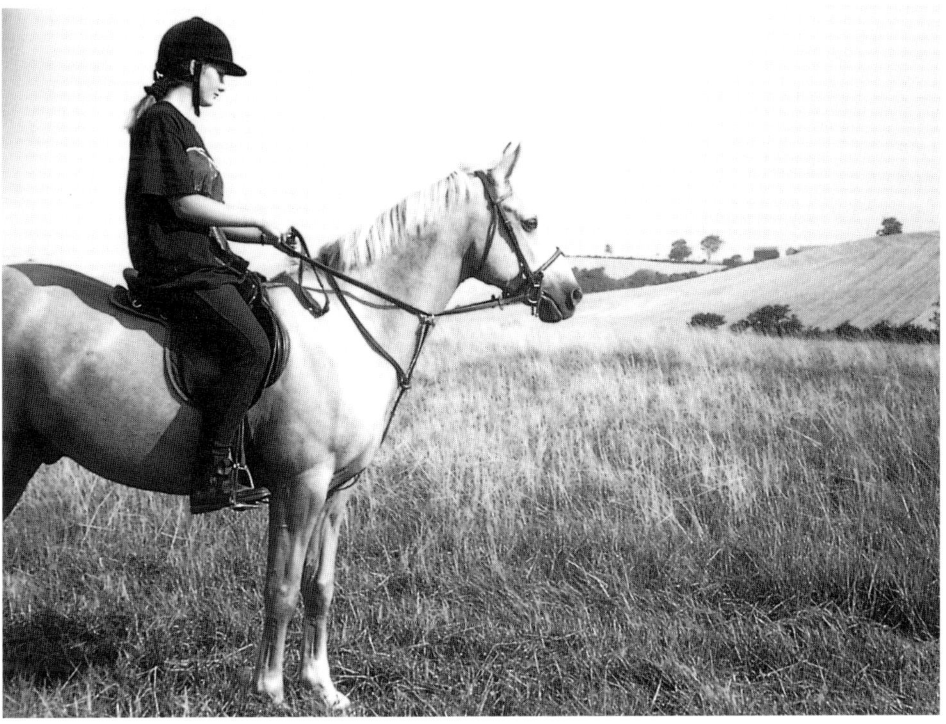

This running martingale is too tight and is pulling the rein down.

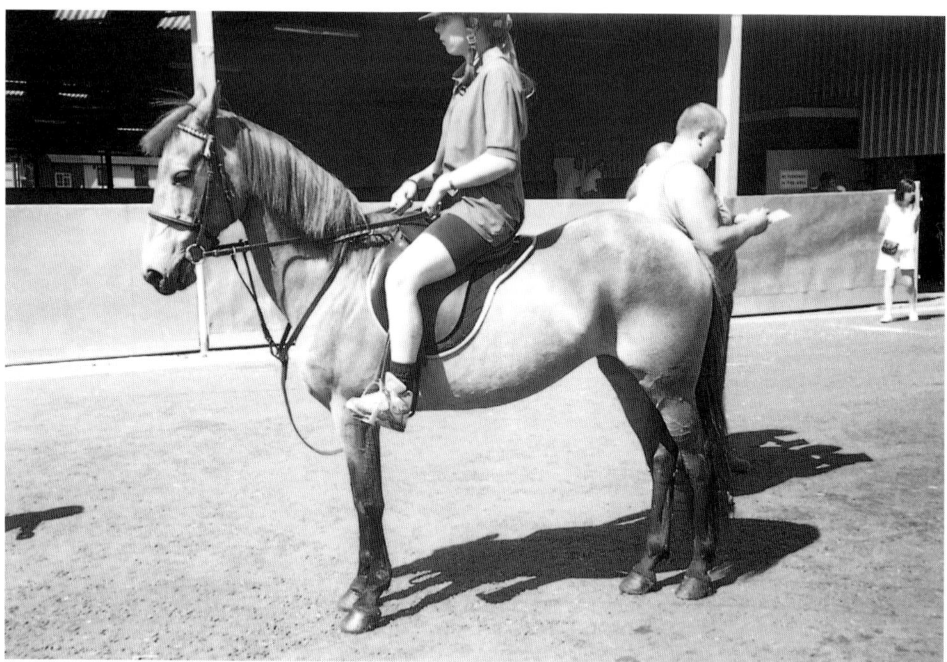

This running martingale is dangerously long and is hanging down between the forelegs. The rider is also sitting behind the movement.

horse's stride in all gaits. The horse will feel that its forward movement is restricted. It may nap, whip round or run backwards. It may be unwilling to approach or go over a jump because it feels it has no freedom to use its head and neck, essential when jumping.

When the martingale is too tight in this way, the reins will be pulled down at an angle, the lowest point being where the rein goes through the martingale ring. The rider now has an indirect contact on the horse's mouth. There is a strong backward and downward pull which stops the horse from going forward freely. The rider is no longer able to have an 'allowing hand' and no longer has a direct guiding contact with the horse's mouth.

A horse which throws its head up can learn to come back towards the rider's face with its head and set its neck against the martingale. In doing this it will become more difficult to control and will develop a large bulge of muscle on the underside of its neck and lose what muscle it previously had on top of its neck. It may become ewe-necked.

Standing martingale

Standing martingales should be fitted so that when one end is attached to the girth and the other to an ordinary noseband, the slack can be lifted up into the horse's gullet. When wearing a standing martingale a horse does not have complete freedom of forward and downward movement of its neck and head. It can learn to lean against the noseband, held by the martingale, develop a bulge of muscle under its neck and lose any muscle that it had on top of its neck.

When looking at a horse to buy, note if it has a bulge of muscle under its neck and not much on top. Feel the bulging muscle and, if it is thick and hard, realise that you are buying a strong horse with a high head carriage. A horse that goes incorrectly in this way is likely to be a problem.

RUGS

New Zealand rugs – slipping and rubbing

Every horse and pony is a slightly different shape and you have to pay for a New Zealand rug before you can try it in the field and see if it stays in place without rubbing the animal's shoulders or withers.

Put the rug on in the stable and do it up at the neck. Pull it back as far as it will go towards the horse's tail. The top of the neck of the rug should still be in front of the withers and should not be pressing tightly on to the top of the horse's neck. If the neck is too big, the withers will get rubbed even with a piece of sheepskin on this part of the rug.

If, as the horse walks, you can see the bulge of the point of its shoulder straining the material, the hair will soon be rubbed off this area. Some rugs are made with darts and a flair or slit here to allow free shoulder movement. If the central back seam is absolutely straight all the way along, the rug is likely to slip sideways. When folded in half along the centre seam, a well-cut rug should appear a little higher at the withers and at the highest point of the hindquarters and should dip down lower at the back. When you put a rug cut in this way on your horse, the curved part designed to sit over the hindquarters should sit snugly in place and the neck and shoulders should not be being pressed by the front of the rug. There should be freedom to move. If this curved part comes in front of the hindquarters the rug is not long enough for that horse.

Now look at the rug from the back. Does it stand out shapelessly away from the hindquarters? If so, it may slip sideways as the horse moves about the field. A well-cut rug should have darts at the back, on each side of the centre seam, so that the shape of the rug follows the shape of the hindquarters and the rug will stay in place.

If your rug has leg straps, they should each do up on their own side of the rug and should be linked together, one passing through the loop of the other, between the horse's hind legs.

If the rug does up at two different levels in front, the top fastening should be slightly tighter than the one below. The lower one needs to be looser to allow for shoulder movement.

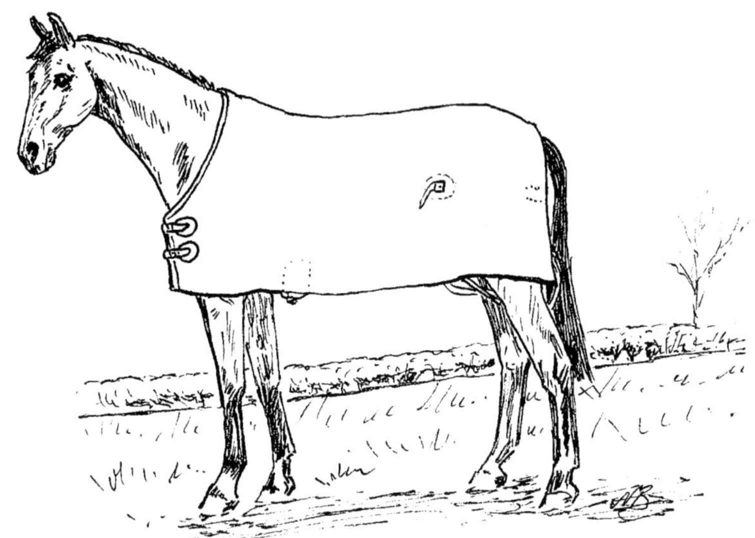

A well-fitting New Zealand rug.

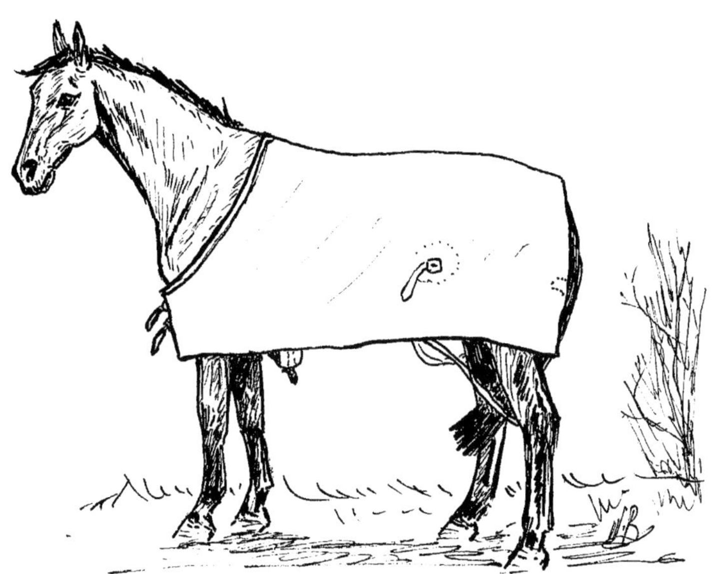

This New Zealand rug does not fit. The neck is too wide so the rug slips back and cuts into the withers and shoulders. The leg straps are too loose.

Modern rugs have several different patterns of straps to keep them on but all New Zealand rugs need to be well cut to stay on. They should be checked and adjusted at least every 24 hours. If a horse lives out permanently in a New Zealand rug, it would be ideal to have two rugs so that a very wet one could be changed and dried out.

Rug tearing

This is a maddening habit and can cost a fortune. Some horses find rugs irritating and set about removing them by rubbing on the stable walls and tearing at the rug with their teeth, ripping it into shreds.

Check for skin irritation. Has the rug been washed in detergent? Has it got a coarse itchy lining? Could the horse be too hot? Is the rug too tight anywhere?

A New Zealand rug made of very strong canvas may defeat some horses.

A stiff leather bib attached to a headcollar allows the horse to eat but prevents its teeth from contacting the rug. Any form of muzzle has to be removed for eating.

A rod with a spring clip at each end, attached to a side D of the headcollar at one end and the roller at the other, prevents the horse from bending its neck to reach the rug with its teeth.

A cradle (made from a series of wooden rods about 60 cm or 2 ft long, connected by two leather straps) can be strapped round the neck to prevent the horse from reaching its rug.

Tearing off bandages or wound dressings

The above methods may also be used to prevent a horse removing bandages or dressings from wounds on its legs.

An additional aid to prevent a horse from removing dressings from a leg wound is a pricker boot. This boot has small, sharp spikes sticking out, which will prick the horse's nose or lips. It is put on over the bandage or dressing.

6 AILMENTS

TEETH

A yearling has only milk teeth. The four corner incisors look very small and for this reason some people confuse a yearling's mouth with of a four year old. A four year old has only the four corner incisor milk teeth left, the other front teeth are permanent ones. If in doubt, look at the shape of the animal. Does it look like a yearling – a bit leggy, narrow and gangly? Look at its tail. Is it full length with straight strong hairs all the same colour? If so, it is probably four. A yearling's tail tends to be above the hocks and have curly, often gingery hairs at the end.

Milk teeth have narrow 'necks' where they grow out of the gums. Permanent teeth have no 'necks'. Compare the shape of the centre teeth where they leave the gums with that of the corner teeth. See if this area is different, as it would be in a four year old, or the same, with all teeth having 'necks', as would be the case in a yearling.

At two and a half years (normally about Christmas time) a horse loses its two central incisors from top and bottom as they are pushed out by the permanent teeth.

By Easter these teeth will have grown up level. About the following Christmas, at three and a half years, the next two milk teeth from top and bottom will be pushed out so that, at four years old, the horse will have four permanent teeth on top and bottom and one milk tooth at each of the four corners.

At four and a half the corner milk teeth are pushed out and at five years the horse is said to have a full mouth.

Between four and five years male horses grow extra teeth (known as tushes) in the gaps between their incisor and molar teeth.

It is not just the twelve incisor milk teeth which fall out and are replaced by permanent ones. The same thing is happening with the 24 back molars but as they are out of sight you will not be so aware of this. A mare has 36 teeth; a male horse has 40 – 36 plus four tushes.

Tushes coming through can make male horses uncomfortable with a bit. Loose incisors and molars can make all horses uncomfortable so be aware of this. If a young horse becomes fussy in its mouth, hack it about on a long rein.

106

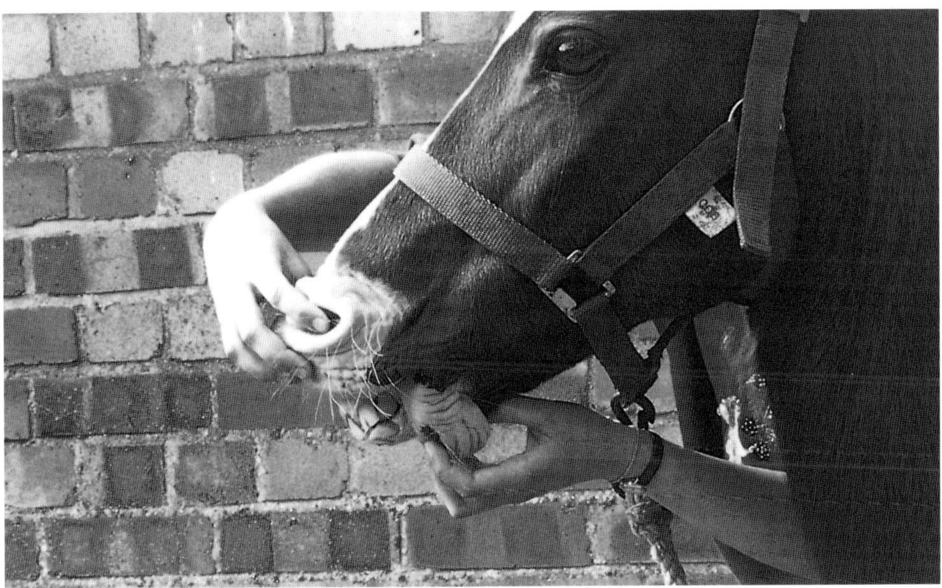

Look at the slope at which the teeth meet and see if there are any milk teeth before opening the horse's mouth wide to look at the biting surface and the marks. This pony has very sloping bottom teeth and is older that it at first seems to be.

Don't insist on schooling it and trying to get it 'on the bit' or you may cause permanent stiffness and resentment in the mouth or make the horse permanently fractious. Be patient and understanding.

Five year olds have a full mouth of permanent teeth but the corner teeth are not up far enough to be in full wear all over. The centres are still hollow. The outside edges may be in wear but the inside edges will not be. Sometimes gum is still visible in the centre of the teeth.

At six years the inside and outside edges of the four corner teeth will be in wear but the centres will still be slightly hollow.

At seven years the centres will be in wear and there may be a hook on the back end of the top corner incisors where they have not yet been worn down by the position of the bottom corner incisors. The 'seven-year hook' is not present in all horses and may sometimes be seen on one side and not on the other. At this age the incisors meet vertical to each other.

As the horse gets older the incisors meet on more and more of a slope. This is an important rough guide to age when first opening a horse's lips to check its age. It is also an important place to check when you see a seven-year hook on the top corner incisor because this hook sometimes reappears at thirteen or fourteen years of age and can be misleading.

The shape of the biting surface of the teeth is long and narrow on a young horse. The marks on the biting surface of a young horse's teeth are also dark, long and narrow. As the horse gets older the biting surface becomes rounder, then more triangular, and the marks become rounder and yellower with age. The slope as the front teeth meet becomes more and more pronounced with age.

A horse's upper jaw is wider than its lower jaw, and so the outside edges of the top teeth and the inside edges of the bottom teeth do not get worn down because the horse chews in a sideways motion. The top teeth give most trouble as their sharp edges often cut the insides of the horse's cheeks. This can cause two problems: the horse is in pain when chewing so it eats less and loses weight; and it may also be uncomfortable with a bit in its mouth. This discomfort can take the form of head tossing, carrying the head to one side, carrying the head high, being loath to go forward on a rein contact, being difficult to turn in one direction or charging off to try to get away from the pain when the rider attempts to steady the horse by feeling on the reins. A horse's teeth should be inspected by a vet or horse dentist at least once a year.

Wolf teeth

Some horses grow a tiny extra tooth in the top jaw just in front of the first molar, sometimes on one side only, sometimes on both sides. This can cause discomfort when bitted. If they are causing problems, wolf teeth can be easily removed by a vet.

Tushes

A male horse grows four extra teeth in the gaps between the upper and lower back and front teeth between four and five years of age. First you will feel or see a bump and the gum may be red and sore. Until the tooth is right through the horse may be uncomfortable and fussy in its mouth when ridden. Some mares may also grow tiny, rudimentary tushes.

Quidding

Perhaps one day you notice large wodges of partly chewed hay on the stable floor or, if the horse is in the field, partly chewed wodges of grass. When the horse is eating its hay, instead of chewing in a steady rhythm – munch, munch, munch – it gives a couple of chews and then half opens its mouth, partly crosses its jaw and spits lumps of hay out. The same may be seen when eating a feed or grazing but it is most obvious when eating hay.

Your horse has probably got sharp teeth which are hurting, and perhaps cutting, the inside of its cheeks when it tries to chew. Because a horse's upper jaw is considerably wider than its lower jaw, the outside edges of its top teeth do not get worn down. The sharpness is accentuated by the sideways motion of the bottom teeth when chewing. For the same reasons the inside edges of the bottom teeth can also become sharp and hurt or cut the horse's tongue.

Problems with the bottom teeth, however, are not nearly so common as problems with the top teeth.

Sharp teeth can also cause the ridden horse to throw its head up, carry its head turned in one direction, pull or dive at the reins, go sideways, hot up or be difficult to control.

A young horse that is losing milk teeth (at two and a half to five years) can also find it difficult and painful to chew and be fussy in its mouth when ridden. When the loose tooth finally falls out, all may be well but it is better not to ride a young horse which is obviously temporarily uncomfortable in its mouth (unless it is quiet and schooled enough to be ridden in a bitless bridle for a few days).

If you notice that your horse is having these problems, ask a vet or a registered equine dentist to rasp your horse's teeth. Every horse's teeth should be checked at least once a year.

PARROT MOUTH OR OVERSHOT JAW

The term 'parrot mouth' is used to describe horses whose upper jaw juts out beyond their lower jaw. This abnormality does cause several problems.

- Normal horses graze by nipping off the grass between their top and bottom front teeth. To do this successfully the two sets of teeth must meet. A parrot-mouthed horse cannot graze in this way and has to adapt by placing its tongue against its teeth to pull at the grass or by trying to nip the grass off between its corner teeth. Whichever method it learns to use, it is absolutely essential to graze a parrot-mouthed horse in a field with long grass so that it can get hold of the grass. A parrot-mouthed horse can almost starve on a very bare field. If the horse loses condition, be prepared to bucket feed it and to provide hay all year round if necessary.

- Because the front top and bottom teeth of a parrot-mouthed horse do not meet, there is no means of wearing them down so they will grow very long. In a gelding the tushes (the four extra teeth which grow in the gaps between the molars and incisors) will not be in the normal position and may interfere with each other. They may come in contact with the bit and make the bit difficult to fit correctly and comfortably. Because the whole jaw is

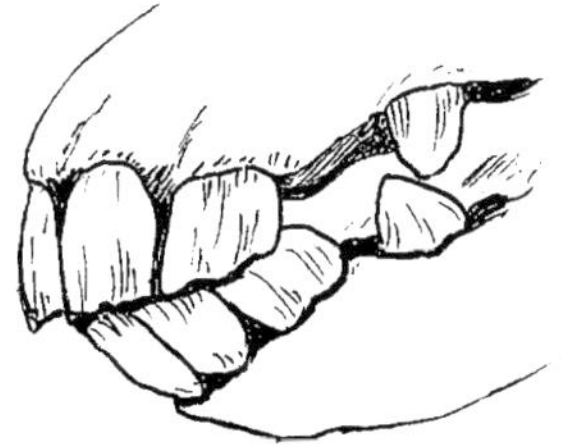

Parrot mouth or overshot jaw.

abnormally positioned, the molars in the top jaw come further forward than the molars in the bottom jaw. The front molar on each side of the top jaw has nothing to meet and wear down against and so these teeth often grow into sharp hooks which can press on the bottom gums. In the same way the back molar on each side of the bottom jaw has nothing to meet and wear down against, so these teeth grow upwards and can press on the gums of the top jaw. Because the jaws are closer together at the back than at the front, there is no room to accommodate this extra growth and it becomes painful for the horse to chew. This situation often goes unnoticed.

The horse may need constant attention from a horse dentist or a vet experienced in these problems.

SOW MOUTH OR UNDERSHOT JAW

This term is used to describe exactly the opposite situation to that described above – the lower jaw juts out beyond the upper jaw. This condition is not so common but all of the problems of a parrot-mouthed horse also apply here. In this case it is the top back molars and the bottom front molars which have nothing to wear down against and so may cause problems.

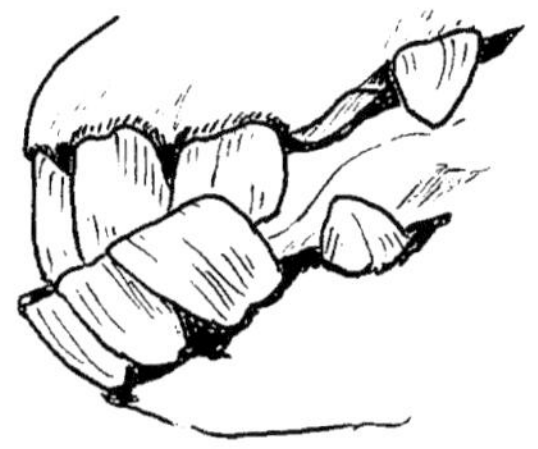

Sow mouth or undershot jaw.

CHEEK POUCHES OF GRASS

Large wodges of grass can get stuck in the cheeks of some animals. They are uncomfortable and difficult for the horse to remove although it can often be seen attempting to do so by rubbing its cheek on the inside of its knee. A missing tooth or malformation of the teeth is the usual cause. The grass ferments, smells horrible and can cause a gum or tooth problem as it decays. Some horses will open their mouths when you rub the outside of their cheeks and you can then push the grass out without having to put your hand in their mouths. If this does not work, you will have to push your index finger between the cheek and the horse's teeth and hook the wodge of grass out. Some horses

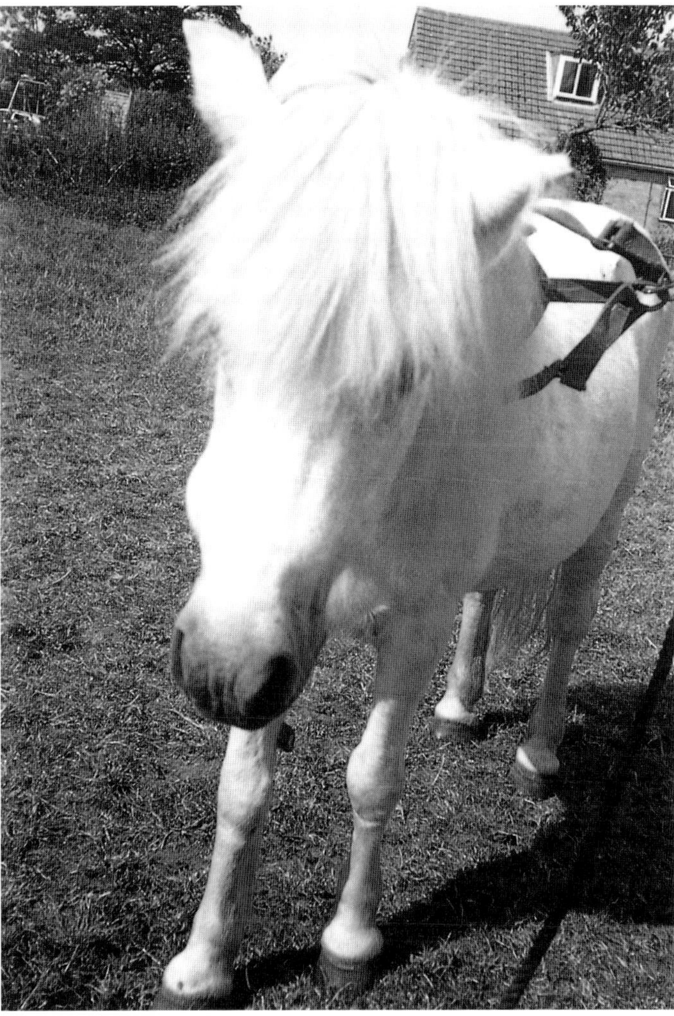

A pouch of grass in a pony's cheek.

seem totally unable to remove such a wodge themselves so you will have to do it for them at least every 24 hours.

Hay and bucket feed rarely cause the same problem in the cheeks as grass.

SPLIT LIP

This condition can go unnoticed because the corners of some horses' lips turn in in almost a double fold and the split is on the inside out of sight.

Young horses with soft-skinned mouths, unused to a bit, will often develop small sores in the corners which can be clearly seen. Use rubber rings to protect the corners if necessary (see page 81) and do not allow splits to form.

Horses which reach and dive their heads down and get frantically excited can often split their lips. Worn, sharp, jointed bits can cause a cut in the corner of the mouth which can become a split.

In any of the above situations, check the corners of the mouth carefully. Open the mouth and look and feel inside it to find out if the inner fold of skin at the corner of the mouth is damaged.

If the skin on the visible corners of the mouth is kept greased with petroleum jelly, it is less likely to split.

A thick bit can drag on the corners more than a thinner bit and may cause a split.

Going from a straight bar to a jointed bit, or vice versa, can help the split to heal. If it is slow to heal and the horse is uncomfortable and fussy to ride in a bit, you may have to rest it for a few days (the mouth usually heals quickly) or ride in a mild, bitless bridle.

Do not allow the condition to become chronic when two thick lumps of skin tissue with a split between them may form in each corner of the horse's mouth. This will open up every time the horse is ridden in a bit and will be very sore. It may even be necessary for a vet to operate, remove the scar tissue and allow the new wound to heal closely.

SORE GUMS

Young horses get inflamed, swollen gums when teething just as children do. If your three- to five-year-old horse suddenly becomes fussy in its mouth, suspect this to be the cause. Lunge it in just a cavesson or ride it in a mild bitless bridle, preferably in an enclosed area, until the inflammation subsides.

LAMPAS

Lampas is a swelling of the roof of the mouth, which can be caused by teething or sometimes indigestion. The area seems to protrude below the level of the teeth. It is uncomfortable for the horse and looks red and inflamed. If it is caused by teething the problem should resolve itself. If the cause is indigestion, change the diet.

SORE EYES

Some horses are so tormented by flies that their lower eyelids sag open, their eyes stream and they get a yellow pus infection.

A fly fringe (see photograph, page 115) is not sufficient protection.

A green vegetable net of the type brussels sprouts are sold in can be fixed to

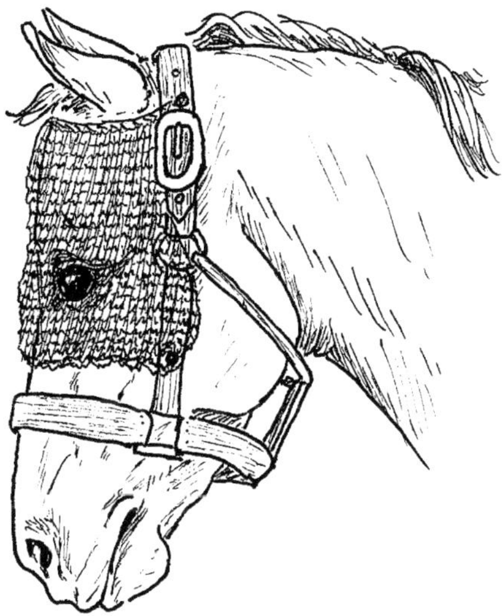

A fly net made from a vegetable net bag.

a headcollar to form eye protection. Cut out a piece of net to cover from just below the ears to halfway down the nose. Put a headcollar on the horse and work out where to punch a hole in it near to the ear on the off (right) side. Remove the headcollar and stitch the top of the net to this hole to stop it slipping down. Stitch the other top side of the net to the appropriate hole in the strap near where the headcollar does up. Sew or fasten the net to the right cheekpiece of the headcollar. Sew a popper on to the lower left of the net so that it can be wrapped round the left cheekpiece and fastened with the popper after the headcollar is in place.

If your horse is to be turned out in a headcollar, this must be made of leather which will break in a crisis if the horse gets caught up when rubbing or when trying to scratch an ear with a hind foot. Nylon head collars do not break and can cause horrific accidents.

HEAD SHAKING

- Horses which have a problem in their ears (mites, warts, a bit of twig or leaf) shake their heads sideways. The affected ear is often carried slightly out to one side and down at an angle.
- Horses which have a sore place on their heads, or ft the bridle or browband is making hairs pull uncomfortably, or if it is too tight, shake their heads sideways.
- A 'head shaker' shakes its head up and down, never sideways. It may carry its head up high or down low for several strides. It may, as it flings its head

right up, bring its forelegs off the ground and give a little skip. It may rub its nose on its knees or rub its nose frantically on the ground almost kneeling down to do so. A bad case of 'head shaking' can make a horse unridable during the summer yet the same horse will show no symptoms whatsoever during the winter.

The cause is a severe allergic reaction to something. Some horses react to bean flowers and nothing else. They are almost unridable near a field of beans in flower but all right as soon as the pods have set.

Other horses are allergic only to rape flowers (as are many people).

Some horses are only affected by pollen. Others react when ridden near trees or hedges where there are tiny insects but not when ridden out in a field well away from trees or hedges. They seem to react to insects near their nostrils but not to pollen.

Horses which have never had a problem in their previous home can produce violent allergic reactions when sold to a different part of the country.

Unfortunately there is no known cure, so what can you do if your horse has this problem?

- Some horses improve if a leather or string fly fringe is attached to their noseband.
- A pair of ladies tights can be cut and shaped to encase the nose and attach to the noseband. These can be worn when show jumping but not in a show class or dressage competition.
- Anti-histamine may help some animals.

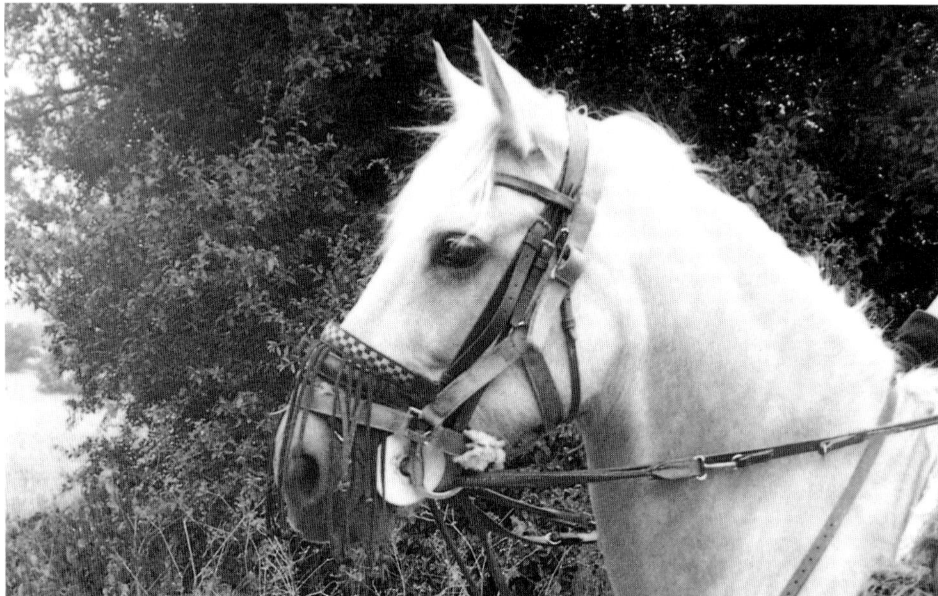

A fly fringe worn over the nose of a head shaker.

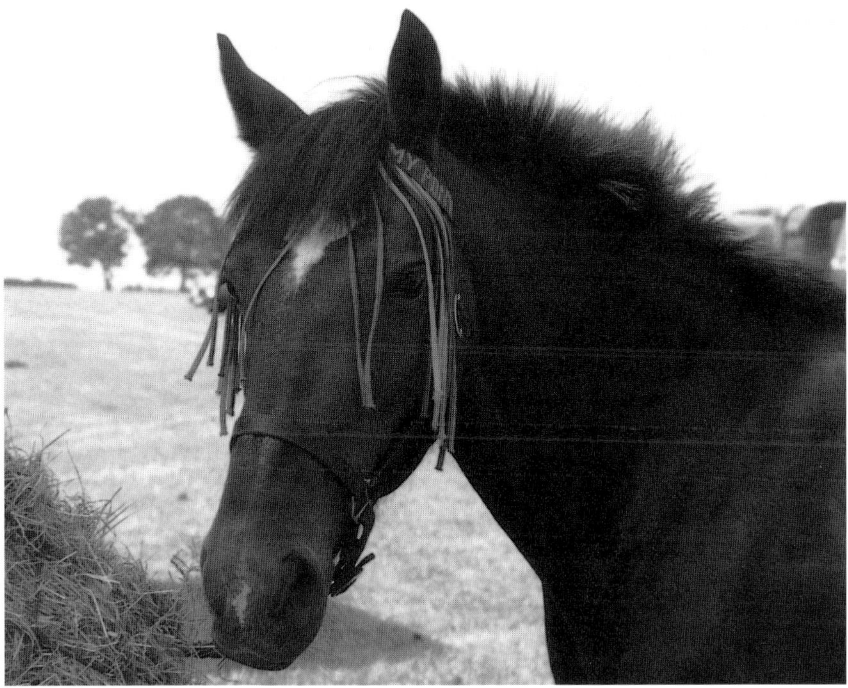

A fly fringe.

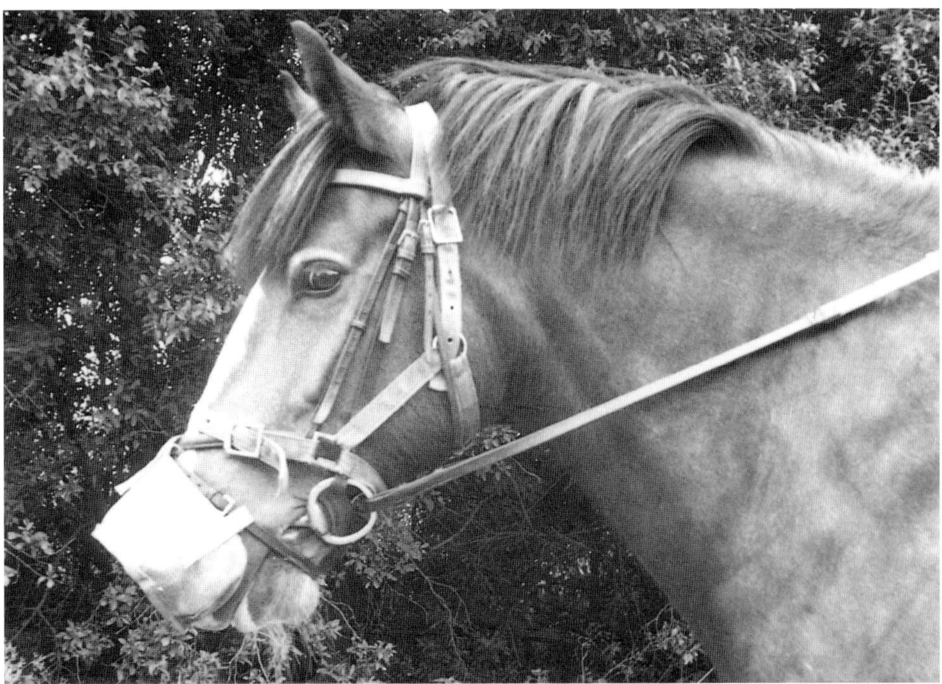

This horse hated rain on its nose and always wore this nose shield. It could also be used on a head shaker or to protect a white-nosed horse from sunburn.

Sadly, if you want to use your horse or pony all year round it is best to sell a head shaker because although the condition may vary from day to day, you are certain to have great disappointment. A home which only wants a horse to work in winter, in the hunting field for instance, will have no problem.

An operation to desensitise the lining of the nostrils helps some horses.

ALLERGIES

Dust allergy

This is probably the commonest problem with stabled horses nowadays. It is not, in fact, dust but the fine mould spores found in some hay and straw which cause the trouble.

Symptoms vary from the occasional cough in the stable, coughing when first trotted on exercise and fast, laboured breathing to a single, long, hollow cough and a double heave of the flanks when breathing out, plus distress when trotting or cantering uphill or for a distance.

Mild symptoms can usually be controlled by bedding the horse on wood shavings or paper (the box must not be connected to neighbouring boxes bedded on straw) and feeding clean hay that has been well soaked in water. More severe cases need treating with additional medication such as Ventipulmin and to be fed specially treated hay such as Horsehage. Horses with mild symptoms, which clear up with soaked hay and dust-free bedding, can usually cope with fast work such as hunting or eventing with no problem.

Horses showing a double heave when breathing out and having quicker, somewhat laboured breathing are unlikely to cope with anything more than light hacking. Actual lung damage is permanent.

Many allergic horse will cough for two or three days if, by mistake, they are given only one small armful of dry hay, so great care must be taken. Mouldy straw is lethal to any horse because when it lies down its nostrils touch the straw, breathing the spores into its lungs. You can damage the lungs of any horse by bedding it on mouldy straw or feeding it mouldy hay.

Wood allergy

Some horses show a skin reaction when bedded on shavings or wood chips. The skin becomes red and itchy in patches and the hair may start to fall out. The horse may constantly rub and roll to try to relieve the irritation. It is thought that some kinds of redwood can cause the trouble. Check the source of your bedding. Some firms use only white wood.

Heel and nose scab in summer

White-nosed and white-legged horses can get large scabby formations on white areas that are in contact with the grass when walking or grazing. These are sore and unsightly and can cover most of the white-haired, pink-skinned area. This irritation is thought to be caused by the plant of St John's wort (*Hypericum* species). The quickest cure is to move the affected horse into another field as the plant seems to be restricted to certain areas. Often only one field will cause the trouble.

Soap powder

Washing girths and numnahs in detergent can cause a skin reaction. The girth and numnah both cover areas where the horse may sweat and any detergent residue left in the material then gets into the pores of the skin and causes irritation. Use only a mild soap when washing anything which will be in contact with the horse's skin. Always rinse such items thoroughly

Nettle rash or hives

Confusingly, this is not caused by nettles.

It is very frightening to come into your horse's stable in the morning and see that its head has swollen up gigantically so that its eyes are almost closed and its nose, lips and nostrils are enormous. It is suffering from an allergic reaction to something in its food. You will probably never find out what caused it but if, the day before, you had just started a new bag of feed, take it back for analysis just in case. Ring the vet immediately and he or she will give the horse an anti-hystamine injection which will bring the horse's head back to normal in a matter of hours. It is essential to call the vet in this case because the swelling may affect the windpipe and make breathing difficult.

A swollen head is the most alarming sight to see but other parts of the body may also be affected by large, soft swellings, varying from golf-ball size to the size of a dinner plate. These are usually on the belly, between the fore and hind legs. Again, an anti-hystamine injection will cure the condition.

Wasp or bee stings can cause a similar reaction.

Nettle stings

A thin-skinned horse which has rolled in a bed of nettles or even fallen into a ditch full of nettles, may hurl itself about in pain or stagger about on stiff limbs giving the impression that it is out of its mind or, in the latter case, that it has damaged its back. I do know of a horse that was very nearly shot after having fallen into a ditch full of nettles because it appeared hardly able to stand, then thrashed about in an uncoordinated manner until it fell down. It was driven mad by the pain of the nettle stings but there was nothing else wrong with it and in 24 hours it was as right as rain.

If this happens to your horse, call the vet who will administer a pain-killing injection.

Sunburn

Some pink-skinned horses can suffer from sunburn. Pink-eyed albinos are particularly at risk but even a dark brown horse with a pink nose can be affected.

Early signs are redness and peeling skin. In severe cases the skin cracks open and clear golden serum runs out. Keep the horse in during the day or use a sun shield attached to a headcollar. Sun block creams can be used but are expensive if you have several horses to treat. When the sun gets strong, check your pink-skinned animals each day – prevention is better than cure.

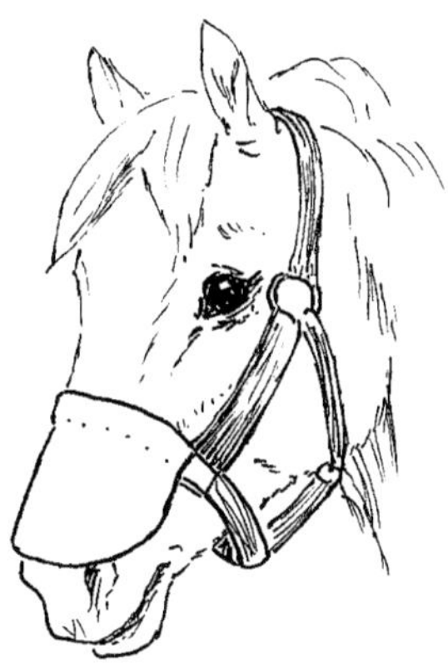

White-faced horses often get sunburnt and need protection from strong sun in summer.

BACK PROBLEMS

The following are all signs which could suggest back problems in your horse.
- When you change diagonal in trot, the horse feels very different on one diagonal. Instead of your body being thrown up and forward as you rise, you feel that you are being thrown up and sideways and that, as you go down into the saddle, you drop sideways in the opposite direction.
- Your horse will always canter leading on the same foreleg and if you do get it to lead on the other leg, it will change back to its favourite leg.
- The horse will always canter disunited (with the legs out of the normal three-time sequence).
- The horse is very much stiffer and more uncomfortable when circling on one rein than on the other. (Most horses show a slight stiffness on one rein.)
- The horse appears to drop its hindquarters when turning or on a small circle in one direction.
- The horse drags one hind toe only, wearing that shoe out quickly.
- When walked on a hard surface, the regular four-time beat is not even. There seems to be either a quicker, shorter step or there is a distinctly louder

beat. The horse is not lame but it is not absolutely level and even in rhythm or sound.

- In trot, look and listen to see and hear if the two-time gait of trot is absolutely level and even. (In trot the legs move in diagonal pairs.) If it is not level and even, there may be a problem.
- A horse, which has had no problems until now with taking the correct lead in canter, suddenly develops a problem.
- A horse which has always jumped willingly, starts to refuse.
- Your horse is difficult to mount or dismount or suddenly becomes so. (This can indicate a problem near the withers or a pinching saddle.)
- In trot the horse keeps giving little 'skips' of canter with its forelegs. (This often indicates a problem near the withers.)

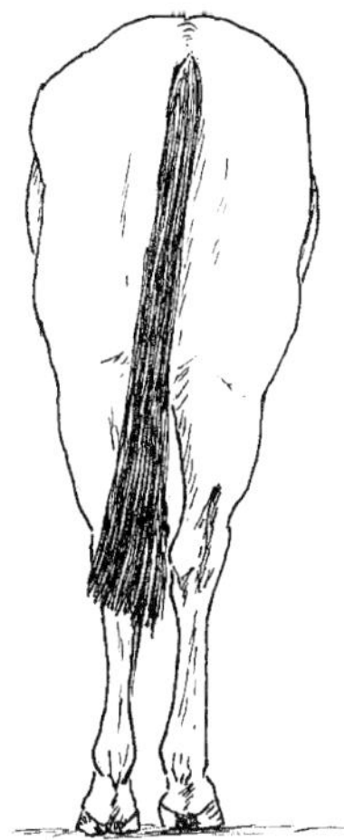

The nearside hip has dropped and there is muscle wastage on that side. The tail is hanging crookedly.

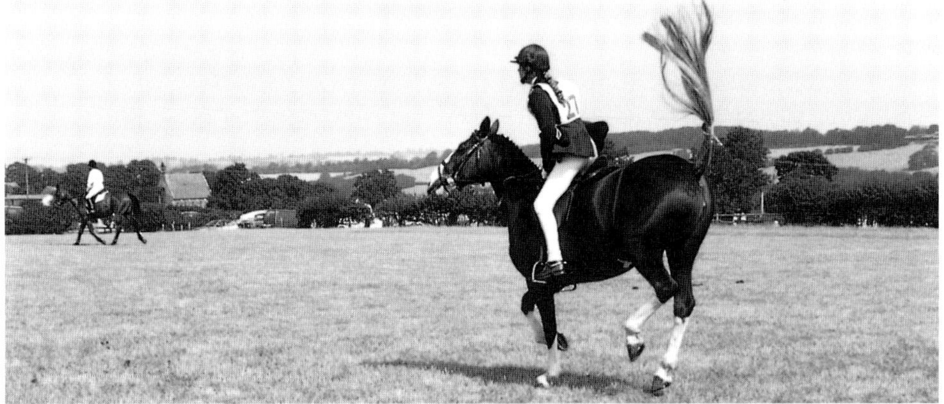

This pony is bucking and looking backward anxiously as if something is hurting or uncomfortable. The saddle or a problem in the horse's back could be causing the reaction.

- When you stand directly behind your horse on level ground and it has both hind legs parallel, you notice that one hip bone is higher than the other.
- When your horse has been cast in the stable, has slipped up when loose in the field or had a fall with you and it feels different when you ride it, or if it moves or turns differently in the stable, or cannot get its head to the ground, there may be a problem in the back.

If you have any doubts, get a registered equine chiropractor to examine your horse as soon as possible.

MAREISH BEHAVIOUR

It is normal for a mare to come into season every three weeks from March/April through to September/October. Some mares show no obvious signs of being in season and their behaviour and competition performance are unaltered. Others can show any or all of the following behaviour patterns for as long as a week.
- Squealing and striking out in front if another horse approaches.
- Squealing and kicking out behind if another horse approaches.
- Squirting small quantities of urine when another horse approaches.
- Going 'wooden' and refusing to move.
- Whinnying and behaving in a hysterical manner.

In a pony any of these patterns of behaviour can be a safety problem where small child riders are concerned. In this case, ask the advice of a specialist horse vet as hormone treatment can help.

Some mares are almost perpetually in season during the summer. If your mare behaves in a mareish way and you want to compete, you are likely to have a frustrating and disappointing time.

COLTY BEHAVIOUR

Perhaps you have bought a new gelding and then noticed unusual behaviour. He may neigh in a different way from a normal gelding, making a 'h–h–h–h–h–h' noise when he sees another horse. He may squeal and strike out with a foreleg if he is near another horse, possibly at the same time exposing and stiffening his penis. When in the field with others, he may show all the above signs and may mount mares and try to serve them.

In the stable he may hold your clothes in his teeth, not with ears back and biting at you but usually with ears pricked and just holding on.

If kept alone he may become very excitable when he sees or hears another horse.

All of this behaviour is normal in a stallion but you would not expect to find it in a gelding which has been properly castrated. Horses which have been castrated late in life, however, may retain some stallion characteristics for a year or so.

Some young geldings show a little interest in mares the first spring after they have been castrated but most change character and behaviour within a few months of castration.

If your gelding shows stallion characteristics he may not have been properly castrated. One testicle may be retained, never having dropped in the normal way. (This gelding is termed a 'rig'.)

The gelding may have been 'cut proud' so that he will retain the pride of carriage of a stallion, but often some of the characteristic behaviour of a stallion also remains. This can be because an insufficient amount of the cord attached to the testicles has been cut off during castration. A further operation to remove more of the cord can transform the horse into a perfectly behaved gelding.

Sometimes the only inconvenient signs of abnormality are that the gelding mounts mares in the field. In this case, if possible, turn him out only with other geldings and do not separate him from other horses by any form of wire fence as he will be likely to strike out at other horses with a foreleg and may get hung up.

(Any form of wire fence dividing horses is potentially dangerous because most horses of either sex are inclined to strike out at each other.)

RESPIRATORY PROBLEMS

A fat or unfit horse will puff and blow when trotted or cantered.

Whistling

A horse is said to 'make a noise' if a high-pitched, almost whistling sound can be heard as the horse breathes in. Technically, this horse can be described as a 'whistler' and this is an unsoundness for which a vet will fail a horse. Some horses whistle all the time, others only whistle when unfit. Some will only whistle on a circle in one direction and not on the other rein. Some will only whistle when arching their necks when ridden or when excited and pulling. Some will whistle for a few days then not do so again for several months. Some will 'whistle' while they have a cold or cough.

Whistling can be a disadvantage to any competition horse, such as race horses or event horses where speed and endurance are necessary, but it has very little effect on the performance of show jumpers or horses used for riding club or Pony Club work. Many horses whistle and still hunt regularly with no problem. A show horse which the judge hears whistling will be put down the order for it because it is an unsoundness but unless the judge actually rides the horse it may be very difficult to hear the noise at all. Many horses with a slight whistle continue to be placed year after year.

The whistling noise is caused by the cartilage and vocal chord (often only on one side of the throat) not moving to the side of the larynx in the normal way when the horse breathes in. They remain partially across the larynx and cause the whistle. Sometimes air passing over the small pouch between the cartilage and the vocal chord accentuates the whistling noise as the horse breathes in.

Roaring

If the muscles controlling the cartilage and vocal chords become weaker, the noise made as the horse breathes in deepens in tone and becomes more of a 'roaring' sound.

If the horse's performance is affected, consult your vet who may recommend the operation known as Hobdaying. This is performed from the outside of the throat into the larynx and usually results in a clear passage of air. There is more chance of success if the operation is done in the early stages of whistling.

Another operation, known as tubing, is rarely seen nowadays. A metal tube is inserted directly into the windpipe, roughly halfway down the horse's neck. This has a 'lid' which is removed to allow free passage of air when the horse does fast work.

Feed horses with wind problems on damped, dust-free food, well-soaked, good, clean hay or on specially treated hay such as Horsehage. Bed them on dust-free bedding such as shavings or paper.

Broken wind – emphysema

The outward signs of broken wind are wide, dilated nostrils, a lot of movement of the rib cage when breathing and a double heave as the horse breathes out with effort. A hard line (heave line) shows along the bottom of the rib cage, which is caused by the muscular effort of breathing out. The breathing is faster than normal for a horse at rest. The lungs are permanently damaged and the condition is irreparable because the walls of some of the air sacs in the lungs have broken down. Watch the horse's flanks for several minutes while it is standing still to check for the outward signs mentioned. If the horse is given a short, sharp canter, all of these signs will become more obvious and the horse may be very distressed.

Wind cough

Horses with lung damage will often give a long, drawn-out, hollow, single cough when ridden or when standing in the stable. If you hear a horse for sale making this noise, be very suspicious.

Many horses will cough the first time that they trot or canter each day on exercise but they will not cough again. It is said that if the horse sneezes after coughing, it is less serious. Some horses may cough a few times at first when ridden in an indoor school but will not continue to cough. Both of these types are likely to have a degree of lung problem but may go on for years without getting any worse.

High blowing

This is not a wind problem but I have included it in this section because it is often thought to be one. It is *not* an unsoundness. Unlike wind problems, this noise is made as the horse breathes *out*. A horse breathes naturally in time with canter, breathing out as the leading foreleg comes to the ground. It is at canter that you will hear the regular, quite noisy sound of high blowing which sounds rather like a cat purring very loudly. Some horses have an enlarged 'false nostril' – a flap of skin inside the nostril – which vibrates and is the cause of high blowing. It is not detrimental to the horse.

Coughing

Many horses will cough the first time that they trot or canter on a ride, and then not cough again. If having had only one bout of coughing they then sneeze, they are usually just cleaning their lungs and bronchial passages and it is nothing to worry about.

Some horses are affected by the atmosphere or dust in an indoor school and will always cough during the first few minutes that they are worked indoors but will not continue to cough.

Horses which live out but are brought into a stable for a short time before a ride may cough in the stable and/or when first trotted or cantered because they have been eating a bit of hay or straw.

All of these types of cough sound as if they come from the throat and may continue for years without getting any worse.

A horse which keeps giving one long, drawn-out, hollow cough which sounds as though it comes from deep down in its lungs usually has a wind problem. It is inadvisable to buy any horse which you hear giving this kind of cough. If you own a horse which coughs like this, damp all its feeds, soak its hay and bed it on shavings or paper. Ride it quietly and steadily and do not put any strain on its lungs by riding it fast or up steep hills.

Some horses will get a dry cough and have regular bouts of several coughs every few minutes. This condition can develop in both horses which are usually stabled or those which live out. The coughing starts suddenly and the horse does not seem to feel off-colour or have any sign of a cold. If the coughing is worse when you ride the horse, then do not do so. If the horse is normally kept out, leave it in the field. If it lives in, turn it out during at least part of the day. If the cough is only slight, exercise the horse at a walk and if the coughing bouts become less frequent as the ride progresses, include short, slow trotting. As it clears up, a cold can lead to a cough. Do not allow a coughing horse to sweat and do not put any strain on its lungs by making it puff with fast work or uphill work.

Coughs and colds spread very quickly. Isolate affected horse. Keep your horse well away from other horses with coughs or running noses when you are riding it.

Horses are much less likely to get coughs and lung problems if they have plenty of fresh air. Shutting the top door of outside boxes at night is not a good idea. If you don't believe this, try taking a deep breath of the fug and ammonia that has built up by the time you open the door in the mornings.

The disadvantage of indoor barn stabling is that coughs and colds spread quickly from horse to horse because they are all breathing the same air. If the horse normally lives out and is coughing, bringing it in is likely to make the condition worse and/or make recovery slower. This is because stables contain dust and spores which irritate the bronchial tubes and lung tissue.

Colds

Horses mostly catch colds through droplet infection from other horses in exactly the same way that people infect each other. If the horse lives out, it is better to leave it out but make sure it is moving about as usual and grazing normally. A horse that is feeling ill will stand about with head low and ears drooping and will not be grazing. Its ears may feel cold and it will look generally dejected. Take its temperature (normal is 100.5 °F). It may be necessary to call the vet if the horse continues to look miserable and does not graze.

Inhaling.

A horse cannot breathe through its mouth so a thick runny nose causes great discomfort. If the horse is not feeling ill, it can still be exercised at a walk but must not become distressed in its breathing or made to sweat. If stabled, feeding it on the ground will encourage the mucus to run out of its nostrils.

Inhaling can help to clear the passages and make breathing easier. You will need help from an assistant if you have not done this before. Put a mat of hay in the bottom of a bucket and add eucalyptus, or some proprietary inhalant. Make sure the steam is not too hot then slowly lift the bucket towards the horse's nose holding one side of a towel over the front of the bucket and close to the horse's face between the level of the horse's nostrils and its eyes to prevent the fumes from rising up and hurting its eyes. Do this two or three times a day. If the horse objects strongly to this treatment, put some Vick on a cloth and hold this near its nostrils.

Most colds and runny noses clear up of their own accord in a few days so inhalants are only needed if the horse is having real difficulty in breathing.

Do not put any strain on the breathing of a horse with a cold or cough because this can do serious and lasting damage to its lungs.

Stabled horses with coughs or colds will benefit from having all food damped, all hay soaked and being kept on dust-free bedding such as shavings or paper. Keep them warm with rugs and stable bandages if they have a temperature but remember that they need plenty of fresh air.

Sudden loss of weight

Possible causes of a sudden loss of weight include:
- Lice which are blood suckers and quickly pull the horse down.
- Pain, for instance an abscess in the foot which persists for some time.
- Sharp teeth which give the horse such pain when chewing that it ceases to eat or eats very little.
- Stress – caused by a change of home, bad treatment in the stable or when ridden – which really upsets the horse.
- Extreme wet and cold; being turned out in an unsheltered field in bad weather having previously been stabled.
- Continual long hours of fast, hard work when unclipped so that the horse sweats profusely. Perhaps also carrying a rider who is too heavy.
- Being worked hard when not fit enough.
- Being worked hard and not given enough food or suitable food.
- Digestive problems – note if there is a change in the quantity, colour, smell or consistency of the droppings.
- Urinary problems – note if there is a change in the frequency, amount or colour of the urine and if the horse strains or shows discomfort when urinating.
- Worms – worm the horse regularly every six weeks. Have a worm count done by the vet.

- Anaemia – if all of the above have been checked, the vet can do a blood test.

AZOTURIA

You have been riding your horse for fifteen to 30 minutes when it quite suddenly becomes stiff in its hind legs and back. It may become reluctant to move at all, may sweat profusely, with little beads of sweat literally leaping off it, and it may start to tremble violently. Try to keep it moving as far as the nearest stable. Get a vet immediately. Keep the horse warm, especially over its loins.

The rapid onset of these symptoms is very alarming. They are brought on by a sudden release of lactic acid into the muscles over the loins, causing them to go into spasm.

A stabled horse which is being fed on a high-protein diet and worked regularly every day may produce these symptoms when it is first exercised after a few days off work. If a horse used to a large amount of hard feed is suddenly given no work, it is essential to cut down drastically on the amount of heating food it is given. This must be replaced with extra hay. If possible, keep the horse exercised by lungeing, leading from another horse or by turning it out if you cannot ride it for some reason.

With some horses azoturia is an ever-recurring problem so their diet and exercise must be carefully managed. This type of horse will benefit from being 'worked' twice a week, as well as being exercised each day. A long canter, a good gallop or energetic hillwork will all help to prevent a build up of lactic acid.

An old-fashioned but very simple prevention was to feed five or six large, chopped-up raw potatoes a day. The starch from the potatoes is thought to neutralise the acid. This does work with some horses and is well worth trying.

Horses running on land where the grass has been treated with a lot of nitrogen, for instance a dairy farm, can develop azoturia when there is heavy rain on the grass after a long dry spell. A lot of nitrogen is suddenly taken up into the grass and eaten by the horse, upsetting its system.

Extreme stress caused by getting caught up in something, or from being in great pain, can produce an acid imbalance which can give a horse azoturia.

LICE

Lice are most likely to occur on unclipped horses that are turned out. From November onwards carefully inspect the fluffy hair round the forelock and ears every week for signs of lice. This is the area in which they first appear. To find them, separate the hairs and look at the skin where you may see tiny, yellowish-grey bodies the size of a pinhead crawling about. The minute, yellowish eggs are laid on the hairs.

Lice are blood suckers and multiply very quickly until they are all over the body. Horses covered in lice lose condition very quickly. Other horses can catch the lice but they do not live for long on people.

Do not be ashamed if your horse has a few lice, just get immediate treatment from the vet. Even fat, well-cared-for horses can get lice. A horse which has lice one winter is likely to get them again. I looked after the same bunch of ponies for several years and every year the same ponies got lice while the rest of the group never did, although they were all in close contact. All the ponies were fat and well. The conclusion is that lice seem to prefer certain blood types.

Do not try to shake louse powder on to your animal's neck and head. Put some powder in the palm of your hand and gently work it in, particularly round the ears and forelock. Keep it out of the eyes.

An old fashioned remedy is to mix one-third paraffin with two-thirds water. Keep this mixture well away from the eyes!

Whatever you use, repeat the treatment every two weeks.

ANGLEBERRIES

These little growths look rather like berries in that they have a neck or stalk and are often marble-shaped. They have a blood supply and when rubbed by saddlery or the opposite limb (if situated high up between the hind legs) they form a horrid, bloody mass. Severe growths need treating by a vet but if one angleberry with a thin neck appears, you can remove it by tying an opened-up elastic band very tightly round the neck. On a larger one with a thicker neck, apply one of the rubber rings, called an Elastrator, that is used for castrating lambs or removing their tails. One puts this on by stretching it open with a special four-pronged metal tool which allows the ring to close as you ease it off. In both cases the blood supply is cut off and the angleberry withers and drops off.

SCALDED BACK

This usually occurs in a soft, unfit horse which has perhaps been turned out to grass for several months. On returning from exercise, you will notice that although the horse is quite dry there are wet, sticky patches on the horse's back under the seat of the saddle. These do not dry off as normal sweat does. When they do eventually dry, a greyish-white deposit is left on the hair. There may be some swelling and the area may be painful to the touch of your hand and very painful if you use a brush. The movement of the saddle has caused friction which creates heat – hence the term 'scalded back'. Check for this condition every time you remove the saddle from a soft, unfit horse. If you see and feel sticky patches, bathe the area then apply surgical spirit or salt and water (1 tablespoon to 0.5 litre or 1 pt) to help to dry and harden off the skin.

Until the horse's back has completely recovered, lunge or ride and lead it for exercise. Check the fitting of the saddle as too much pressure towards the back can contribute to the problem. If the saddle sits on the horse cocked up in front and sloping to the back, your seat will slide to the lowest point in the saddle and cause undue pressure there. If necessary, use a different saddle.

GIRTH GALLS

Girth galls can be caused by:
- a very wide girth;
- a hard girth with a sharp or rough edge;
- lumps of mud or sweat on the girth;
- a fat, soft horse;
- mud or sweat left on the horse under the girth;
- a very fat horse whose enlarged stomach will push the girth forward too near to the elbow.

Having discovered the cause of the problem, bathe the area with salt and water, then:
- if the horse is always stabled, lunge it or lead it from another horse for exercise until the area has healed;
- use a girth which has narrower sections behind the elbows, such as a Balding or Fitzwilliam girth;
- use a different girth to the one which caused the problem and thread it through either a scooter tyre rubber inner tube or a sheepskin or nylon fur tube. These tubes must be kept clean and dry;
- make certain that the girth area is clean and free from sweat or mud.

Prevention
With a new horse, or a horse in soft condition, check the girth area on both sides every day after you have ridden so that you will notice the very first signs of girth galls, such as soreness or hair rubbed off.

SWEATING

As individuals, horse vary enormously as to how much they sweat. Obviously, a fat, unfit or woolly-coated horse will sweat more and all horses sweat more in hot weather.

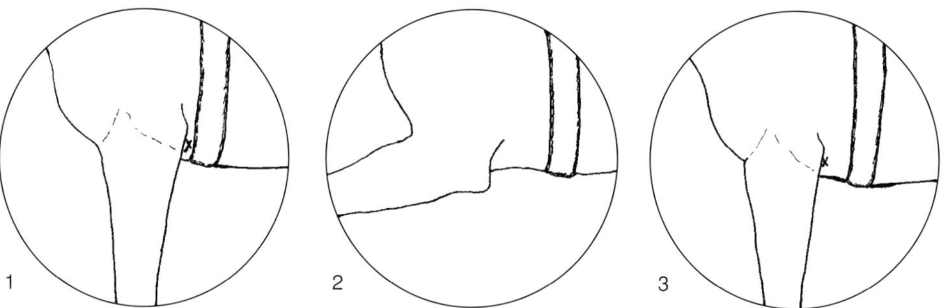

Gently pulling each foreleg forward (Fig 2) will make the girth sit further back from the elbow, smooth wrinkles of skin and help to prevent girth galls.

Clipping (see page 73) will help to stop animals sweating when worked hard during the winter.

Patches of sweat always to be found on the same, uncovered part of an otherwise dry horse are an indication of injury or pain.

Cold sweat

An overtired horse will break out into a cold sweat after a long day's hard work; after hunting, for instance. The horse feels cold and clammy; its ears are wet and cold. Do not take the rugs off and walk the horse about outside to dry it off or it may get a chill. Dry its ears with a towel if it will let you and rub them to get them warm. Keep the horse rugged up. Use a sweat rug 'thatched' with straw under the stable rug. Remove rugs that are wet with sweat and replace them with warm, dry rugs. Rub the legs to get the circulation going and bandage them with woollen bandages. Give the horse a warm feed. Go back last thing at night. If the rugs are again wet with sweat, replace them with dry ones.

MELANOMA (LUMPS ON A GREY HORSE)

Many grey horses have little lumps on the hairless part underneath the top of their tails or round the anus or vulva. These are often only pea sized and may never give any trouble. Sometimes the lumps grow as big as an orange or even larger and can be seen on any part of the horse. The larger lumps can cause problems, particularly if they develop internally. They are more usually found on older horses but even young horses can be affected. If you are going to buy a grey horse, check under and around its tail for small lumps. Melanomas are a form of cancer so think carefully before buying a horse with obvious lumps and be aware that even very small ones can progress.

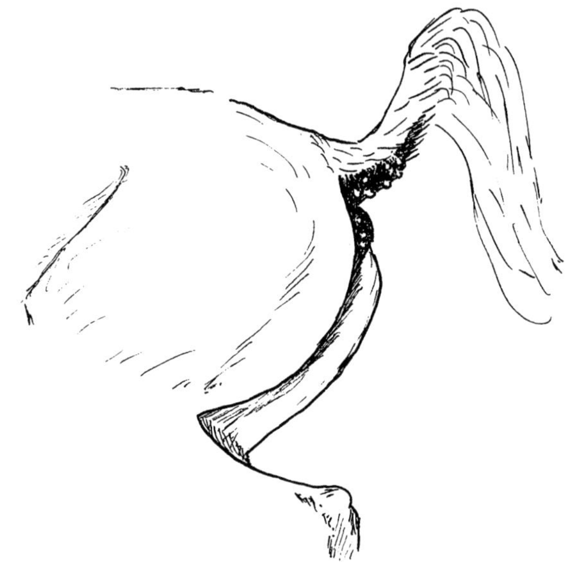

Melanoma.

These lumps may form anywhere outside or inside the horse's body and may be no problem for many years. If they are in a position where they interfere with bones, muscles or important organs in the body, the condition can be very serious, even fatal.

If you own a horse which develops melanomas, don't panic as many horses go on working happily for years with melanomas the size of cricket balls. The seriousness of the situation depends entirely on where they form and how quickly they grow.

TAIL RUBBING

Why does a horse rub its tail?
- It may have worms. In this case, it is trying to rub the irritation round its anus but its tail gets rubbed instead. Sometimes yellowish traces can be seen round the anus. Tell your vet and obtain a suitable wormer. Wash the area every day.
- If the tail is scurfy and itchy, wash it with a mild shampoo and rinse well.
- Sometimes putting a tail bandage on will make the tail hot and itchy. This will make the horse rub the tail bandage off and then continue to rub its tail. A tail bandage put on too tight or left on too long can start the habit.
- Some horses will rub their tails in spring and autumn when changing their coats, and at no other time.
- A horse which starts to rub its tail in the spring and continues to do so all summer, often rubbing the skin of the tail and sometimes the hindquarters above the tail until they are bleeding, has most probably got sweet itch.

SWEET ITCH

In the winter beware of buying an animal which has a hogged mane and short hairs bushing out at the top of its tail. It may have sweet itch every summer and even rub itself raw. This is now thought to be an allergic reaction to the saliva of midges. This allergic condition can be hereditary so think of this when breeding from a mare with sweet itch.

Anti-histamine injections, benzylbenzoate and various proprietary brands sold for the purpose can be used but must be started well before the first midge appears. A cheap, rather gooey preventative is liquid paraffin. This seems to prevent the midges from getting in close contact with the skin and biting the horse.

Feeding garlic regularly, starting well before the midge season, can make the horse smell faintly of garlic all over. This can discourage midges which dislike the smell. Alternatively, crush a small amount of garlic each day and either rub it directly on the mane and tail and the areas immediately surrounding them, or mix the crushed garlic with a little petroleum jelly and apply it to these areas.

Early mornings and evenings are the worst times for midges. The bright sunlight of midday can often be the best time for the horse to graze.

The hoods sold to keep horses' manes free of mud when turned out can also protect a horse from midges. A lightweight rug with a piece of material coming right down over the hindquarters (as in the Rambo design) can protect the tail and hindquarters.

The condition will occur every spring but may vary in intensity from year to year.

Sweet itch often does not appear until a young horse is rising three years of age.

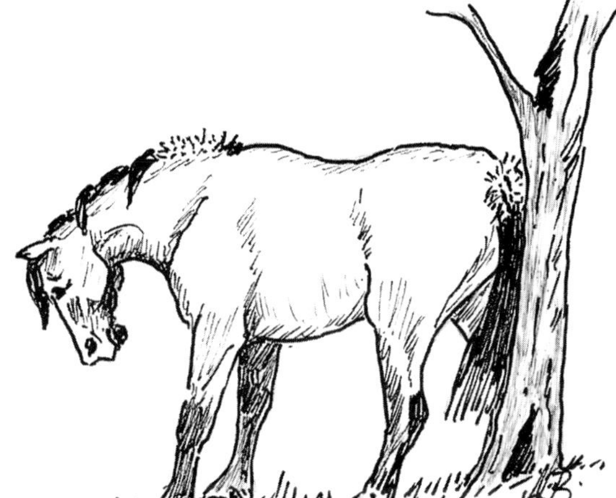

A pony rubbing sweet itch.

ABSCESSES

The commonest site of an abscess is in the horse's foot. Unshod horses sometimes get a bit of dirt or grit in the open-grained area between the wall of the foot and the sole, known as the white line. This often works inwards and causes infection. The foot becomes hot and inflamed and a pocket of pus forms. The pressure of the swelling within the hard hoof is agonising and the horse may stand on three legs, holding up the sore leg. It will be hopping lame, reluctant to move and may be trembling with pain.

The condition is exactly the same as the infected and very painful type of swelling that people often get under a fingernail but it is much worse for the horse because the hard hoof makes the pressure of the swelling within desperately painful.

Wash the foot off and see if you can find a tiny hole or crack oozing a black, smelly substance. Ask your farrier to see if he can find the place where it will all come out. If he can, he will open up the underside of the foot, allowing the pus to run out. The relief for the horse will be almost immediate. Keep it in, keep the foot poulticed for two or three days, then plug the hole with a small wodge of cotton wool covered in Stockholm tar. Do not put the horse in a wet, muddy field until the hole has healed. If a small pocket of pus has remained, the infection may recur in exactly the same way so the treatment will need repeating once more.

If the pus does not burst out at the bottom of the foot, it may work up to the weakest point, the edge of the hard hoof near the coronet. An abscess here is known as a quittor and is very difficult to drain completely as it cannot run uphill. For this reason, it often does recur. It is much better to try to get the pus to come out at the bottom of the foot.

Abscess on the withers – fistulous wither

This can be caused by a hard object cutting or pressing into the withers when the horse is rolling or if the horse falls. A pocket of infection may form. The area will be sore, hot and swollen. A vet should be called as a drainage tube may be needed because, here again, the exit is uphill.

Abscess under the jaw or on the cheek

An abscess under the jaw may be caused by the infectious and contagious disease of strangles (see page 133).

Abscesses on the lower jawline or on the cheeks may be caused by a broken or diseased tooth. Call the vet to investigate as surgery may be necessary.

STRANGLES

This is an infectious and highly contagious disease. The first signs are that the horse looks ill and slobbers. It usually develops a very hard swelling which can be felt on the outside of the lower jaw between the cheeks. This abscess may burst. There may be a thick discharge from the nose, causing difficulty in breathing.

The horse may have a high temperature.

Call the vet. Isolate the horse. Burn all its bedding. Disinfect its clothing. Wash and change your clothes before going near another horse.

LAMENESS

Stumbling

Your horse may stumble simply because it is naturally unbalanced and uncoordinated. Very long, overgrown feet will cause a horse to stumble, as will weakness, tiredness and riding a young or unfit horse too fast at walk or trot.

If your horse is unshod, how long is it since its feet have been trimmed? This should be done every six weeks. Is the horse stumbling because it is footsore? Worn-down feet will make walking or trotting on rough stony ground painful, so the horse may need shoeing.

An unbalanced horse will hurry along with its weight on its forehand and may well trip. Walk and trot the horse slowly and work on smooth ground, steadily decreasing and increasing the size of your 15–20 m circles. Use serpentines and, if the horse can cope with them fairly easily, 10-m circles at walk and slow trot. At a slow speed in each gait the horse has to step under its body further with its hind legs, get its centre of gravity further back and carry itself. If you allow it to go fast it will continue to run along on its forehand and never improve.

If your horse is shod, how long is it since it was last shod? If it is more than six weeks, long feet may be the cause of the stumbling. Is your horse in good condition? Are its ribs covered? Has it got a firm crest or can you only feel two bits of skin between your finger and thumb when you take hold of its crest? A horse which is thin and weak may stumble.

Are you working your horse too hard for the amount of food it is getting? Are you working your horse too hard for its state of fitness? Are you working your horse too hard for its age? (This question applies equally to young and old horses.) Are you too heavy for your horse?

If, having considered these questions, you still cannot decide the cause of your horse's stumbling, ask a knowledgeable person to look at your horse and to watch you riding it.

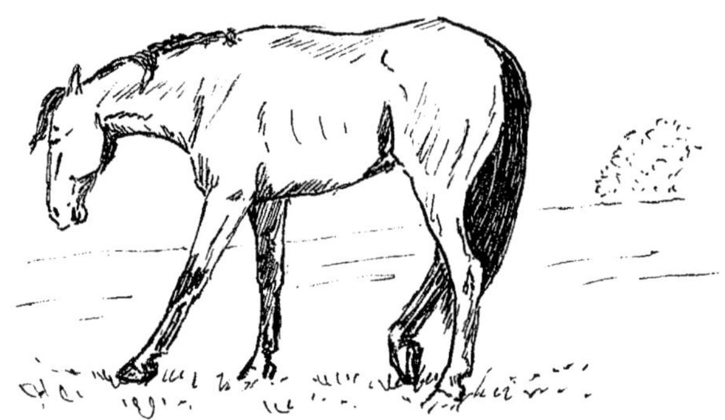

This horse has learnt to rest two legs at once. It may change over and rest the other diagonal pair. It is not a sign of unsoundness but it can be an indication of tiredness and overwork.

Which leg?

When a horse is lame on its near (left) foreleg, it nods its head down as the sound off (right) foreleg goes to the ground and slightly raises its head as the lame leg goes to the ground. It does this because it is trying to put less weight on the lame leg and more on the sound leg.

If a horse is lame on its off (right) hind leg it will drop its head down as the lame hind leg goes to the ground because it is trying to put more weight on its forehand. Viewed from the rear, it will appear to carry the hip of the lame leg slightly higher and drop on to the sound hind leg.

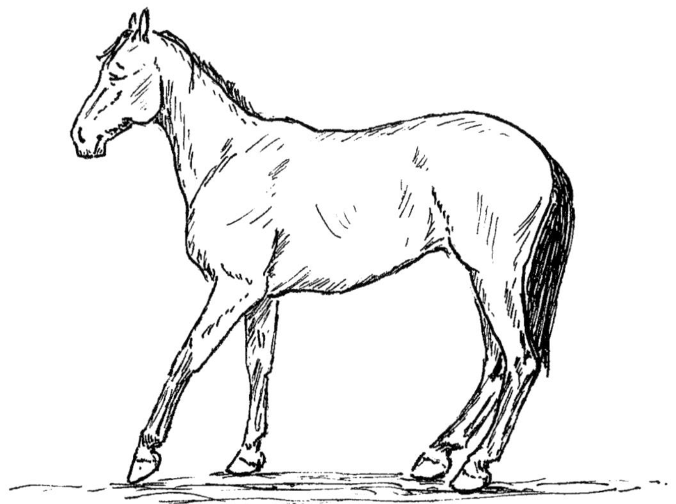

This horse is pointing its front foot. This is a sign of unsoundness in that foot. The horse's weight is carried on the other three legs.

The lameness will be more obvious at trot and usually more obvious on a hard road than on grass.

Listen to the hoof beats on hard ground at walk. Are they a regular one, two, three, four, or can you hear an uneven beat?

Listen to the hoof beats at trot. Are they a regular one, two; one, two, or can you hear an uneven beat? (Trot is a two-time gait, with the legs moving in diagonal pairs near fore and off hind together, then off fore and near hind together.)

Sudden lameness when riding

You are riding along when, suddenly, your horse goes very, very lame. It may even hold a foot up.

Dismount at once and pick up the foot.

- The horse may have trodden on a sharp stone which is still lodged firmly in the foot, in which case remove the stone using the hoofpick you always carry in your pocket, a stick or another stone as a lever if necessary.
- The horse may have trodden on something sharp which has badly bruised or even cut the sole, in which case a white mark or line may be visible on the sole.
- The horse may have trodden on a nail or sharp object which is still in the foot. Look carefully. If it is small, try to remove it yourself. If it is large or long and has gone in deep, it is probably better to try to send for a vet because removing the object could cause serious bleeding.
- The horse may have hit a fetlock with the edge of the shoe on the opposite foot. This type of lameness lasts only a few seconds but the cause must be investigated. The shoe may be protruding beyond the hoof, or a clench may be sticking out. There may be a small cut where the horse has knocked itself. (See Brushing, page 139.)

Even if the horse is not holding up a foot, you should still be able to tell whether it is lame in front or behind but, to be safe, pick up and check all four feet.

Unless something is still in the foot, lead the horse at walk for a few minutes, then lead it at trot. If it is sound, remount and continue your ride.

If it is still lame, lead it home. Check the site of the injury when you get home and again next day. A horse which is lame on the way home may be sound again next day if the cause was only bruising or knocking a joint.

If something like a nail or sharp object has punctured the sole, put the injured foot in a wide, flat tub containing salt and warm water (1 teaspoonful to 0.5 litre or 1 pt water that has been boiled and allowed to cool) for fifteen minutes twice a day and make sure your anti-tetanus injections are up to date.

If there is more heat, or if the horse is lame next day, call the vet.

LEGS

Get to know the look, feel and temperature of every lump, bump or swelling on your horse's legs. Only by doing this will you notice quickly when something is different. Feel your horse's legs every day before you ride it, perhaps while you are picking out its feet.

Sprained tendons

If there is heat or swelling, try to think what might be the cause. Swelling and heat in the tendons are likely to mean a sprain. Even if the horse is not lame, if you ride it or jump it just as usual you may make a sprain much worse. Sprained tendons are nearly always found in the forelegs. Galloping over rough ground, galloping or even cantering over ground which is firm in some places and very soft in others, turning suddenly, landing on rough ground after a jump, or an uphill landing after a jump can all cause sprained front tendons. A tired horse losing rhythm can sprain a tendon. A horse with even a slightly sprained tendon should only be bought if it is very cheap and then only if the leg is cold and hard.

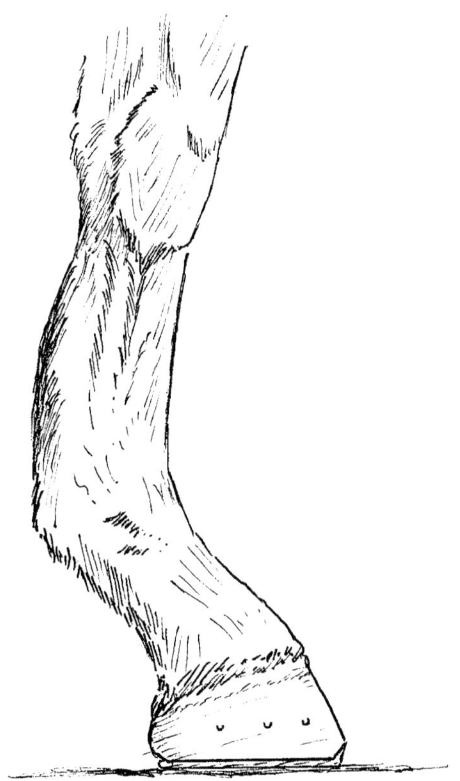

A badly sprained tendon.

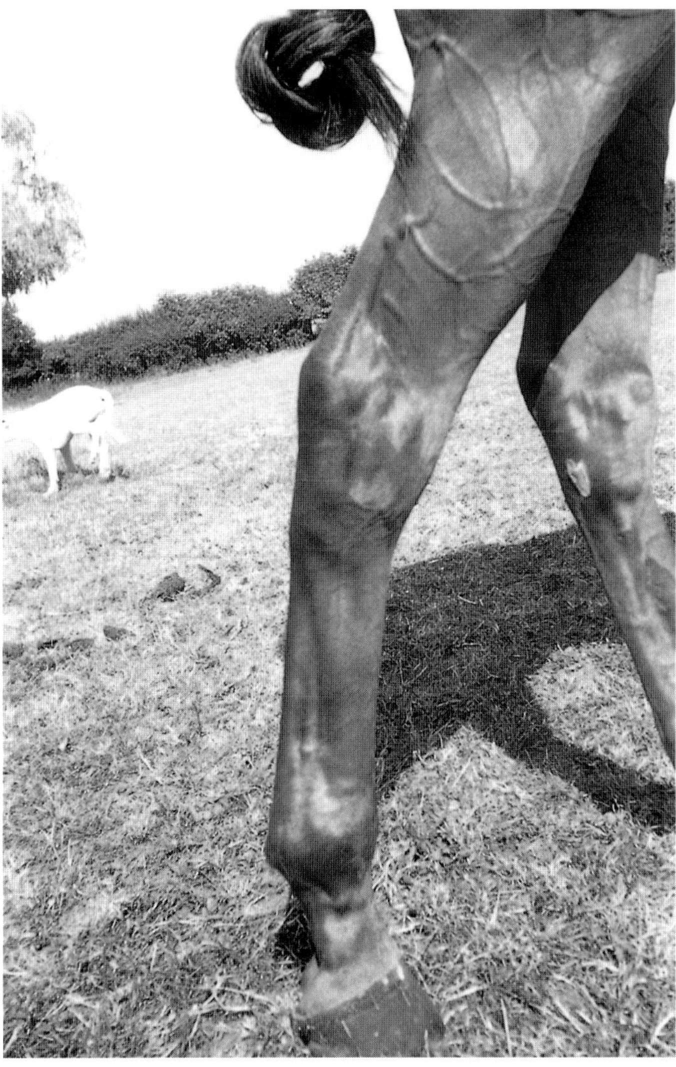

A curb.

Curbs

A curb is a sprain of the hind leg below the back of the hock. It is most noticeable when you stand sideways on to the horse and can see the bulge of the curb.

A curb can be caused by a weak hind leg with sickle hocks (see page 9) or by the hind legs suddenly slipping forward underneath the horse. Curbs reduce a horse's value.

A horse with a cold, hard curb may stand up to competition work but be wary of buying a horse if the curb is soft and warm as you are likely to be buying trouble.

Sprains

Sprains can be serious even if the horse is not lame. A slight sprain may go unnoticed by a careless or ignorant owner. If they continue to work the horse as usual, however, the sprain may get much worse, lame the horse and necessitate long rest.

If you notice a slight sprain and the horse is not lame, work it at walk until several days after the heat and swelling have gone and resume normal work very gradually, checking carefully for the slightest reappearance of the problem.

Sprained tendons are a serious problem and, if visible as a bowed swelling (see page 136), it would be inadvisable to buy such a horse except for light hacking. This obvious damage would lessen the animal's value considerably.

Some horses do hunt and compete with bowed tendons but when you feel them they are hard and cold. Swollen tendons which feel soft and warmer than the other foreleg are a sign of trouble still present.

If your horse produces any sprain which is large and hot or which does not go down and cool down after rest or just walking, get expert advice even if the horse is not lame.

Thorn wounds

After you have been jumping hedges, always examine your horse's legs very carefully for thorns. If the horse has made a mistake and gone *through* a hedge, also examine its chest, forearms, stomach and right up inside and outside its hind legs. Even if blackthorns are found that same day, the wounds can still become infected. If they are not found until next day they very often cause trouble.

Feel slowly and carefully over every inch with your fingers. If the hair is long, wetting it can make the tiny bump of a thorn show up. When you feel a thorn, try to grip the end with your fingernails, noticing the angle at which it went in before attempting to pull it out at the same angle. Be very careful not to break the thorn as the little piece left in the leg is almost certain to give trouble.

If you feel only a bump where the thorn is, but are unable to get hold of it with your fingernails, trim off the hair round it with scissors and try to get hold of the thorn with a pair of tweezers (eyebrow tweezers are ideal). Carefully pull the thorn out at the same angle that it went in.

Poultice or use hot fomentation on the thorn wound (unless it is on a joint where there is the danger or drawing out joint oil if the thorn is long and has gone in deep).

Make sure your horse is up to date with its anti-tetanus injections as puncture wounds are the most dangerous cause of this often fatal problem.

If you find hot, sore or swollen areas next day, consider the possibility of thorns as the cause. Obviously, sprains also cause pain and swelling but their positioning will probably be different.

Buffing

When a horse brushes low down on the coronet of the opposite foot a white line shows where contact has been made. This is called buffing. It is most common behind and it is noticeable when an animal has been worked on turns and circles in a confined area for several days. A typical example would be after two or three days of Pony Club Camp where everyone had been regularly working in rides in 20 x 40-m areas. The problem may also show up on horses being lunged. A slight mark is of no consequence but if the coronet becomes bruised and sore or if the area buffed becomes deeper and sore, action must be taken.

A ring or sausage boot worn round the pastern of the affected leg may prevent the trouble continuing. If not, an overreach boot will protect the area.

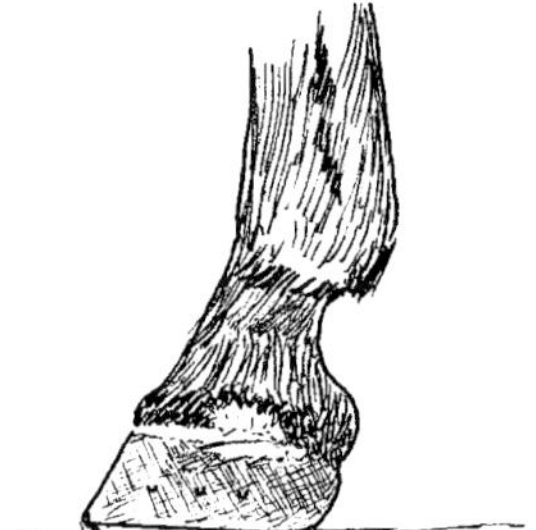

Buffing.

Brushing

In slight cases of brushing, the only outward sign is a patch of mud on the inside of the fetlock joint. There may also be some bruising, slight filling and

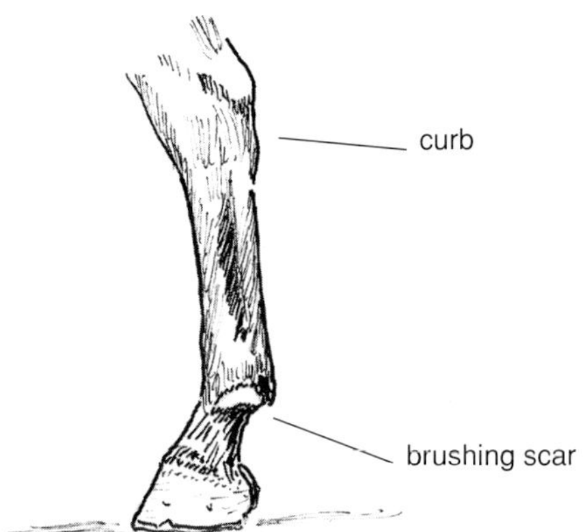

A hind leg showing a curb and an area on the underside of the fetlock which has been damaged by brushing.

warmth in that area. If ignored, the hair may be worn off and, as the area fills and protrudes more, it will be hit even harder by the opposite shoe, often until it is sore and bleeding. The horse may go lame for a few strides when its opposite foot hits the sore place.

Horses which brush usually stand with their fore and/or hind toes turned out slightly. In action, their feet move in a sideways, inward-curving flight instead of straight. Even an unshod horse may brush but a shod horse is more likely to do so and the shoe will do more damage to the opposite leg when the inside of the shoe hits the underside of the opposite fetlock joint. The horse is more likely to brush on a circle because turning accentuates the curved flight of the foot.

Reasons for brushing include:

- conformation;
- deep, heavy ground;
- overgrown feet (the horse needs shoeing);
- a risen clench sticking out on the inside of the wall (the horse needs shoeing);
- a tired or weak horse;
- a young horse being given too much work for its age;
- the horse's head and neck are bent too much to the inside when it is ridden on a circle.

Brushing boots are not the only remedy. The cause must also be treated. Get your farrier to watch the horse's action in walk and trot. He can then shoe the horse to alleviate the problem.

- He may put on a feather-edged shoe, which is narrower than a regular shoe and chamfered on the inside, with only one nail hole at the front beyond the toe clip on the inside. There may be an extra toe clip on the outside to support the shoe. The hoof will protrude slightly beyond the shoe on the inside.
- He may put on a three-quarter shoe (with no metal on the inside other than near the toe).
- If the brushing is only slight, he may simply shoe the horse under and chamfer the inside edge. The inside of the shoe will then be tucked in under the hoof wall.

Boots should be worn as an added protection. Boots alone are not the answer, however, because their bulk makes the horse brush even more and the constant concussion on the fetlock joint is bad for it and may cause swelling.

When you groom the horse, regularly feel the inside of the lower part of the fetlock joint, slightly towards the back of it. If you feel the slightest hardness of the skin, if the hair is worn or broken or if there is even the tiniest cut, your horse is brushing and the shoeing needs changing.

You should also consider whether the horse is fit and strong enough for the work it is doing.

Brushing above the fetlock joint

This high brushing is not very common and for this reason is often mistaken for a sprain or a low splint forming.

Horses with high, round action and toe-out conformation may knock themselves above the fetlock joint if their feet have grown long and wide or if they are worked on heavy or rough ground or in long grass. Both of these tend to make a horse pick its feet up higher than usual.

You will notice patches of mud, soft swelling, slight heat, broken hair or broken skin anywhere from just above the inside of the fetlock joint to the lower half of the inside of the cannon bone.

Lead your horse out on level ground and observe how close its front feet go to the opposite leg. Watch to see if the flight path of the foot is straight or in an inward curve.

An interesting experiment can be tried, which will prove whether the horse is knocking itself and show exactly which part of the opposite foot/shoe is causing the damage. Put an old boot on the filled leg and spread bright coloured or white paint thickly on the part of the boot which is covering the filled area of the leg.

Lead the horse out in hand at walk and trot, first on level ground, then on rougher ground. Check all the time to see if there is any paint on the inside of the opposite foot/shoe. If no paint is showing, tack the horse up and ride it in circles on both reins at walk and trot on differing ground.

Notice exactly where the paint is picked up on the opposite foot. Ask your farrier to come and show him that area on the shoe.

● Putting on lighter shoes may help as the horse's action will not then be so high. It is also likely to move straighter in lighter shoes.

● Ride on good, level going and do not do any circling until the swelling has gone down. The swelling will have made the leg stick out more than usual so it is possible that, when carefully shod, the horse may no longer knock itself once the swelling has gone down.

● Special shoes which can be used include:
  – feather-edged shoes which are much narrower on the inside and set under the foot so that the hoof protrudes beyond the shoe. They have only one or two nails on the inside and these are near the toe. Sometimes there is a second toe clip on the outside to help to stabilise the shoe;
  – aluminium shoes;
  – three-quarter shoes which only cover the front and outside area of the hoof. There is nothing on the inside quarter so if the horse has been hitting itself with that part of a normal shoe, it may cease to do so.

● Protective boots make the legs thicker so the horse will knock them even more. They alone are not the answer but, used in conjunction with careful trimming of the feet and special shoeing, they can prevent further damage being done.

The horse may not be lame even though the inside of the foreleg is considerably swollen. The horse may, however, flinch if the area is pressed and, if it suddenly knocks itself hard when you are riding, it may go lame for two or three strides then go sound again.

It is inadvisable to buy a horse which goes very close in front because this will often cause brushing problems.

If you notice a horse standing with its toes out, watch it carefully from the front and from behind at walk and trot. This conformation makes a horse go very close and it will be inclined to brush.

Brushing boots

There are so many different types of brushing boots on the market that I am not going to advise you what kind to buy, but the correct fitting of any boot is essential.

A horse usually brushes the lower areas of the inside of the fetlock joint, catching it as the opposite foot passes it in forward flight. For this reason, the boots must cup snugly round the lower area of the inside of the fetlock joint.

Loose-fitting boots can collect mud and grit if you are riding in deep going, so check the horse's legs afterwards in case there are sore, rubbed areas.

Splints

Splints are a bony enlargement on a splint bone. The splint bones are two pencil-like bones running down one on each side of the cannon bone.

Splints are mostly found on the forelegs and are caused by jarring on hard ground. Too much fast trotting on hard roads can produce splints. They develop most often in horses between four and six years of age but can sometimes suddenly appear on much older horses.

Splints occasionally appear on a hind leg but here they are usually caused by a knock.

The position of a splint determines its seriousness. One growing towards the back of the splint bone near the tendons can cause problems, as can a high splint growing near the knee. A splint on the inside can be knocked by the opposite foreleg.

If your young horse goes slightly lame in front on hard ground or perhaps just on a circle, check to see if a splint may be forming. Pick up the foreleg and feel for the splint bone. Starting at the top of the cannon bone near the knee, pinch and press hard on the splint bone, working very gradually down to its tip. If the horse flinches at one place, recheck and if it flinches at that same place again, you have probably found a splint that is forming.

If the horse is not lame in walk but is lame in trot, continue to work quietly in walk and the splint will be likely to settle down and harden. This may take several weeks. Many people advise complete rest but, in my experience, if you do give the horse complete rest, the inflammation returns once more when

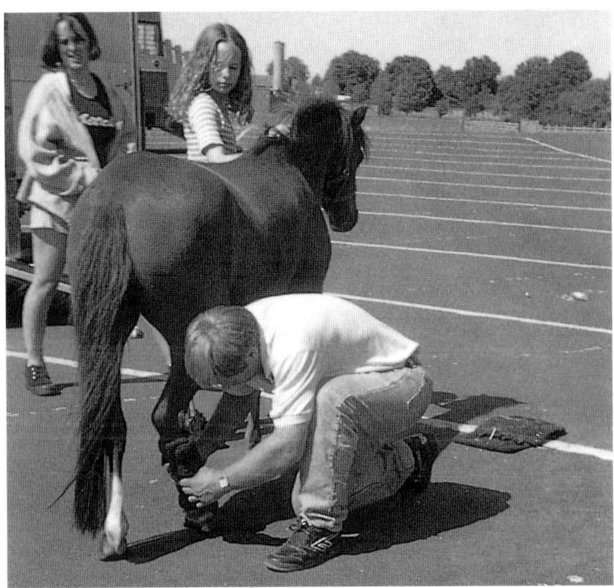

Putting on brushing boots. It is dangerous to kneel down to do this as you will be very vulnerable if the pony kicks.

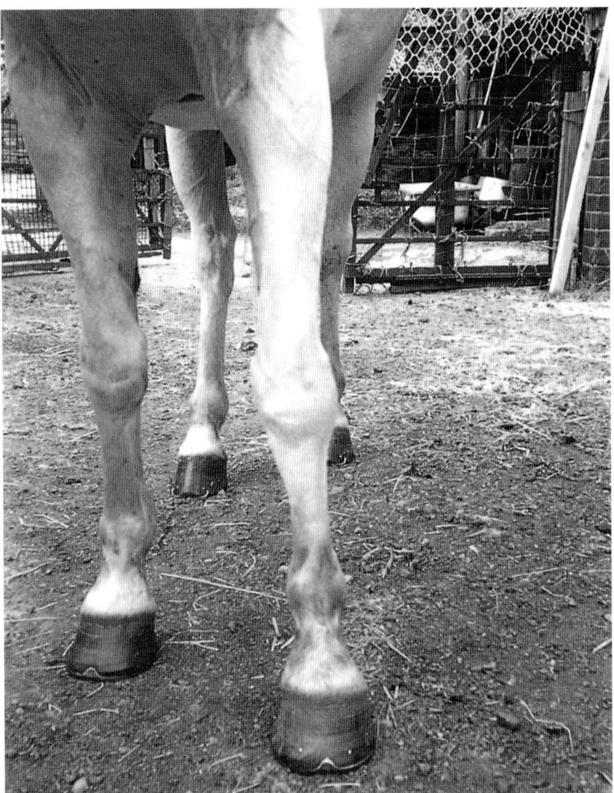

A splint high up on the inside of the near foreleg.

you bring the horse back into work and I have found that working a horse through it at walk is more successful.

Once formed and cold and hard, a splint rarely causes trouble, the exceptions being if it is touching the tendons, interfering with the knee joint or being knocked by the shoe of the opposite foreleg.

In some cases it is possible to have a splint surgically removed.

Windgalls

Windgalls are the soft, puffy fillings often found just above and towards the back of the fetlock joint in horses which have been worked hard. They can be found in front or behind but are probably commoner behind. They are unsightly and would be counted as a fault in the show ring. They slightly detract from the value of a horse but rarely cause problems. They are caused by general wear and tear in older horses.

Young horses with windgalls have usually been worked too hard for their age or done too much work on hard ground. The bursal sac has stretched and enlarged and cannot be repaired. Pressure bandages with padding put on over the windgalls can make you think they have done some good because when you take the bandage off it can seem as if there is now no filling. In practice, as soon as you use the horse, up they come again.

Occasionally, a very large, tightly bulging windgall will cause unsoundness but the small ones found on very many animals of middle age are of no consequence.

A windgall.

FEET

Laminitis

Small ponies, bred to live in mountainous regions and to search for each mouthful of grass, are too often kept in lush green fields. They stay fat all winter and when the flush of spring grass comes, not surprisingly, they get laminitis or 'fever in the feet'. This swelling of the laminae inside the hard, unyielding case of the hoof is extremely painful. To try to relieve this pain, the animal stands leaning back, with as much weight as possible on its heels.

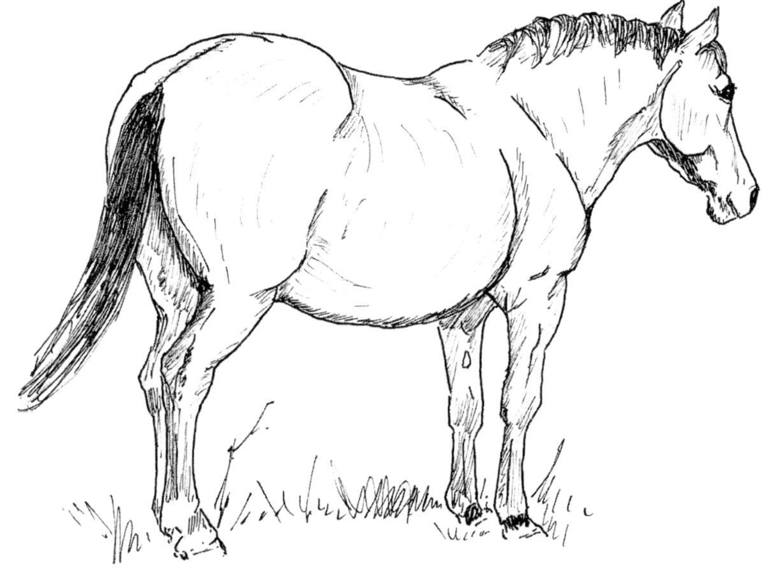

This pony is too fat and is likely to get laminitis.

Prevention is better than cure. Take the opportunity during the winter, when there is not so much grass and when what there is has less food value, to slim your animal down. Keep it in a small field or fence off a small part of a field with electric fencing (see page 23), making sure in both cases that there is some form of shelter from cold winds. Feed clean straw, which has less food value than hay (unless the hay is of extremely poor quality). When the spring grass comes continue carefully to control the area the animal grazes.

If you do not have a small paddock or an electric fence, it will be necessary to restrict the number of hours during which the animal grazes, either by turning it out in the field for only four or five hours out of 24, or by letting it out to graze for two hours night and morning. Try to keep the animal in a large yard or on a bare patch of ground between grazing times rather than shutting it up in a small stable. It must have constant access to clean water and should be offered a couple of sections of clean straw also. If you keep a horse without food all day and all night, there is a danger of a twisted gut which is nearly always fatal. In nature a horse grazes for approximately eighteen to twenty hours out of 24 and its gut is designed always to contain some food. A totally empty gut collapses and can 'twist' round itself, so be aware of this danger when rationing an animal inclined to get laminitis.

Any animal that has had laminitis once is more likely to get it again so take precautions to slim the horse, or more likely pony, during the winter and do not wait for the first signs of laminitis – the animal walking more slowly than usual, lying down more, standing with its weight back on its heels – before doing anything about it.

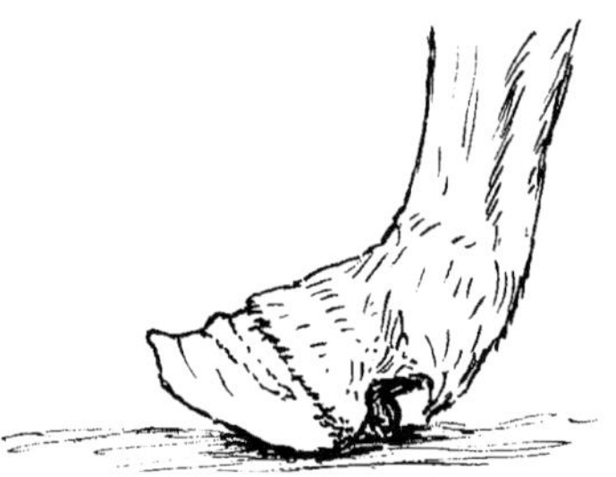

Chronic laminitis.

Laminitis is not only caused by overweight and too much rich grass. An animal which has never had laminitis before in its life can also get it from stress. This can be caused by:

- suddenly being ridden hard and fast when the animal is fat and unfit and has not been worked for months;
- a long and difficult foaling;
- an animal that has been struggling for hours to get up after it has become entangled in a fence or has got a hind foot stuck in a headcollar.

In these cases the laminitis appears suddenly, either almost immediately or within two or three days of the incident. The animal will often lie flat out on its side and be in extreme pain. Call a vet immediately.

The more normal form of laminitis comes on gradually and there is no excuse for allowing it to happen. Prevention is better than cure.

Animals with laminitis can often be bought very cheaply because the owners do not want to have to cope with the problem. I have obtained many ponies in this way and some were in such a bad state that they were *given* to me. Two were standing back on their heels with such long, curled-up feet that you could see their soles. It took two years of care, foot trimming and special shoeing but neither got laminitis again and both led useful lives as active Pony Club ponies. Another had to be practically lifted into the trailer and one of the worst was lying flat out and was carried into the trailer where it continued to lie flat out during the journey home. Neither got laminitis again and the worse one was later successful in the show ring and became a brilliant hunting pony.

The saddest case was a friend's pony which, having never had laminitis or been overweight, got laminitis from stress after thrashing about in the field all night, having got the overlong heel of a hind shoe stuck in the narrow ring of its nylon headcollar. Its head was cut and swollen, it was lying flat out and was unable to stand. It was going to be shot. It was not old and was a particularly nice little pony so I asked if I could try to get it right again. It recovered completely and never got laminitis again but for the first few weeks there was only slow progress.

Many cases need the help of a vet. Painkillers, bran mashes, soft hay in small quantities, clean straw, careful foot trimming, hosing feet, standing in streams, standing in wet mud, leading out at a walk, very frequently and gradually increasing the distance, will all help. When the animal is well enough it can be ridden at a walk and the work time and pace increased very gradually. Ever-watchful care must be given for the rest of its life to be sure that there is no opportunity for laminitis to recur. The animal must be kept slim and in regular work. Careful attention must be paid to foot trimming and shoeing.

Animals prone to laminitis must *not* be half-starved of food. Their food and work must be sensibly controlled and balanced.

Corns

Shoes which are left on too long can cause corns as the foot grows and the heel of the shoe digs in. In extreme cases the hoof grows round the heel of the shoe. If a horse is consistently shod with shoes that are too short in the heel, pressure where the short heel finishes can cause corns. If you buy an animal with corns or the farrier finds signs that it has had them, they may continue to cause problems. Even special shoes cannot work an instant miracle.

Special shoes for corns
Three-quarter shoes have no metal covering the area where a corn is sited. Set-heeled shoes have the heel under the corn cut away from the road surface to ease pressure on the corn. Seated-out shoes are hollowed out below the corn on the surface nearer to the foot to ease pressure on the corn.

If you have a good farrier who comes every six weeks, a horse is unlikely to develop corns.

Dishing

Horses which naturally stand 'pigeon toed' (toes turned in) in front tend to 'dish' (move with their forelegs swinging in an outward arc from below the knee). While this may look ugly and be marked down in the show ring it is of no importance in the ordinary 'jack of all trades' horse or pony. An animal which dishes has one great advantage – it never brushes! (Brushing is when the horse knocks the inside of one foreleg with the opposite shoe.)

In a foal, careful and frequent trimming of the feet by a knowledgeable farrier can improve the animal's action. Young horses can also be improved by a good farrier who will adjust hoof and shoe very gradually. Any sudden alteration would produce discomfort and even lameness. (See page 148.)

Dragging toes

If a horse drags both hind toes it is likely to be for one of the following reasons.
● It is tired and perhaps doing too much work for its age or its state of fitness.
● Its rider is too heavy for it.
● It is not getting enough food for the amount of work it is doing.

- It is a lazy horse (and perhaps the rider is lazy too and letting it slop along).
- A novice is riding the horse and so it is not being ridden forward and made to use itself.
- Its feet are very long and it needs reshoeing.
- A young horse which has only been ridden for a few weeks may begin to drag its toes when it has done enough work for its age. It may need a rest and time to grow and strengthen.
- A rider sitting too far back, 'behind the movement', may make a horse drag its toes.

If your horse drags one toe only, it is usually a sign of discomfort in the horse's back or in any of its hind-leg joints or muscles. It is likely to be going unlevel in its stride behind. It may even be slightly lame. There is something wrong which needs to be checked. This action will not improve until the cause is discovered and treated. Dragging one toe only is potentially more serious than dragging both toes. (See Back Problems, page 118.)

The click of dragged toes can be heard distinctly when the horse is ridden on a tarmac road. It is normally most obvious at trot, the click being heard at every stride of trot if it is dragging both toes and at alternate strides if it is dragging only one toe.

If the horse is dragging its toes so badly that it is wearing the toe of the shoe away and wearing the hoof off square, it can be shod with rolled-toe shoes in which the metal comes a little way up the wall of the hoof at the toe and so protects it. A very hard metal called borium may be added to the toe of the shoe so that it will not wear out so quickly.

These are only temporary measures, however, as the cause of the problem must still be discovered and rectified.

Trimming feet

If you have unshod young horses or ponies which do not need shoeing, their feet must still be rasped regularly. Foals and young horses which do not stand correctly must have their feet rasped and shaped by a very knowledgeable farrier who knows exactly where to take off some horn and where to leave it to grow to improve the horse's stance. To have a lasting effect without doing any damage, these corrections must begin as soon after the birth as possible and continue for three years if necessary. It is very difficult to change what has become the natural incorrect stance of a mature horse because, even if done a very little at a time, it will still affect the horse all over to some degree. Have you ever hurt your little toe and changed your weight towards your big toe when walking so that it would not hurt so much? If you have you will have noticed that this change in your way of walking affects your whole body, right up into your neck. The same is true when you try to change the stance of an adult horse.

As long as a good farrier trims the feet of horses and ponies with no foot problems every eight weeks, there is no reason why you can't help to care for their feet by running a surform plane round any small chips and smoothing them off. This plane is made of lightweight metal and looks a bit like a cheese grater. It is easy to use but quite sharp so at first you will probably grate a bit of your own knuckles off by mistake!

Small ponies, and young horses when first being ridden for only a short time, may not need shoeing behind. After each ride, examine the hind feet and rasp any slight chips immediately. Animals with really hard feet may not even need shoeing in front but if the ground gets hard be prepared to get them shod if the chips or breaks become longer or more frequent.

Pick the foot up and look at the wall of the hoof. Is it wearing evenly or is there more growth on one side than on the other which is more worn down? Many horses walk with more weight on the inside or the outside of their feet, just as people do. This is particularly true of hind feet. You should observe the way in which each of your horse's feet is worn and, if you trim them yourself sometimes, you should be aware that you must leave the worn side to grow and take more off the long side. Unless you are very knowledgeable and have been properly taught by a good farrier, however, it is unwise to undertake the trimming of your horse's feet yourself. A good farrier still needs to check on your work every three to four months.

Brittle feet

If your horse's feet break or crack easily, keep it shod in the summer (even if it is turned out to grass) if the ground is hard. Badly broken feet take a long time to recover and when you bring your horse into work at the end of the summer the farrier may have difficulty in keeping the shoes on it because broken walls are weak.

You can improve the condition of your horse's feet by rubbing Cornucrescine well into the coronets (this is the area from where the horn grows) every three days all summer. Start the treatment before the ground begins to harden. If you find that your horse's feet tend to break even in winter, continue the treatment all the year round.

Really severe cases can be helped by feeding a tablespoonful of gelatine every day. The cheapest way is to buy a really large catering pack of it. Feeding one tablespoonful of cod liver oil every day will also help to promote sound horn growth. A nutritional supplement known as Farrier's Formula is said to improve the growth of sound horn. Obviously, all of these treatments will take three to six months to show results. Dry feet become brittle, so keeping the horse in a boggy field or creating an area of wet mud inside a loose box where the horse is tied up each day can help. Get the farrier to visit every six weeks or more often. Long feet tend to break round the nail holes.

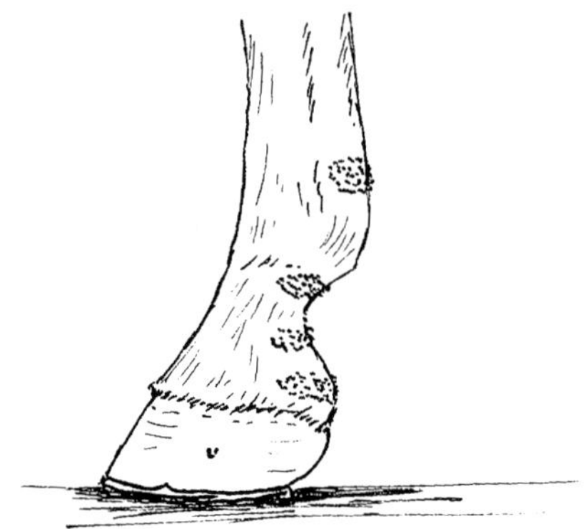

Cracked heels at the scabby stage.

Cracked heels and mud fever

Horses with white socks are more likely to get cracked heels because their pink skin is more sensitive than that of horses with black or brown legs. Trimming or clipping the long feather off the heels can help to cause this problem because you are removing the natural drainage route for water which normally follows the long hair to the ground and does not run down into the heels. Removing the feather also allows mud and grit to get close to the skin and into creases in the heel where it may rub and will irritate the skin as the horse is exercised or walks about in the field grazing. If the skin is broken, infection may get in and in no time you will have a running scabby crack right across the back of the pastern (often at two different levels) or several moist scabby spots of mud fever in the heel, pastern and fetlock area. These are very, very painful and even a quiet horse may really fight, kick and strike out at you if you attempt to treat the condition.

Prevention is better than cure and meticulous attention to the heels, feeling them daily really carefully with your fingers so that the tiniest scabby place will be found immediately, is essential. Keeping the heels greased with petroleum jelly will help the skin to stay supple and keep water off it. Petroleum jelly is the best thing to use as, not being too sticky, it does not collect so much mud as other creams.

If you do find even a tiny scab, scratch if off so that you can treat the mud fever infection underneath, either with a purple spray or an anti-bacterial cream, both obtainable from the vet. Wash the area with warm water and a gentle soap first to clean it and soften the scabs, so making their removal less painful for the horse. The area must be kept dry afterwards so bandage a pad of gamgee over the area when the horse is turned out or exercised and avoid mud and wet places. If you catch mud fever soon enough you may prevent it from spreading up the legs and under the stomach. In two or three days, the one tiny scab will disappear as long as you continue to remove it before applying your dressing of spray or cream. If it does spread or if you only discover the condition when there is a large scabby area, you must still remove all the scabs before applying spray or cream and rubbing the latter well in.

It is a great help to teach your horse to stand tied up really short – with just 15 cm (6 in) of rope between its headcollar and the knot you tie it with – to make it easier for you to treat any problem. If the horse strikes out or kicks so much that you can't cope, get an assistant to hold up the foreleg on the same side as the infected heel if this is on a hind leg, or the foreleg on the opposite side if the infection is on a foreleg (see page 155).

Some horses always seem to get cracked heels; others never do. Feeding a tablespoon of cod liver oil a day does seem to prevent the problem, perhaps by making the skin more supple.

Mud

Before riding in muddy conditions, smear baby oil or cooking oil on your hands and rub this all over the horse's legs, belly and up inside its hind legs. The mud will not stick and will fall off easily when dry. This also helps to prevent cracked heels and mud fever.

Clicking and forging

Clicking and forging are both names given to the noise made when the toe of the hind shoe catches up with and clicks against the toe of the front shoe. It mostly occurs during the two-time diagonal action of trot but can sometimes be heard in walk.

There are several possible causes.

- The horse is unbalanced and probably trotting too fast. Its centre of gravity is too far forward, therefore it is on its forehand and its front feet are not picking up quickly enough. As the front foot is coming up, the hind toe moves in under the front foot and they catch toe to toe.
- Its feet have grown long and it needs shoeing.
- It is a sloppy, lazy horse or a tired and weak horse.
- It has got a sloppy, lazy rider!

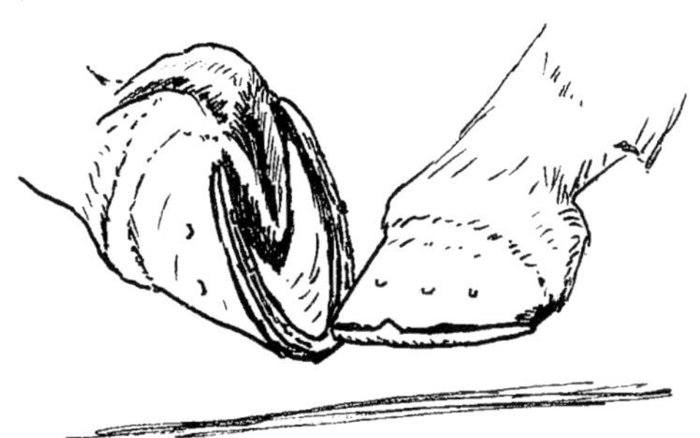

Clicking or forging. The toe of the hind shoe hits the toe of the front shoe.

Overreaching

Overreaching can occur in deep going when the forefeet are held by the ground fractionally longer than normal and the toe of the hind shoe catches up with the heel of the front foot and makes a downward cut in it.

A horse can overreach if it is going too fast and becomes unbalanced by a change of terrain or a sudden change of direction. Moving from firm going on to a soft patch of ground can cause the problem. Jumping where the landing is deep will often make a horse overreach.

A tired or weak horse may overreach because it is easily unbalanced and loses the normal rhythm of its stride. Riding over undulating ground across country, where the bottom of any dip is often deeper and the going heavier, is a very likely occasion on which to get an overreach.

In very many cases the rider can prevent overreaches by steadying and rebalancing the horse by check, check, checking it to shorten its stride and move its centre of gravity further back. This lightens the horse's forehand and enables it to get its forefeet out of the ground more quickly so that the hind shoes will not catch up.

It is the inside edge of the toe of the hind shoe which makes the overreach cut so the hind shoes could be set back a little under the hoof. The whole toe area can then be rounded off so that there are no sharp edges.

An overreach cut slicing into the heel often forms a pocket in which dirt and grit lodge. If there is just a thin flap of skin, cut if off (or get the vet to). In any case, clean the area really well and if the flap of flesh is too big to cut off, make sure that it heals from the inside outwards by keeping the outer edge of the skin open to allow drainage. Keep it clean. If it heals quickly from the outside, infection may set in and a pocket of pus may form. It will then take much longer to get your horse back into work.

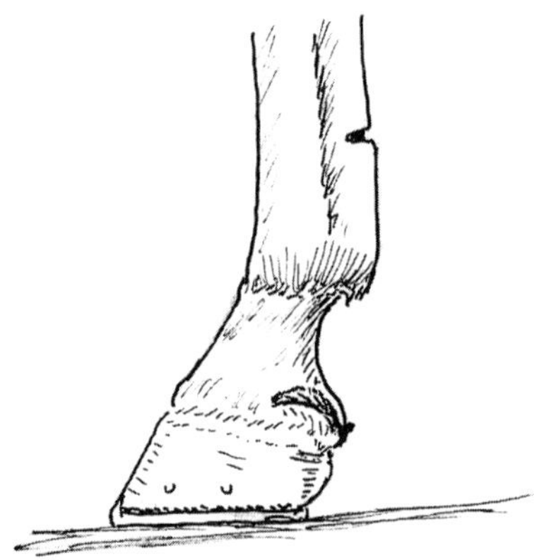

Overreaching and striking into the leg (a high overreach into the tendon). These are two of the wounds that can be made on a foreleg by the toe of a hind shoe.

Overreach boots may be worn to protect the heel area. There are two main types: open or full closed circle. The closed circle ones are put on by turning them inside out so that the horse's toe is put into the widest part first before the narrow area is pulled over the hoof. Once on, the wide area is turned over and pulled down to cover the hoof. If this type of boot is tight and difficult to put on, soak the boots in hot water for a few minutes first, to soften them. The open type are fastened round the coronet.

All overreach boots must fit so that the back of the boot around the heel is just clear of the ground and the boot fits fairly close around the hoof. If the boot is too long at the back, the toe of the hind shoe will tread on it and pull the boot off, possibly making the horse stumble as it does so.

Thrush

If your stable is allowed to become wet and soggy by being filled with dirty straw, droppings and urine, your horse will constantly be standing in filth and is likely to develop thrush, a foul-smelling infection of the foot. This is most often found in the cleft in the centre of the frog but sometimes also appears on each side of the frog if there is a deep groove there to hold moisture.

Keep the horse in a clean, dry stable, pick up droppings regularly and remove wet patches of straw so that the horse's feet are kept dry. Pick the feet out thoroughly, cleaning out all clefts and grooves carefully. Scrub the feet well with soap and water. Leave them to dry off then, if necessary, pick them out clean before lifting each foot up in turn and pouring neat hydrogen peroxide into every cleft and groove. Hold the foot up for a minute or so if possible, to allow gravity to pull the hydrogen peroxide right down into the deepest part of the clefts and grooves of the foot. Treat the affected feet twice a day. It is not easy to cure deep-seated thrush which can occasionally lame a horse if it becomes badly infected and inflamed.

Many horses always have slight thrush, which usually causes no problems, but do try to prevent a horse contracting thrush while in your care by regularly picking out its feet and by keeping the stable floor clean and dry.

GIVING A HORSE MEDICINE BY MOUTH

Some horses will not eat anything strange put in their food, however well disguised it may be with grated carrots or black treacle.

- Using a syringe-type wormer it is usually possible to get the dose into the horse's mouth if you tie it up very short and put the tip of the syringe into the corner of the lips. If the horse does not like being tied up, back it into a corner so that it cannot run backwards. Make sure it has not just been eating a feed or hay or it will spit this and your expensive wormer out at the same time.

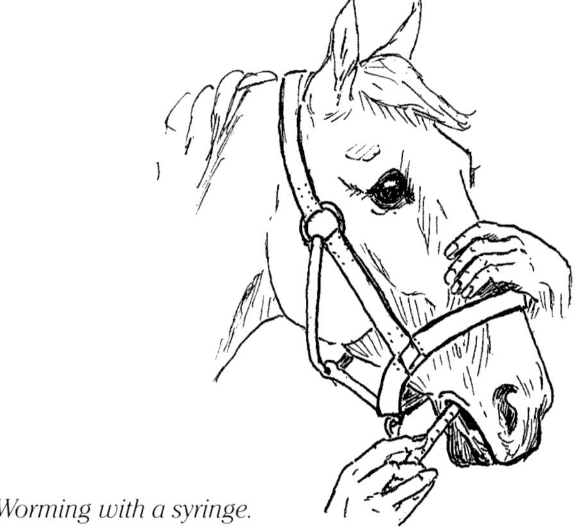

Worming with a syringe.

- Powders can be mixed with a little golden syrup (stickier than black treacle). Use a wooden spoon to get the mixture on to the back of the horse's tongue. (Use a wooden spoon for cough paste too.)
- Liquid medicine can be drawn up into a rubber bulb with a narrow tube-like nozzle. Insert the nozzle into the corner of the horse's mouth and squeeze.
- A plastic bottle can be used – *never* glass. Tip only a small amount into the corner of the horse's mouth to allow only one swallow at a time or the horse will cough and choke and may panic. Raise the horse's head a little but do remember that if you hold its head really high the liquid will go down its windpipe instead. (You try swallowing liquid with your head tilted right up and you will feel exactly what happens!)

RESTRAINING A HORSE IN ORDER TO TREAT WOUNDS

It is often necessary to keep a horse as still as possible for its own safety and yours, perhaps when being clipped or shod or when you are trying to dress a wound.

Tying a horse up short with its head raised a little will restrict its movement to some extent. NB: some horses panic when tied up very short and may then be an even greater danger to you and themselves.

To treat a foreleg

Tie the horse up short, if possible, and get a capable assistant to hold up the opposite foreleg to the injured one, holding the hoof near the toe and pressing

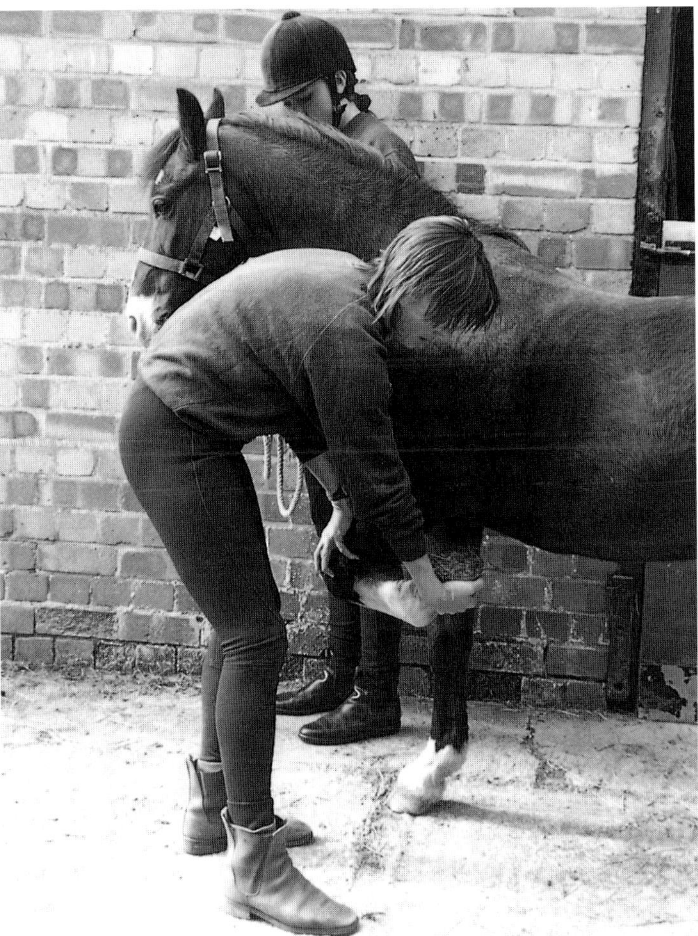

Holding up a foreleg.

it tight towards the horse's elbow with one hand while pushing down just above the horse's knee with the other. The assistant should be facing the horse's tail and leaning against its shoulder. They must try very hard not to let go, even if the horse hops about on the other foreleg. No one should stand in front of the raised foreleg.

Dressing a wound on a hind leg

Tie the horse up short.

Pick up the front foreleg on the same side as the injured hind leg. Have one hand on the front hoof near the toe and pull the toe up tight towards the horse's elbow. With the other hand push down just above the horse's knee. If it hops about, hang on tight. If there is a third person to help, they can turn the horse's head towards the foreleg that is being held up. This will help to make it more difficult for the horse to swing its hindquarters towards the person dressing the wound and perhaps kick them. This person must stand facing the horse's tail, as close to the girth as possible, rest their hand nearer the horse on its back and use their other hand to reach the wound. The hand on the back acts as an early warning feeler in case of a kick because the preparatory muscle movement will be felt. If the horse swings round and tries to kick, the person treating the wound must move closer to the horse and nearer to the shoulder. Be aware that, besides kicking out behind, a horse can cow kick forwards under its stomach.

Some horses will behave better if they cannot see what is happening so you could try cupping a hand round behind the horse's eye.

Twitching

All twitches are potentially dangerous for inexperienced handlers to use.

The commonest type of twitch is a strong round piece of wood about 90 cm (3 ft) long with a hole drilled in the smooth, rounded end through which a 15-cm (6-in) loop of soft, thick rope is threaded. This loop is put round the horse's top lip so that it does not interfere with its nostrils and the stick is twisted until the loop is tight on the nose. This is often easier said than done because a horse which has previously been twitched knows what is coming and will do everything in its power to avoid having the loop of rope put on its nose. It may rear, strike out at you, try to knock you over or panic and go berserk so do not attempt to twitch a horse unless there are two very capable people present who have dealt with this sort of problem many times before.

Once the twitch is on, the person holding the pole must keep their hands well apart and concentrate one hundred per cent on the horse's expression and tension because it may explode at any second. A loose twitch flying around still attached to a panicking horse's nose is a very dangerous item!

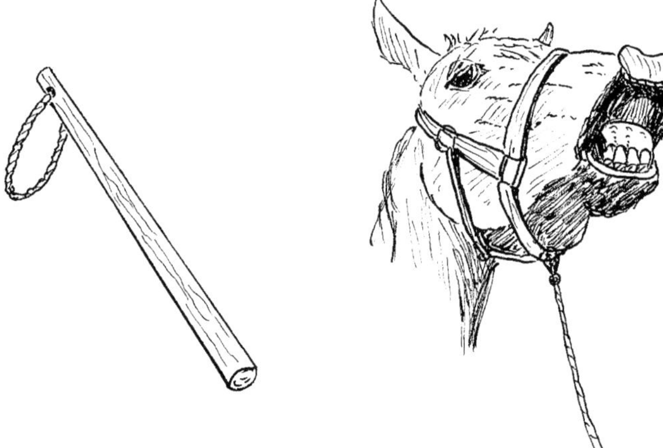

Old-fashioned restraining twitch.

Keep the twitch on for as short a time as possible and only use one if all else has failed. Avoid using a twitch on a young horse if you possibly can. For instance, when clipping for the first time, leave the head or ears if they cause a problem. You do not want a young horse to associate clipping with being twitched.

Humane twitch

The old-fashioned form of humane twitch was two pieces of wood about 36 cm (14 in) long with notches carved in them. They were hinged at one end and the two rounded ends at the other end could be joined together and tightened up with a leather strap.

The modern version is made of two rounded, shaped pieces of curved metal.

Both types are intended to go across the top lip and be tightened on it.

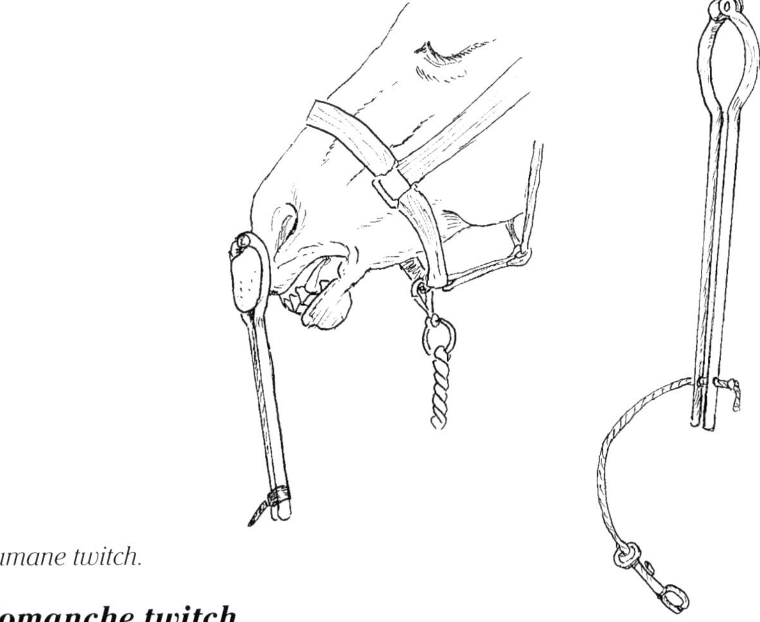

Humane twitch.

Comanche twitch

A strong metal ring and a thick piece of soft cord approximately 1.8 m (6 ft) long can form a twitch to distract a horse's attention without really hurting it.

Always put a headcollar and lead rope on first. You need a strong metal ring about 5 cm (2 in) in diameter. Attach the ring securely to one end of the cord. Keeping the ring on the near (left) side of the horse's face, halfway up its cheek, pass the end of the cord over the horse's head and bring it inside the mouth between the top teeth and the top lip so that it is resting on the gums above the top teeth. Bring the end of the cord out of the left corner of the horse's mouth and thread it through the ring. There is a little central flap of skin connecting the top lip to the gum here (you have this too) and it is a very sensitive area. As you pull down on the loose end of the cord you put pressure

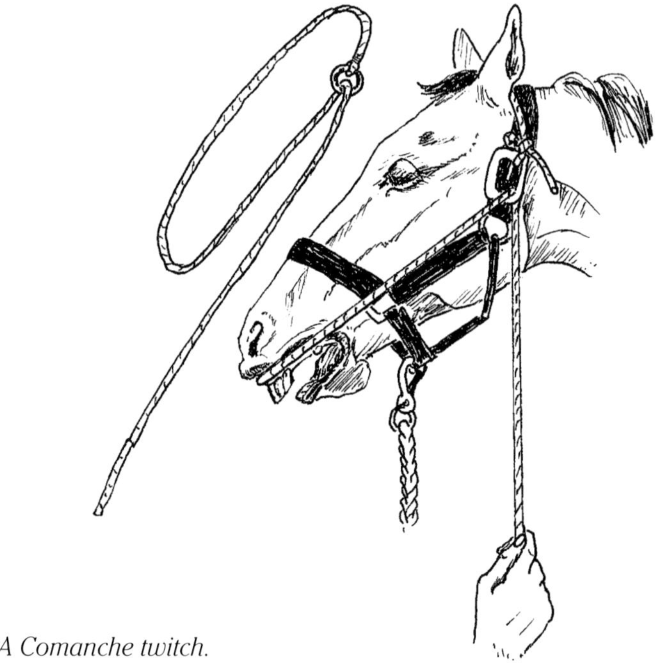

A Comanche twitch.

on this area. If used severely the skin may tear and bleed. Slight, gentle movements of your hand on the end of the cord are often sufficient to keep the horse still.

NB: *never* wrap the headcollar rope or the loose end of the cord round your hand.

BANDAGING WOUNDS

If it becomes necessary to bandage the knee, hock, forearm or thigh, it is essential to bandage from the coronet upwards first. If necessary, use several bandages going almost up to the wound. Apply the chosen wound dressing then bandage it in place using the lower bandages for support to keep the last bandage up. Your final bandage will go over the top bandage and overlap the support bandage.

A knee or hock should be bandaged with a figure of eight bandage to allow it to bend.

It may be necessary to cross tie the horse so that it cannot move about too much or lie down if it is essential to keep a dressing and bandage on.

Travelling boots can help to support bandages and keep everything in place.

A slight wound is better left exposed to the air.

7 TRAINING

REWARD

Constantly giving horses titbits from your hand tends to make them pushy and can make them bad tempered.

Rewards of food should be reserved for horses which are difficult to catch and horses which are nervous of approaching people, even in the stable.

Animals do not 'pat' each other. They rub or scratch each other for enjoyment. Horses enjoy being rubbed on the forehand, ear roots, withers, crest, chest, in between the cheek bones and round the root of the tail. See which place your horse seems to enjoy most and use a rub there and gentle words as a reward.

If a horse has worked hard and well, dismount and lead it, running up your stirrups and loosening its girth as a reward.

Allow your horse to graze for a few minutes after good work but only when you are dismounted. Allowing horses to graze when you are on their backs leads to snatching and diving for grass or foliage.

Do not go on and on trying to get something perfect or the horse will become tired, bored or confused and you may get frustrated and bad tempered. If the horse has tried and succeeded even a little, stop and reward it. Always try to finish on a good note.

PUNISHMENT

A horse only understands any form of punishment if it receives it within seconds of misbehaving. If you are going to punish your horse, try to do it as it begins to do wrong.

Do not punish it unless you are absolutely certain that it was deliberately misbehaving. Do not punish it unless you are absolutely certain that it will know what you are punishing it for.

Could it have misunderstood what you asked it to do? Could it have been frightened to carry out your request? Did you give it enough time to listen or feel your request, understand it and carry out your wishes? Was your request clear and easy for it to understand?

Unnecessary punishment and punishment for something the horse has not understood or is frightened of causes many problems. Your horse may no longer trust you, it may become jumpy and nervous or become bad tempered towards people in general.

If you are going to hit the horse when you are riding it:

- Make sure that it is facing in the direction in which you want it to go.
- Hit it really hard, *once*, and use your legs to ride it forward.
- When you hit it behind the saddle you must put both reins in one hand and use the whip in the other hand. (If you keep the reins one in each hand as you hit it, you will jerk its mouth if you are using a short whip.)
- Hit it as it starts to misbehave or the very second it has done so.
- If you hit it hard to ask it go forward, sit so that you will be in balance and 'go with it' if it shoots forward. Be ready to push your hands forward so that there will not be a pull on its mouth, as this will only cause more problems.
- If a horse is shying from naughtiness, you can use your whip down its shoulder on the side further away from the spook.
- If you want a horse to go forward, you must hit it behind the saddle.
- Use of the whip on the lunge must be very accurate or the horse will not go where you want it to. You must be in an enclosed area. If you use a whip in an open area, you may lose the horse!
- Punishment in the stable should be with the voice or a thump of your fist, not with a whip. A horse must feel safe and confident in its stable. A horse which is constantly hit in its stable becomes a mental and often physical wreck.
- If you growl at the horse as you hit it (mounted) or thump it (in the stable), it will associate your tone of voice with punishment and may learn to respond to just a growl of your voice.
- Some animals buck, refuse to move on and become 'piggy' when hit with a whip. Hitting them more and harder is not the answer. Sometimes blunt spurs work with horses which react to a whip in this way.

Be firm and consistent. Do not allow your horse to do something one day and then hit it for doing it the next day.

Be certain that your horse knows why you are punishing it.

Be certain that your horse has understood what you asked of it.

Be certain that it is not misbehaving from fright.

Do not take it out on the horse because you are in a bad temper or have had a row with your husband/wife/boyfriend/girlfriend/parents!

LUNGEING

If you have never lunged a horse before, you cannot teach a horse to lunge nor can you correct a horse which is difficult to lunge.

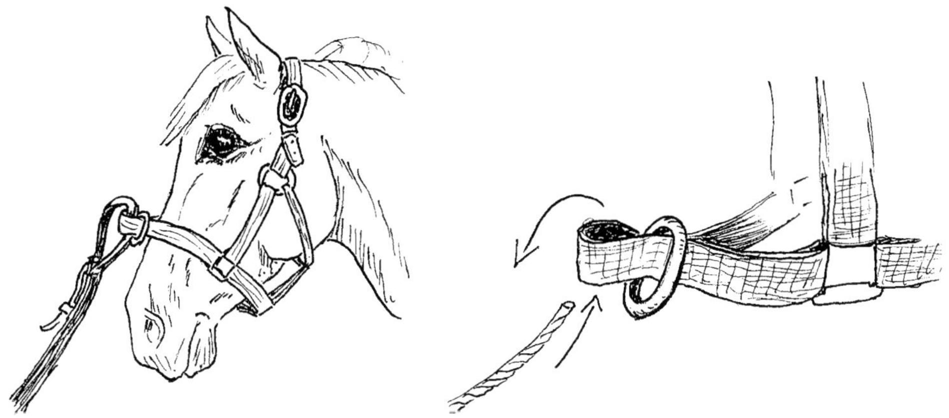

If you have no lungeing cavesson, use a webbing headcollar with a ring.

Before you even think of lungeing yourself, watch an experienced person and have a few lessons so that you are sure you have grasped the basic principles.

Practise on a quiet, sensible animal. Use an enclosed or fenced-off area or make a lungeing circle from barrels and poles. If you do not have a lungeing cavesson, use a strong headcollar and push the centre front of the noseband through a strong metal ring to form a loop. Attach your lunge rein to this loop. Most horses prefer to go round to the left so start in this direction. Carry the lunge rein in your left hand so that the loops fall off in sequence and are big enough not to entrap your hand. Carry the lunge whip in your right hand, pointing away from the horse.

Start off with the horse parallel to the side and facing into a corner. Step sideways a little towards the horse's quarters and use your voice to encourage it to go forward at walk. Your body must always be in such a position that you feel you are driving the horse forwards – not leading it. There must be a straight line from your hand through the lunge rein to the horse's nose. The lunge whip must be used carefully because some horses are very frightened of a long whip. To encourage the horse to go forward, bring the point of the whip towards the horse's tail, keeping the tip of the whip low on the ground. If the horse does not respond, raise the whip a little and move the tip up and down or in a circular motion. Use your voice in a quick, higher tone to encourage the horse forward. To slow the horse down, bring the tip of the whip low to the ground and turn it behind you, using your voice in a slower, deeper tone.

If your horse just races round and round flat out on the lunge, it is essential to have an enclosed area. Pulling at the lunge will not slow the horse down. Use a calm, quiet voice, stand as still as possible, try to keep the lunge line clear of the ground (many horses will try to cut across one part of the circle) and wait until the horse eventually slows down. Only calm repetition several

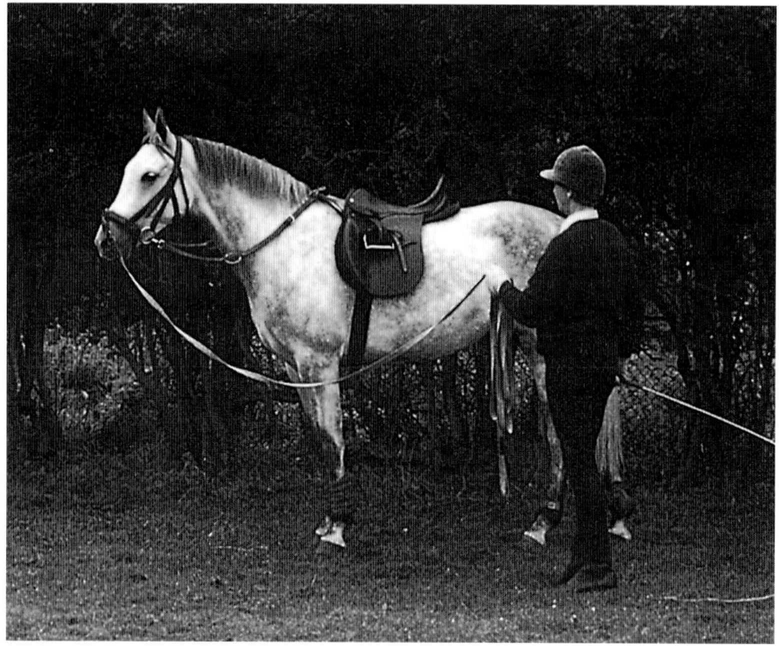

Ready to ask the horse to walk forward.

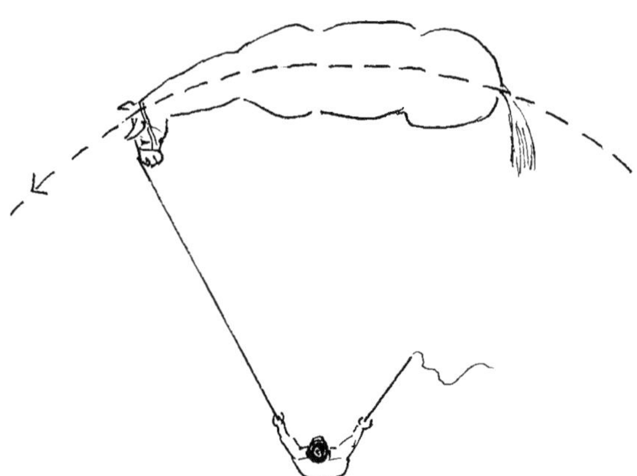

The correct position for the lunger.

times a day will slow down a horse which is frantic on the lunge.

Sometimes such a horse will calm down more quickly if loose-schooled because it is then not attached to the lunge. A very strongly fenced small area of approximately 20–30 m (22–33 yd) diameter is necessary for loose-schooling. Having calmed down when loose, the horse may then be calmer when lunged.

A normal horse can be controlled somewhat by the lunger's body position. If they step towards the horse's tail, they can send it forward more easily so this

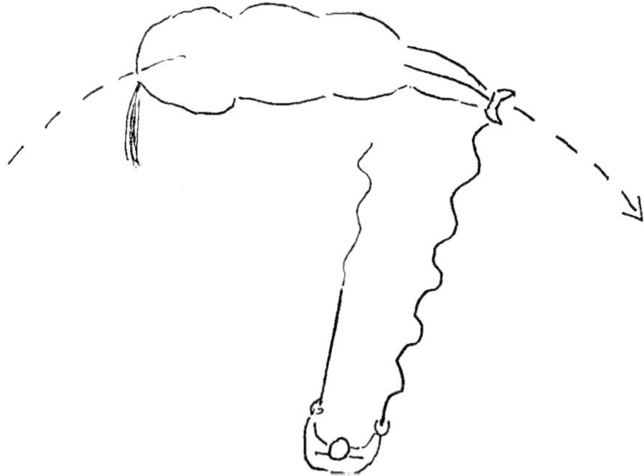

Snaking the lunge line and pointing the whip at the horse's shoulder to prevent it from cutting in on the circle.

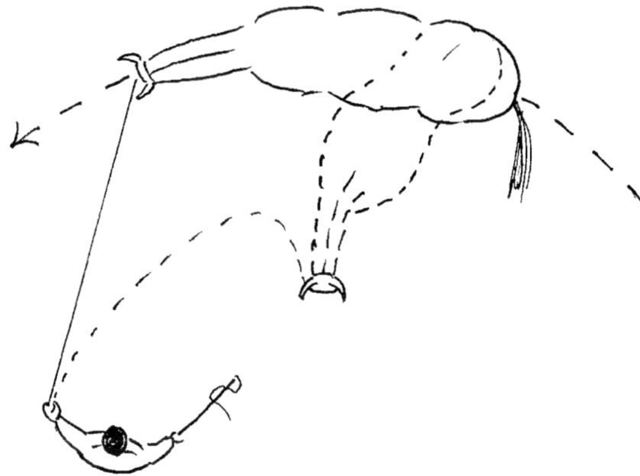

The wrong position for the lunger. She is trying to 'lead' the horse round with her left arm out to the side. She is standing in advance of the horse which is likely to turn inwards and go in the opposite direction.

position would be used with a horse which constantly tried to whip round inwards and go the other way. If the lunger steps towards the horse's head, they can slow the horse down. This would be combined with putting the tip of the whip low and behind them.

Some horses are very quick to evade the lunger by whipping round inwards and changing direction. The lunger must never take their eye off the horse's eye and must be very, very quick to anticipate the turn, step towards the horse's tail and use the whip to drive it forward.

Correcting a horse which is bad to lunge is a job for an expert. It is almost impossible in an open field. The most common evasion is whipping round inwards. To cure this a second rein can be attached and passed round the horse's hindquarters as in long-reining. Again, this is a job for an expert because perfect co-ordination is essential to control the horse by keeping the correct amount of tension on both reins.

Whipping round outwards

Horses usually attempt to do this when you are trying to lunge them in an open field. You cannot control a horse which does this in just a headcollar or cavesson, not even if you are in an enclosed area. Lungeing from the bit (preferably with side reins to prevent the horse from throwing its head up as it whips round) is essential.

The horse which whips round outwards uses the full strength of its neck and body to drag you along. It may dive off straight out of the circle so that you are behind it and it can tow you along quite easily. It may whip round and go in the opposite direction, leaving you with the lunge rein coming from the wrong side over its withers or round its hindquarters to your hand. In an open field you have very little hope of controlling or correcting a horse which has learnt either of these tricks. An enclosed area and a very experienced person to lunge it are essential.

Ways of attaching the lunge rein

A lunge rein can be attached:
- to the front of a headcollar;
- to the front of a cavesson;
- to the front ring of a Wels cavesson. (This cavesson fits lower on the nose, very like a drop noseband);
- to the side ring of a cavesson or side D of a headcollar, together with the ring of a snaffle bit. If you attach a lunge rein only to one ring of a snaffle bit, it is likely to pull through the mouth. Attaching the lunge line to the bit ring *and* the headcollar or cavesson prevents this from happening (and makes it less severe because some pressure is taken by the nose);
- from the far ring of the snaffle bit, under the chin and through the near ring of the snaffle bit. (It is not so easy to turn the horse inwards and there can be a nutcracker action on the lower jaw.);
- from the far ring of a snaffle bit, under the chin and twice round the near ring of the snaffle bit. (This gives a more direct feel on the near side and helps to prevent the nutcracker action.);
- from the far ring, over the top of the horse's head and down through the near ring. (This gives an upward 'gag' action which is helpful in controlling a horse which tries to dive its head down.) It is not so easy to turn the horse inwards;
- from the centre ring of a leather strap or chain attached under the chin to the two rings of a snaffle bit;

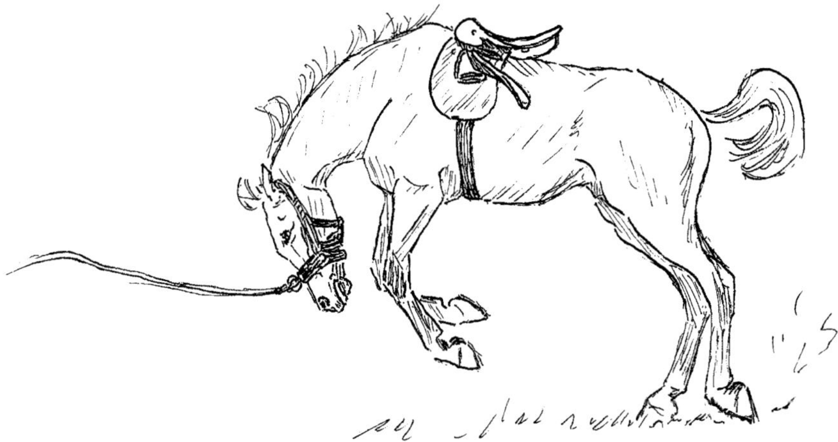

This is quite the wrong way to lunge. The horse should be lunged in crossed side reins for more control. It should be wearing boots. The irons and leathers have not been safely secured. There is nothing to stop the saddle slipping back.

- from the roller or saddle through the nearest snaffle bit ring. (The bit must be attached firmly to cavesson or headcollar on both sides or it will pull through the horse's mouth.) This method is very severe and must only be used by an expert but it will help to control a horse that is really determined to get away from the lunger, or to restrain one which has constantly succeeded in getting away. It will control a horse which tries to take off forwards or one which tries to whip round outwards away from the lunger.

Attaching the lunge rein to the front of a cavesson is the simplest and mildest method. There is nothing to alter when you change the rein. All the other methods of lungeing from the bit (except attaching it to the centre of a leather strap or chain under the chin) involve altering the attachment of the lunge rein when changing direction.

When lungeing from the bit, it is safer to attach the bit to each side of a headcollar or cavesson to ensure that the bit stays in place.

Safety when lungeing any horse

- Wear a hard hat. Horses can kick you or strike out at you. Wear gloves as your hands can get rope burns from having the rein pulled through them.
- Never loop the rein round your hands. You can get your fingers broken or be dragged along the ground.
- Never wrap the lunge line round your waist. If the horse whips round, the rein can encircle you and pull you over. You could be trampled by the horse.

Safety for the horse

Always check the following points:
- boots should be worn all round;
- field gates should be shut;
- no barbed wire;
- no loose horses in the area;
- use an enclosed/fenced small area.

Side reins

Side reins can be attached to a saddle or a roller. The other ends can be attached to a headcollar, a cavesson or a snaffle bit. Always start with them quite loose. (See also page 88.)

To prevent a horse from grazing while being lunged

Attach the side reins to girth or roller, cross them over the horse's withers and tie them together where they cross. Attach the other ends to the headcollar, cavesson or bit. If attached to the bit, make sure they are not so tight as to affect the horse's head carriage. They only need to be tight enough to stop the horse reaching the grass.

To help to control a horse which dives its head down or bucks with its head down, use the side reins as above.

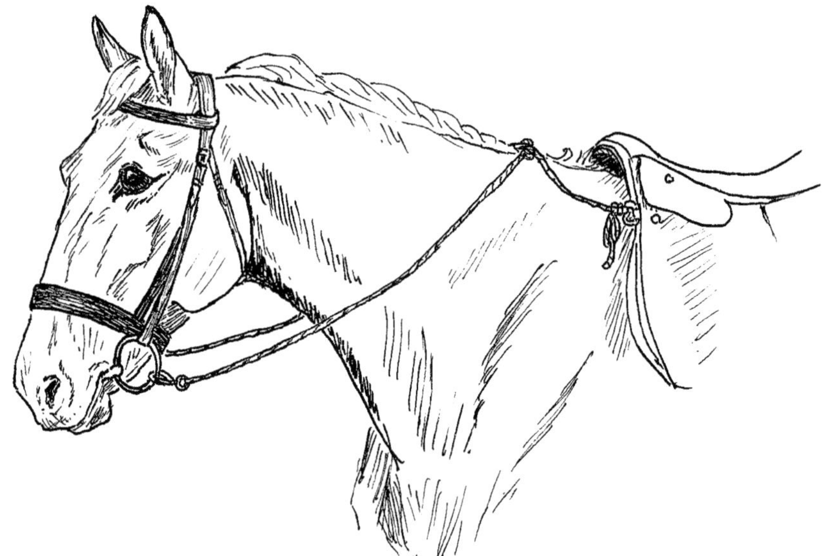

Side reins will give you more control. Loose, crossed side reins will prevent the horse on the lunge from grazing without interfering with its natural head carriage. The side reins can be attached to the side rings of a cavesson or headcollar if the horse is not wearing a bridle or you do not want to attach them to the bit.

Using side reins to control a horse that whips round

Attach the side reins to the girth or roller and then directly to the side rings on the same side of a headcollar, cavesson or bit ring. If attached to the bit, do not have them so tight that they affect the horse's head carriage.

Always fit side reins loosely at first to see how the horse reacts. Be aware that side reins that are fitted too tight can:

- shorten a horse's stride;
- make it go hollow-backed with head up;
- make it go overbent with head low;
- put pressure from the bit on the tongue, which can make the horse try to get its tongue over the bit to avoid this;
- make it run backwards and even fall over.

If you are not experienced with side reins, ask advice before using them.

Lungeing is hard work for a horse. It is constantly on the turn and is likely to brush behind (knock the outside hind fetlock with the inside hind hoof/shoe). Check for this. Thirty minutes is enough for a fit horse. Ten to fifteen minutes is enough for a young or unfit horse. The horse can be lunged twice a day for these lengths of time, depending on its age and condition and assuming that this is the only exercise it is getting. Use large circles of about 20 m (22 yd) in diameter.

Lungeing over poles and jumps

First teach your horse to lunge calmly and obediently (see page 160).

An enclosed area or even the corner of a field will make things easier for you and the horse. For jumping, have the lunge rein attached to the cavesson *not* to the bit. Do not use side reins because the horse must have complete freedom to use its head and neck to jump properly. Put protective boots on in front and behind. (Get the horse used to boots and Velcro in the stable first.)

Always wear gloves to prevent your hands from rope burns if the lunge rein is suddenly pulled through them.

Never wrap the lunge line round your hand. If the horse pulls away, the loops will tighten and you can be dragged along the ground quite unable to free yourself.

Lungeing over poles or jumps necessitates increasing your own speed of movement to go with the horse; lifting your hand to allow the lunge line to clear the curve you have made over the wings and jump stands; and skilfully allowing your hand holding the lunge rein to follow the horse so that there is never a pull on its nose when approaching or going over the jump.

You have to be very experienced or you will do more harm than good. Practise on a quiet old pony; you may be surprised at how difficult this exercise is.

The lungeing rein will get caught up on wings and uprights unless you plan and prepare carefully. You must work your horse equally on both reins so your wings and uprights must have a smooth, rounded top for the lunge rein to slide over from both directions. Your jump must have wings and uprights which are higher than the pole to encourage the horse to go over the jump. Build the jump against a wall or safe, existing fence or hedge. Two long poles, each with one end on the ground and the other two ends meeting at the highest point of the jump stand, can be tied in place where they meet. Wrap a plastic bag round the two ends and tie this down to form a smooth, rounded surface on which nothing can catch.

Lead the horse several times in each direction through the gap in which you will build your jump, then lunge it through the same gap. Now put a pole on the ground in the gap and lead the horse over this before lungeing over it. (See Trotting Poles, page 281, for distances and procedure.)

You now have a choice of either lungeing on a true circle to include the poles or jump or moving forward with the horse so that it goes straight just before, over and just after the poles or jump before coming on to a circle again. (Be careful never to get in front of the imaginary line running from you to the horse's shoulder or you will stop the horse.)

If you work on a true circle, your horse may rush in anticipation of going over the poles or jump again. If you work on a circle over several poles on the ground you will need to lay them in a slight fan shape so that the distance between them, from the centre of each pole to the centre of the next pole, is correct for the horse's steps on a circle.

If you work in a straight line, you can bring the horse on to a circle after the jump and, if necessary, continue on this ordinary circle, missing out the poles or jump, until you decide to work your circles progressively nearer to the poles or jump so that they once more include them.

A few low jumps, taken quietly but willingly in a nice rounded style, should be your aim – not to see how high the horse can jump.

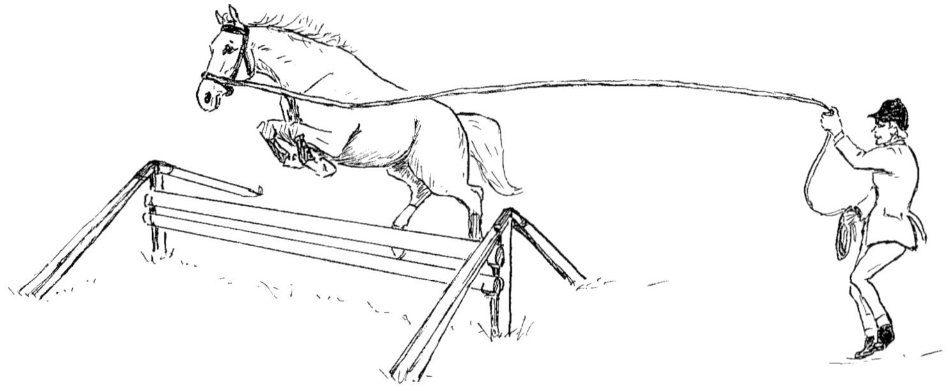

Lungeing over a jump.

LONG-REINING

- Wear gloves.
- Never wrap the reins round your hands in small loops. They will tighten and you may get dragged along if the horse takes off.
- Introduce the horse to the second rein round its hindquarters in the stable first because some horses object strongly to it.
- Do not try to correct a problem by long-reining unless you are an expert at the job. If you are not, approach someone who is and watch and learn from them. Practise on a quiet, amenable animal.

Long-reining can be used when breaking in young horses and for reschooling older horses.

It can help particularly with horses which nap, or cut in or turn in on the lunge.

You can only improve a horse, young or old, on long reins if you are an expert who has learnt to long-rein properly on quiet, steady animals and has progressed to coping with horses which are very lively and very badly behaved. If you are not an expert, don't attempt to retrain a problem horse on long reins because you are likely only to make matters worse.

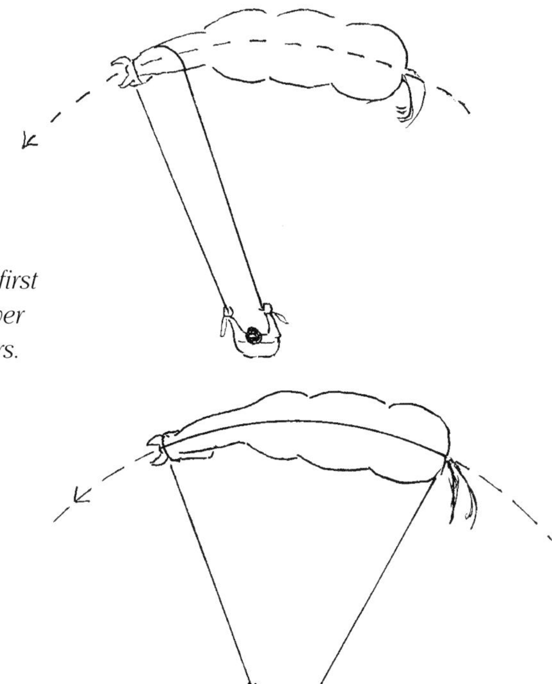

Long-reining on circles – the first stage with the second rein over the neck in front of the withers.

Long-reining on circles – the second stage.

Long-reining requires absolute concentration and the ability and knowledge to pick up minute signals from eyes, ears, muscles and head and tail carriage which tell you what the horse is about to do next so that you can anticipate and, if necessary prevent, its intended actions. Your hands must be able to follow and control the horse's head movements and use the reins against its sides or round its hindquarters to control its backward or sideways movements. You need very supple elbows and shoulders and a good eye for timing the movement and sequence of the horse's legs so that your rein aids are applied at the best moment for the horse to co-operate with you.

Some problems can be helped by long-reining.

- It can be used with a horse which always cuts in on the same part of the circle, usually towards home.

  Gently keep the bend with the inside rein and, well before the horse even gets to the part of the circle where it begins to cut in, feel, feel, feel on your outside rein while holding the long whip pointed towards the horse's shoulder.

- In rearing, napping or jibbing when the horse is refusing to go forward. It will rear up, go sideways, try to turn round, go backwards or just stand still, seemingly immovable.

Have the mildest possible bit in its mouth and put the rein through both the bit ring and the ring of the headcollar or cavesson, or, if the horse is not a tearaway, don't put a bit in its mouth at all. Have the reins on the cavesson. Adjust the cavesson as low as possible but well clear of the nostrils as when it is lower you have more control. Better still, use a Wels cavesson which fits like a drop noseband. You want the horse to go forward so the less you have in its mouth the better, as long as you can control it. To win this battle you need to be able to keep the horse's hindquarters straight or at least to reposition them straight each time the horse tries to turn around. It will be easier to do this if you have your stirrup irons down and securely tied together and also to the girth under the horse's stomach. Thread the reins from the horse's head through the stirrups irons and back to your hands.

You can stand directly behind the horse, out of kicking range, driving it forward with your voice and by flicking your wrists, moving the little fingers inwards towards each other to vibrate the long reins against the horse's sides and hindquarters and using your whip if necessary. Alternatively, you can stand behind it but a little out to one side, so that the rein on the side to which you are standing comes from the horse's head through the stirrup to your hand and the other rein, having passed through the stirrup, comes round the horse's hindquarters just above its hocks and back to your other hand. It is this rein which you will use on the horse's hindquarters to drive it forward, with the help of a long whip if necessary. Some horses always nap in the same direction so if, say, your horse always turns to the left, you should stand a little over to its left so that the right rein can be used strongly round its hindquarters to prevent

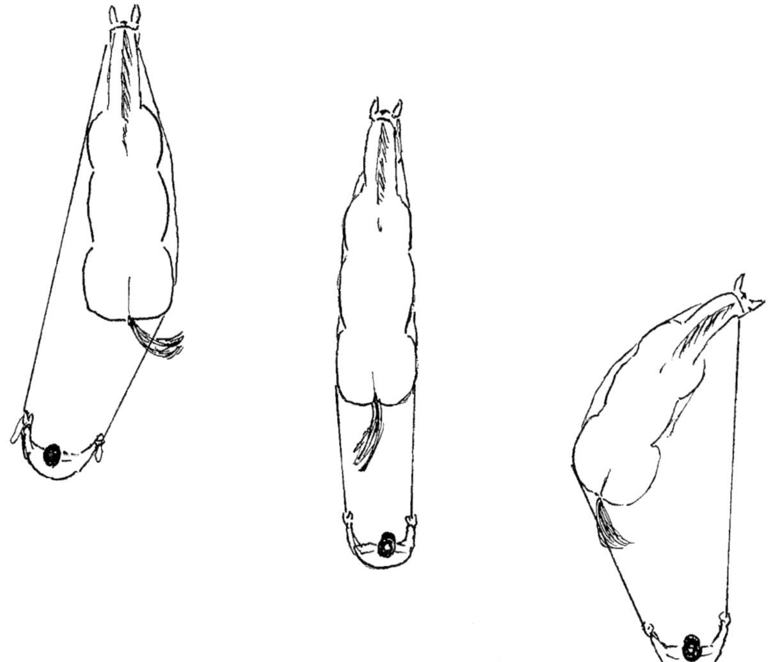

Driving on long reins. Walk to one side of the horse. When turning, move behind the horse then over to the other side.

them from swinging right as the horse tries to turn left, and thus prevent its head turning left.

A standing martingale (see page 102) can give you more control with a horse which rears or a horse which puts its head right up as it whips round. The martingale should be used for only a short time as a correction in a situation such as this.

Watch the horse intently and read the signs that will tell you it is beginning to think about playing up. Get after it quickly and fiercely, driving it forward with voice, reins and, if necessary, whip. The horse *must* feel that you are allowing it to go forward. If it tries to turn round you have to correct it but must then instantly ease your hand forward so that there is absolutely no backward contact on its mouth or nose as you ask it to go forward. This is not easy to do but it is essential if the horse is to understand what you are asking it to do, which is insisting that it goes forward.

A second person may be needed behind the horse to encourage it to go forward.

Perhaps the horse has always played up at exactly the same place when you were riding it. If so, get it going obediently and willingly on long reins in a circle and in several places where, hopefully, it will not play up, before you take it to the place where you have had a problem.

Problems when long-reining

Contact

It is essential to have a consistent and steady contact on both reins so that the horse is not wandering about bewildered on a contact which goes loose, tight, loose, tight. As in schooling, when riding you must have a constant contact so that your horse will go forward smoothly exactly on the track that you wish it to be on.

Stopping or slowing down

If your horse won't halt when you ask it to by feeling mostly on the outside rein, face it up to a wall or thick hedge, something *unjumpable*, so that it has to stop. Use your voice and reins. Don't pull it to a halt but feel, feel on the reins. Practise this several times before trying once more on a circle. As soon as it halts, ease the contact.

Working

Work on a circle until the horse understands and obeys your aids. If you then take it out, do not walk directly behind it because if something frightens it or if it does not want to stop, you will simply be towed along.

Walk out to one side or the other, changing sides regularly so that the horse gets used to the sight and feel of you on both sides. If you have a problem, you can then turn the horse on to a circle to gain control more easily.

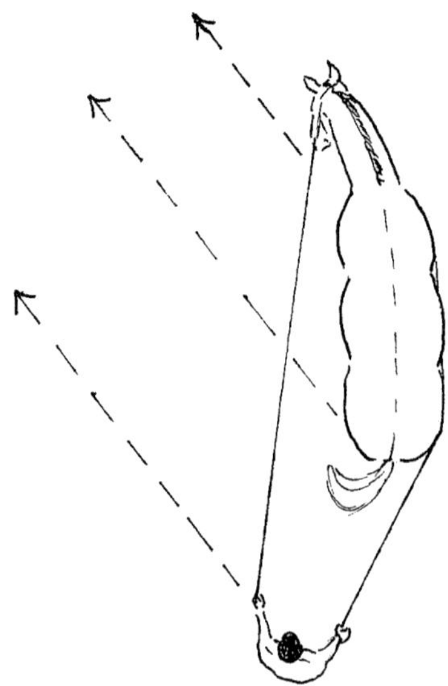

Going forward and sideways. As the horse's off hind begins to come off the ground use your right rein to ask the horse to move that leg forward and under. Use the rein in rhythm with the horse's strides.

Turning the horse on a circle in long reins

Obviously, you must always turn the horse outwards away from you when turning it in long reins. If you are working in the open corner of a field, you can turn the horse when you are in the open half, away from the corner, in which case the horse will be turning out beyond the perimeter of the previous circle.

If you are turning within an enclosed, circular, lungeing area, you must bring the horse in towards the centre of the circle so that it will then have room to turn smoothly away from you.

Always practise everything at walk until the horse understands exactly what you want it to do.

If the horse is going round on the left rein and you want to turn it outwards to the right, steady it with a half-halt with the reins then feel, feel, feel on the outside rein round the horse's hindquarters. As it turns, step forward with it. Quickly put your left hand across on to your right rein and reef in one loop on to your right hand. The right rein, which was the longer one going round the horse's hindquarters when on the left rein, now becomes the shorter rein, going to your right hand. As the horse turns, quickly let out one loop of rein from your left hand. (This is now going to be the longer rein, passing round the hindquarters.)

You have to be very quick and very co-ordinated in your actions, and smooth, not jerky with your hand movements and contact. It is not at all easy to do and really does need a lot of practice and experience if you are to do it correctly.

The horse will soon learn and be ready to start turning as it feels you beginning to make your preparations. When the turn at walk is going smoothly, try turn at trot. Now your movements really do have to be extremely quick and well co-ordinated if the horse is to turn smoothly and maintain the same rhythm of trot throughout. Half-halts are needed and a smooth change of bend just as when ridden.

What to do if the rein slips up over the back

By mistake, the rein may come up over the hindquarters, probably of a smaller animal, so that it now lies near the withers. If this happens only once, you can sometimes get the rein back in place by moving over behind the horse, lifting that rein hand as you do so, and passing the rein back over the hindquarters to its correct position before returning to your own original place.

If this happens several times, as it often does with small ponies, pass the reins through the irons of the let-down stirrups. Tie the irons together underneath the pony and also tie them to the girth to keep them in place.

If you are working on a circle and don't like the feel of the indirect contact given by the inside rein coming through the stirrup to your hand, or if you feel that this slightly backward tension is shortening the horse's stride, you can take the inside rein only out of the stirrup iron.

What to do if the rein drops down

If the outside rein drops below the hocks, raise the hand, holding it as high as possible with just enough contact for it to move back up into place above the hocks.

If the outside rein drops down and the horse gets a hind leg over it, drop the outside rein and bring the horse to a halt, shortening the rein in your hand as you walk towards its head. Either back the horse over the loose rein so that you can pick it up and start again or, if you have accustomed the horse to the feel of this in the stable, pull the rein forward past its legs and then start again.

Bucking

If the horse bucks and kicks, the outside rein may go up under its tail, whereupon the horse will clamp its tail down and shoot forward fast. Hold on to the inside rein and keep the outside rein quiet and slack. With any luck, the horse will relax, lift its tail and the rein will drop down. If this does not happen and the rein remains firmly clamped under the tail of a frightened horse, stop it with the front rein as you walk towards its head. The rein is still under its tail so, standing as close to its shoulder as possible, reach back to its tail and try to lift it so that the rein will drop. Be aware that a frightened horse will kick without thinking.

Attaching the long reins

- They can be attached to the side Ds of the cavesson. This is the mildest way, putting pressure on the nose only.
- For a little more control, which gives nose pressure and a little pressure on the mouth, attach the reins to the bit ring and the side D of the headcollar both together.
- Attach the reins only to the bit. Be very sure that you and the horse know what you are doing and that you are both happy and confident with this more severe arrangement.

Eating grass

If the horse keeps putting its head down to eat grass, attach side reins from the cavesson Ds or from the bit rings so that the reins cross over just in front of the withers and are tied together where they cross. Attach the other end of each rein to the Ds on each side of the front of the saddle or to the side Ds near the top of the roller if you are using one. They must not be so tight that they influence the horse's head carriage in any way but they must be just tight enough to prevent it from getting its head down to graze. If the side reins are not tied together where they cross near the withers they tend to open out when the horse reaches down and it can then reach the grass more easily. (See the illustration on page 88.)

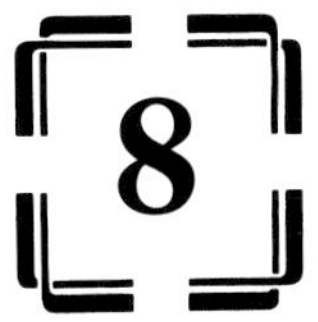

8 LOADING AND TRAVELLING

LOADING

Why some horses are bad to load

- They have been driven too fast and swung round corners. The driver has stopped and started off too suddenly.
- They have had an accident and come off a ramp, perhaps getting a leg over the edge or even falling while being loaded.
- They have travelled next to a horse which has constantly bitten or kicked them.
- They have travelled next to a bad traveller which has gone down in the box.
- They are claustrophobic in small spaces.
- They have learnt that they need not go in. People have been frightened of them, let go of them or failed to succeed in loading them.

A young horse needs time, care and encouragement, as does a horse which has been frightened. An older horse just 'trying it on' will very often go in as soon as a person of strong character gets hold of it and gives it a sharp jerk on the nose with the headcollar and a good thump in the ribs with their fist before asking it to walk up the ramp!

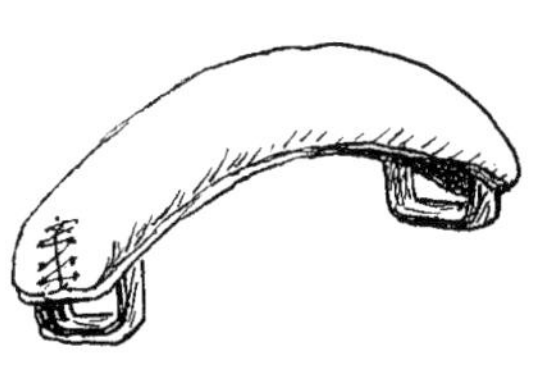

A poll guard.

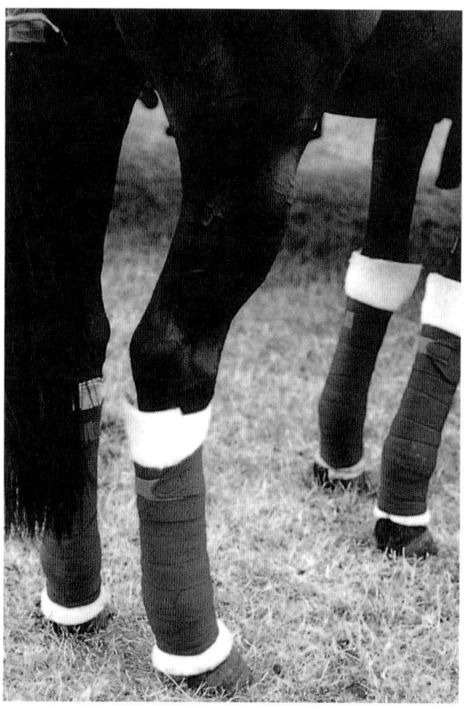

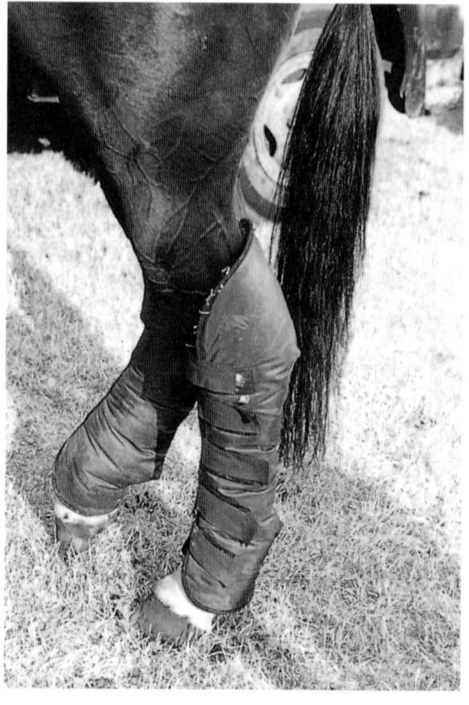

Travelling bandages with felt or gamgee. The bandages should be high enough to protect the knees and tendons and low enough to protect the coronets.

Hind travelling boots must be high enough to protect the hock area.

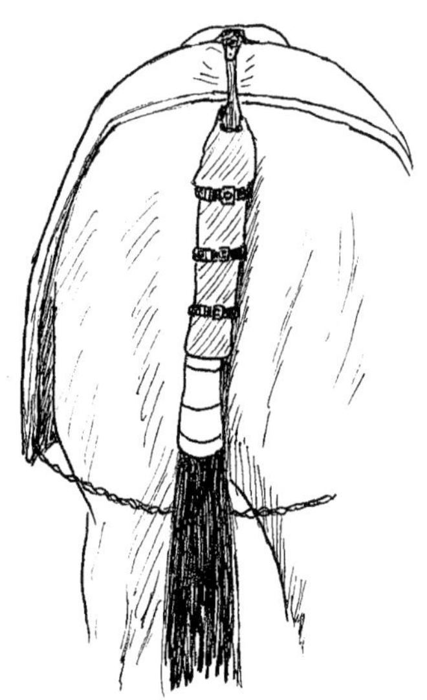

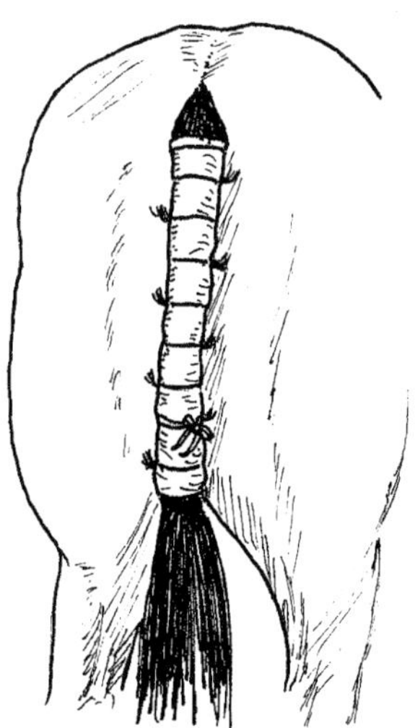

A tail guard over a bandage.

How to bandage for a long journey. Normally only a little bit of hair shows on each side. Here this is exaggerated to demonstrate how this is done.

Think ahead when loading

- Have everything ready before you bring the horse out.
- Put a bridle on over the headcollar so that you will have more control of the horse.
- Give the horse as much space to go in as possible.
- Open the side ramp or groom's door to let light in.
- Use walls, hedges or gates to form a passageway.
- Park a lorry so that the ramp is not too steep.
- Make sure the ramp is very stable, not wobbly.
- Use a ramp with a mat or put straw down so that the ramp is not noisy when stepped on.
- Tempt the horse with food, give it time and encourage it quietly before you try other methods.
- Regularly give the horse its feed in the trailer or horsebox.
- Go on short, very slow journeys at first.
- Drive as if you have a bucket of water in the back and don't want to spill a drop.
- Try travelling a short distance in a lorry or trailer yourself without holding on with your hands or leaning against the sides. You will then begin to understand horses' problems when travelling!

TRAVELLING

Why some horses are bad travellers

Some horses will load perfectly well but then, at some point during the journey, sometimes as soon as the vehicle moves, they will scrabble and panic and even throw themselves down.

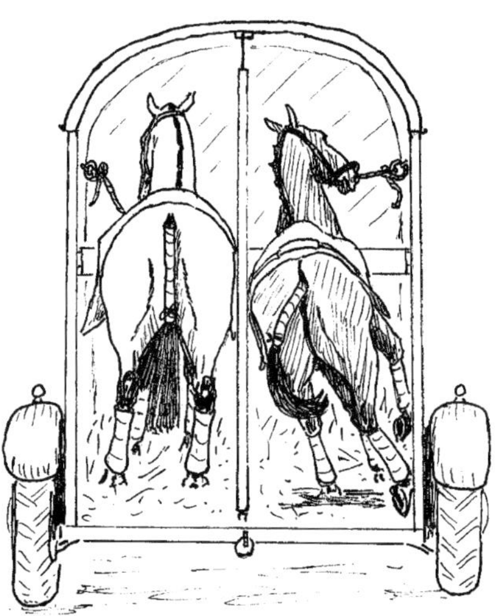

Leaning and scrabbling.

There are two completely different reasons for this as well as two completely different methods of panicking.

1 The horse does not feel safe in a narrow stall. This horse will lean its body against one side of the partition or against the side of the box or trailer while scrabbling its feet against the bottom of the partition or wall on the opposite side. In other words, it is leaning sideways at an acute angle. Initially, this is often the result of a driver cornering too fast or too suddenly. The horse loses its balance and panics, often actually falling to the ground. It is difficult to get a horse up again in a narrow division, so the horse becomes terrified of falling down. Once this habit has begun, you will only cure it by travelling the horse in as wide a space as possible so that it cannot lean on one side while scrabbling with its feet on the other side. You must also drive exceptionally slowly and carefully to regain the horse's confidence. Do not tie it up with a short rope but give it enough length to enable it to use its head and neck to balance. The rope must be long enough for its hindquarters to touch the back of the trailer before the rope pulls on its head. For the same reason, in a horse box give the horse a double section or travel it loose in half of the box.

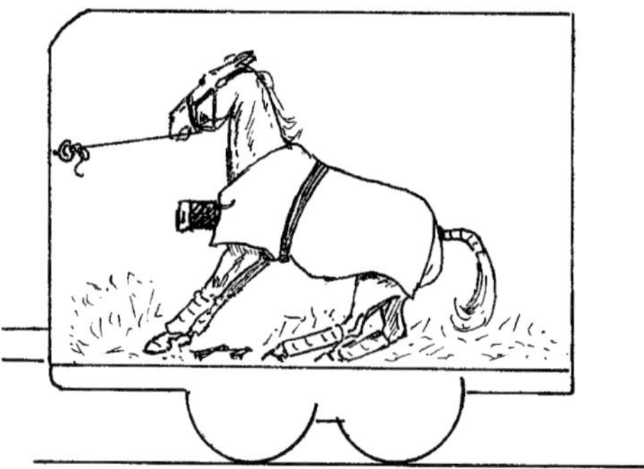

If the horse is tied too short it may pull back or put its head up. Its hind legs will slide forward under it. It is likely to fall down.

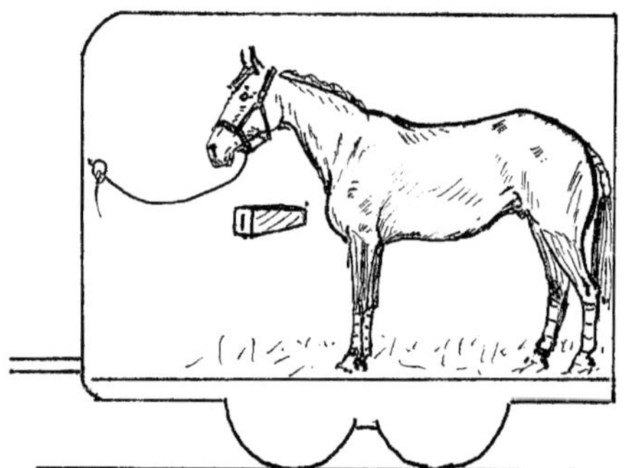

The horse's tail should touch the back of the trailer before there is any pull on the headcollar rope.

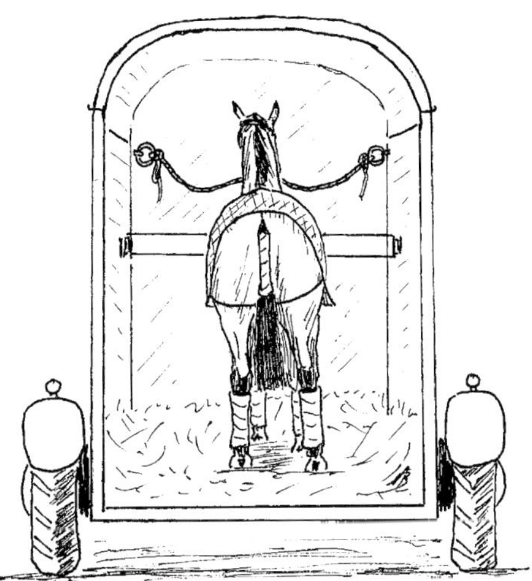

Cross-tie a horse travelling in a trailer without a division to prevent it from turning round. Note that the ramp should always be up before the horse is tied up (omitted from this drawing to give a clear view).

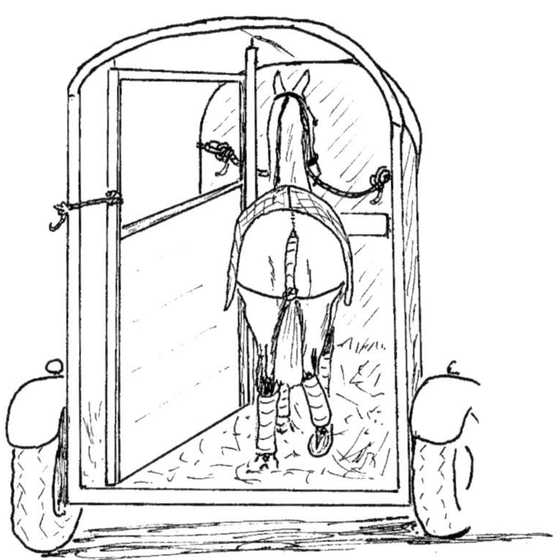

If a horse scrabbles when travelled with the division in place, it may travel happily like this as it will have more space. It may be impossible to travel such a horse safely with another.

2 The horse has been tied up too short. When it panics, it tries to put its head up and pulls against the rope while bracing its back. This causes its hind feet to slip forward underneath it until it practically sits down. If there is only the very slightest feel on the lead rope, it will panic, sometimes even before the vehicle has moved. Both of these forms of panic can be not only upsetting but also very dangerous for any horses next to the panicking one.

Occasionally travelling this horse loose in a division without even a headcollar on will work as, this way, there can be no pull on its head. However, the only certain safe way to travel such a horse is to take all the divisions, including the breast bar, out of the trailer and leave the horse loose, without even a headcollar on. Do not move the trailer. Allow the horse to turn round and look out of the back if it wants to. If it has no headcollar on, it cannot get caught up on anything and there cannot be any pull on its head. When the horse has settled, drive slowly and carefully, for just a short journey the first time. It does not matter if the horse prefers always to travel backwards with its head out over the ramp. If you continue to travel the horse in this way, you will have no more trouble. After several months of regular travelling, it may even regain confidence enough to travel loose in a stall, although still with no headcollar. (When moving a trailer division across and tying it in place to give a horse more room, protect the trailer roof from the spike in the end of the division by putting a cloth and a plastic cup or metal bottle top over it.)

Kicking when travelling

Some horses have the habit of just standing there kicking with monotonous regularity. The cause can be tension, frustration or sheer boredom but they can damage themselves or the vehicle. If travelled completely loose, without even a headcollar on in a trailer, lorry or horse box, most horses which have had any sort of problem will travel quietly. A hunter can turn round in a double trailer and will often choose to travel facing backwards, looking out over the ramp. Be aware, however, that if a horse does this, it can alter the balance of the trailer and thus the towing vehicle, putting more weight on the tow bar and possibly making the steering light.

If the kicking horse has to travel with others, leaving it loose is not practical. Sometimes leaving the headcollar rope as long as possible, so that there is never any pull whatsoever on the horse's head, can make a difference. Standing next to a different horse, travelling in a different position, facing a different direction are all worth trying. Some horses like travelling backwards and will only settle in this position – others will hate it.

To protect the horse and your vehicle, fix a large, thick rubber mat to the area which the horse kicks. Put on hock and long hind travelling boots and use overreach boots behind to protect the horse's coronets. Some horses kick when wearing boots and bandages but not if there is nothing on their legs.

Drive slowly and carefully. Stop, start and corner smoothly.

CONTROLLING THE HORSE WHEN LOADING

If your horse is difficult to load, it will be easier to control it in a bridle. Put this on over the headcollar so that you can remove it when the horse is loaded.

If you only have a headcollar there are two ways in which you will gain more control:

1 Form a loop with the headcollar rope around the horse's nose just above its nostrils. (See page 58.)
2 Take the headcollar rope round and in through the front of the headcollar from the off side (or through the headcollar D if it will fit), through the horse's mouth and out over the noseband in front of the cheekpiece (or through the D on the near side). (See page 58.)

Many older horse will cease to argue with the extra control and will load without any further problem so it is one of the first things to do with a horse that is pulling you about, turning round and dodging round the edge of the ramp.

I do not advise the second method for a very young horse as it may not yet have learnt to respect the control of a bit and, if it panics, its mouth, lips or tongue could be damaged.

It can help to keep a horse's head straight if you guide it with your hand in the noseband at the back of the headcollar.

TRAILERS

Some horses will go up into a lorry with no problem but refuse to go into a trailer.

The head up high problem

Sometimes a horse will not load into a trailer because it feels the roof is too low and thinks it is going to hit its head. It looks down at the ramp and then up

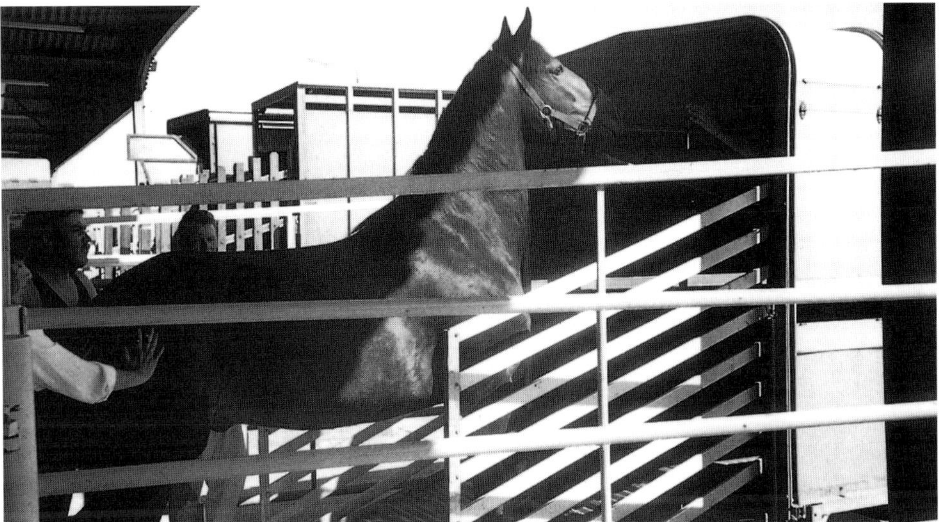

The head up high problem.

at the roof, puts its head up and backs off the ramp or rears and swings round. Some horses stand there with their heads held as high as possible as if to say, 'Look, I can't possibly fit in there'. In both cases, if you try to drive or chase the horse in, it is almost certain to throw its head up, hit it on the roof and make matters even worse.

Obviously, you must take the division out so that there is as much space as possible. If the trailer is a front unload, take all the fittings out and drop the front ramp also. It can help if you park the trailer in the doorway of a barn or garage so that the trailer appears to be a passageway to the outside. Also, the line of the roof is not then so obvious. Any gaps at the sides of the trailer can be filled by gates with horse rugs over them or with straw bales. Ask an assistant to lead another horse or pony into the trailer and go on straight through, then attempt to follow closely with your horse. Do not pull on the lead rope as this will make the horse put its head up high. If necessary, bring the other animal round again and into the trailer. If your horse will not follow, turn the lead horse so that your horse can see its head through the gap at the front of the trailer and feed that horse with a scoop of coarse mix or nuts, then offer the scoop to your horse, almost immediately putting the scoop down on the ramp. Do not try to lead the horse forward. Allow it to drop its head to the scoop and have a mouthful then gradually move the scoop further and further up the ramp so that the horse has to a take step to reach the food.

Some horses will allow you to pick up a foreleg and put it on the ramp (the end of the ramp must be on level ground, very stable and covered with straw or fixed matting as the slightest wobble or noise may make the horse back off). If the horse will allow it, pick up each front leg in turn and place the foot a little further up the ramp so that the horse can reach the scoop of food if it

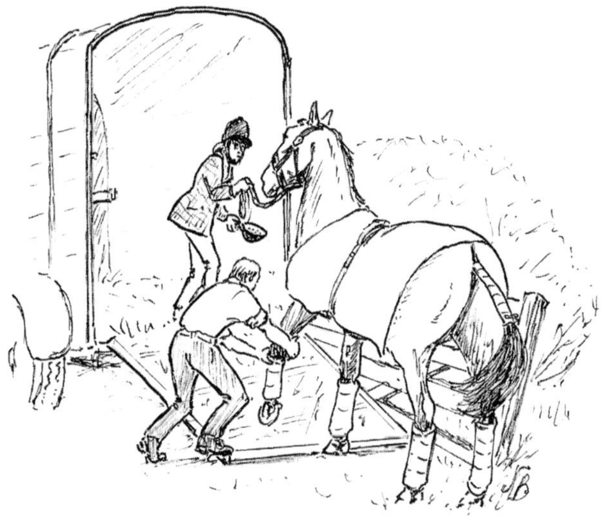

Lifting a foreleg on to the ramp. Note the gate positioned on the right of the ramp.

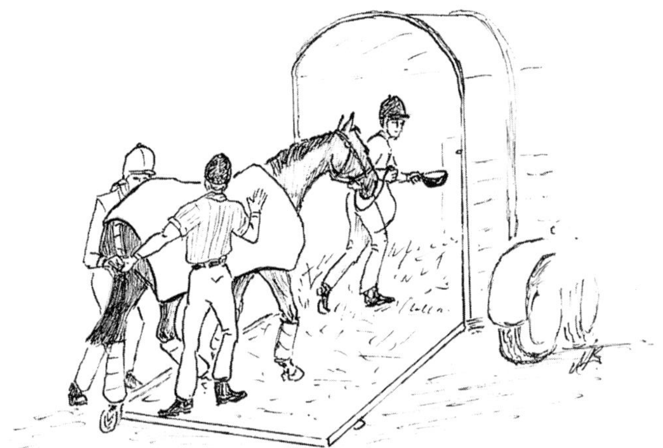

Two helpers with their hands linked round the hindquarters.

takes a step forward. Putting the scoop down on the ramp and then on the floor of the trailer distracts the horse from thinking about the low roof. Even if the horse suddenly shoots backwards, do not pull on the lead rope. Go with the horse with an allowing hand and, very gradually, start again from the beginning.

Encourage the horse to walk on straight through the trailer as the idea that the exit is forward takes its mind off the thought of running back. Repeat all of this several times a day, with no pulling on the lead rope and no encouraging it from behind, both of which tend to make such a horse put its head up high and run back.

Some horses which put their heads up high will load if an extra lead rope is fitted from the headcollar down between the forelegs to a roller or surcingle, (rather as a standing martingale would be). Others may fight the restriction of this rope.

A front-unload trailer is almost essential to retrain a horse which has a really bad trailer-loading problem.

Gradually progress until your horse will walk through without following another horse, will stand still inside, will load with the breast bar in and will load with the division in (but moved across at the back to make the access wider). If you have any trouble, go back one or two stages. If you only want to travel one horse, don't put the division in, as all horses load more easily into a wider space. If you are travelling one horse without the division, cross-tie it with a rope to each side of its headcollar so that it cannot turn. Tie the ropes loose enough so that its hindquarters will touch the back of the trailer before the ropes pull on its head.

Other things that can help include:
- Parking on a bank so that the ramp is less steep.
- If you have no suitable building to back into, use a narrow passageway or driveway.

- Park tight against a wall on one side and form a solid-looking wall with gates covered with rugs on the other side.
- If you have a rear-unload trailer, open the groom's door to let light in. The disadvantage of a rear-unload trailer is that the horse's thoughts are always 'backwards' as it knows that is the only way out. To load successfully, the horse must think 'forwards'.

Some horses will load better if there is another horse already in the trailer. Others are frightened of going in second because they think the horse already in may kick them as they come up beside it. Some are just frightened of being trapped in the seemingly narrow section left for them.

Refusing to load but not because the roof is low

Various methods may work.
- You will need three people, one leading the horse, two holding the ends of lunge lines which are attached on each side of the trailer and crossed over above the horse's hocks. The person leading has a bowl of coarse mix to tempt the horse and only feels on the lead rope if the horse attempts to turn round. Pulling on the lead rope just makes a horse run backwards. The leader must stand to one side of the horse, not in front of it, and must not face the horse. The two assistants pull on the lunge lines to keep the horse straight and encourage it in.
- Lie the loop at the end of the lunge line over the horse's back near its withers to hang down near the horse's elbow on the leader's side. Pass the other end right round its hindquarters, back through the loop at the withers

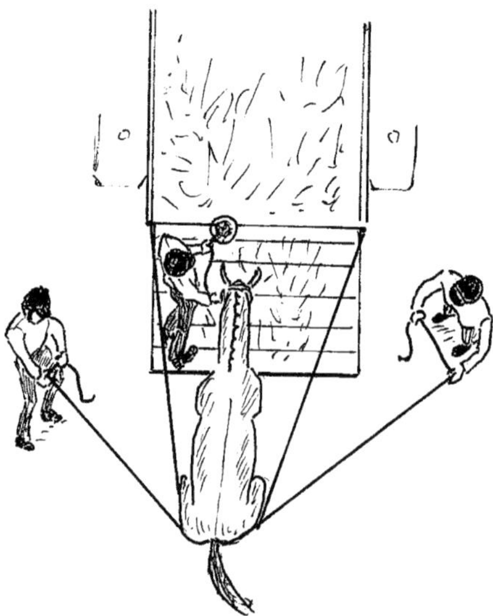

Two helpers with lunge lines crossed round the horse's hindquarters.

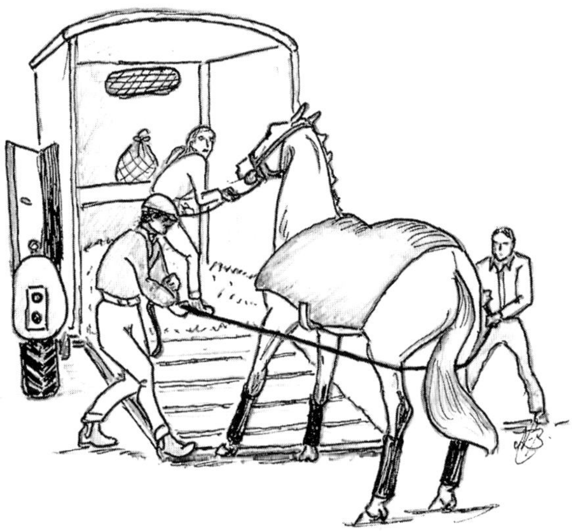

Loading with a simple rope behind the horse.

and through the throatlash and noseband of the headcollar to the leader's hands. The leader holds the lead rope and the lunge line and pulls on the lunge line to encourage the horse in. Because the lunge line goes through the throatlash- and noseband of the headcollar, it helps to keep the horse straight.

- The loop of the lunge line can be moved back to form a 'crupper' round the horse's tail. With some horses this method is more successful in making them go forward than putting the loop round the hindquarters. Others may just buck and kick at the feel of the 'crupper' and not think forwards at all. If the horse is frightened by the feel of something round its tail, be very careful that you do not get kicked when you release the 'crupper'.
- Use four assistants, one leading the horse, three holding up horse rugs as high as possible to form a solid-looking 'wall', one behind the horse and one at each side, shaking the rugs if necessary.
- Rattly plastic bags used in the same way.
- Stable brooms, applied bristle end to the hindquarters, hocks and heels.

Try never to frighten a young horse in as you will be asking for trouble in the future. A young horse is often genuinely frightened of being loaded; it does not understand what you want it to do. A trailer looks like a trap and it is against all its instincts to go in. Have patience, give it time and encouragement.

Many older horse have learnt that they can 'get away with it' and need to be loaded using some of the suggestions above.

A crupper with a rope attached can be used to encourage a horse to load. The kind which opens up with a buckle is the easiest to put on. This method is very useful when you are alone and the horse needs some encouragement from behind. Try it out in the stable first, however, as the horse may buck and panic if you suddenly put it on for the first time when trying to load it.

When the horse refuses to go forward, give little tugs on the rope attached to the crupper.

Attach a lunge line to the front of the rug or to the girth on the off (right) side and bring it round the horse's hindquarters to your hand. Tweak the line to encourage the horse forward while guiding it in with your other hand. This safe and simple method often works well.

In all cases put the ramp up as quickly as possible after the horse is in and do not tie the horse up until the ramp is up in case it runs back.

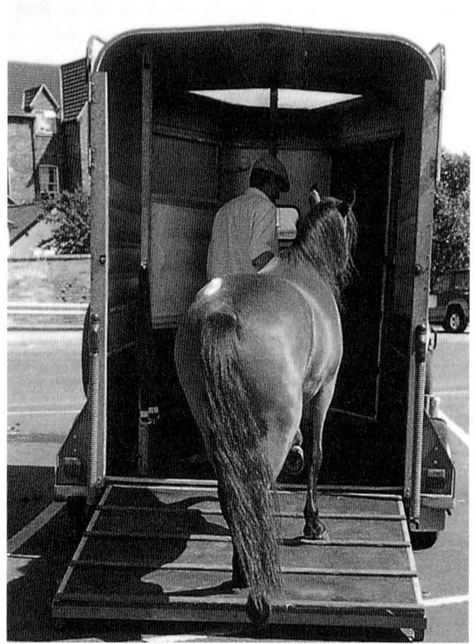

Moving the partition across gives the pony a wider space to walk into.

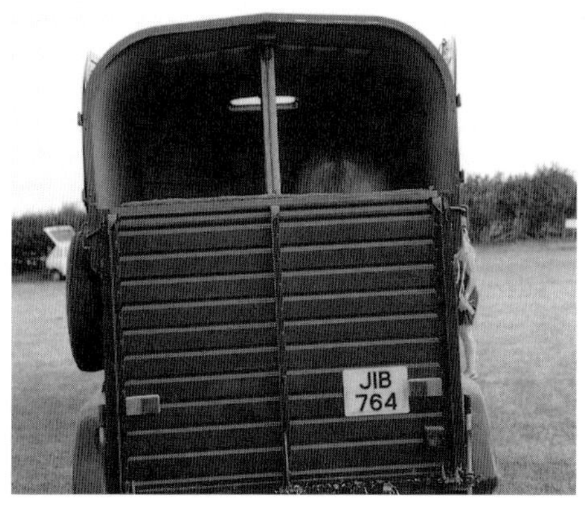

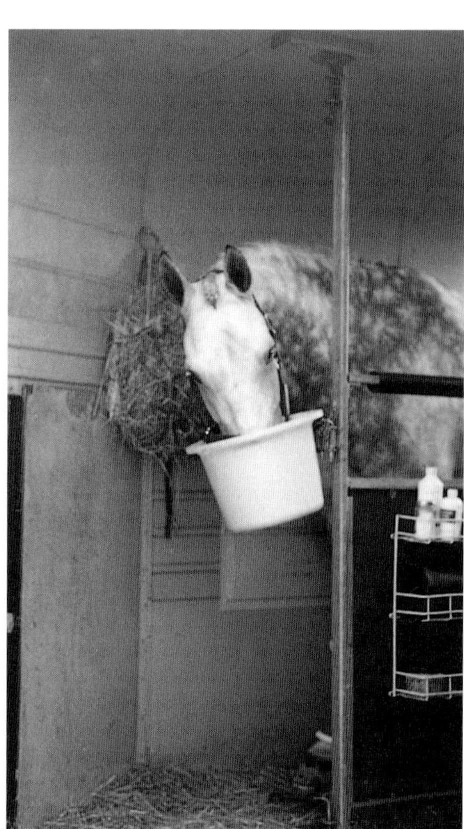

Food can be used to encourage a horse to load.

If travelling one horse in a trailer, put it in a section behind the driver as it will be able to balance better here where the camber of the road is not so steep. (In the UK this would be on the right-hand side of the trailer.) The trailer also tows better.

Some horses do not trust people enough to follow them up into the narrow stall of a trailer. They feel they are going to be trapped by the person in front. When leading a horse into a trailer with a division in it, however, it is normal for the person to go in front of the horse and this can be a problem with some horses.

Try lying the head collar rope safely over the horse's neck and lead it in with your guiding hand on its headcollar. Walk well back beside its shoulder so that it has a clear passage into the now empty space where it will travel. With some horses this works like magic and they walk confidently in alone. Quickly put the breeching strap across and put the ramp up before going in by the jockey door to tie the horse up.

If the horse will load in this way it is an excellent method to use when you are loading without an assistant.

Some people successfully long-rein a difficult horse into a trailer.

Back straps on trailers

When travelling one horse in a double trailer without a partition in it, clip the two back straps to a strong metal ring so that you have something to prevent the horse from running back.

Some full-size double trailers allow you to alter the height of the back straps so that they will go lower for a pony. If they are a fixture and will only go at horse height, it is safer not to use them for a pony. If a pony runs back when they are across, the strap will probably catch on its neck and frighten it. It is very dangerous to travel ponies with saddles on when the back straps are done up at horse height as, if they do run backwards, the back strap can get caught under the saddle and cause a serious accident, besides terrifying the pony.

Unloading from a trailer

1 Untie the horse.
2 Drop the ramp.
3 Undo the backstrap if used.
4 Keep the lead rope slack and allow the horse to back out. If you pull on the rope to try to slow the horse down, it will charge out and probably hit its head on the roof. This can then cause loading problems. Trying to hold on to a horse to prevent it from running back can actually *cause* the problem of running back.
5 If your horse runs back really fast out of a trailer, be ready on its side of the breast bar before the ramp is dropped or the backstrap is undone and always give it a really long rope or put it on a lunge line so there is no pull on its head whatsoever. Over time, it may cease to run back so fast. A horse going back fast usually goes back straight.

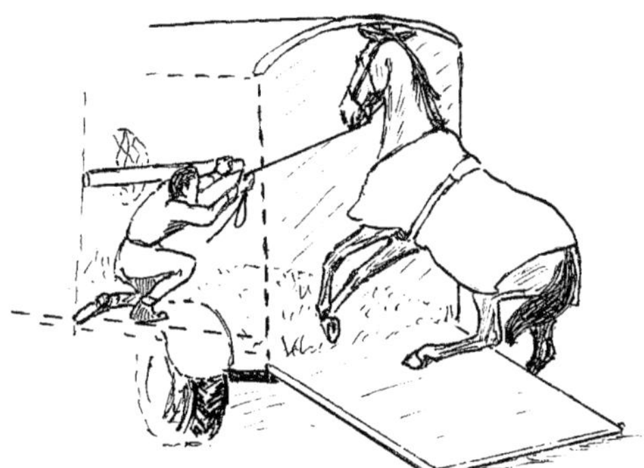

If the horse tries to run back when unloading and the handler holds on tightly to the rope, the horse will throw its head up and bang it on the roof of the trailer. This will make it even more frightened next time. (The horse should be wearing boots and a tail bandage.)

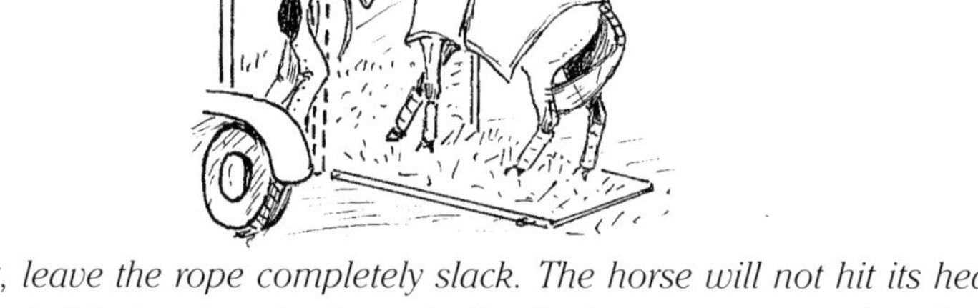

When unloading, leave the rope completely slack. The horse will not hit its head and may get out of the habit of rushing backwards. Put the horse on an extra long lead rope or on a lunge line so that there is no pull.

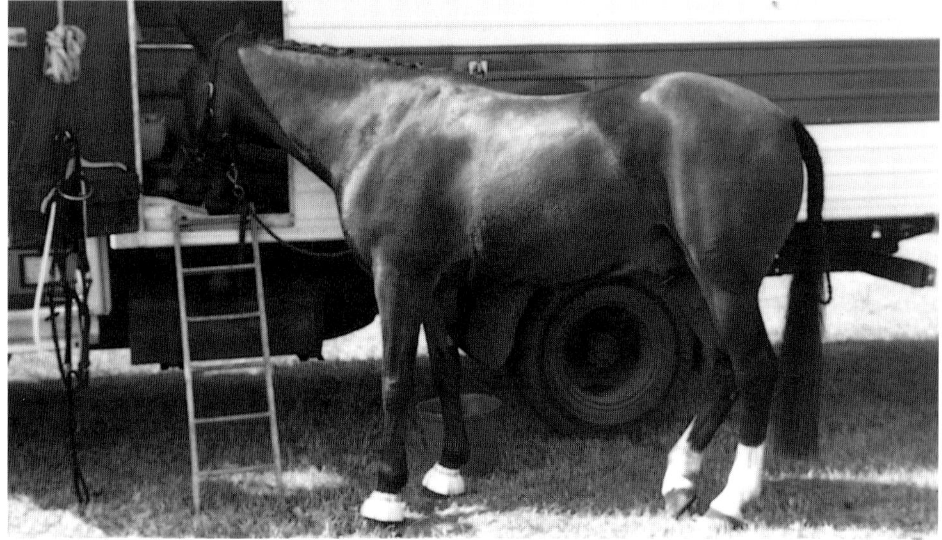

This is not a safe place to tie a horse.

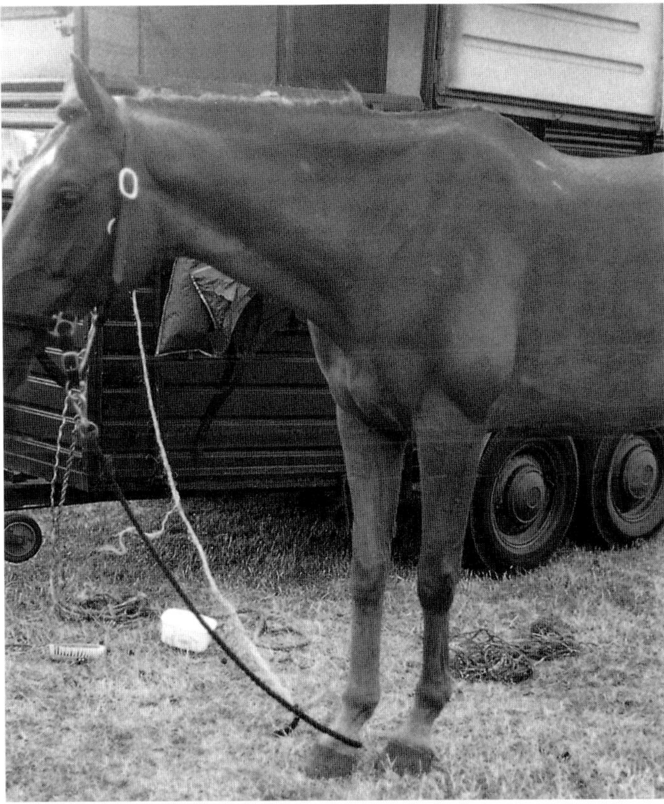

Do not tether your horse like this.

6 If your horse goes back slowly but crooked, with its hind legs towards the right side of the ramp, you can keep it straight by pushing its head to the right, thus moving its quarters to the left away from the edge. Again, don't hold it back, just try to control the path of its hindquarters by moving its head sideways.

LOADING INTO A LORRY

Most problem horses load more happily into the wide open space of a cattle truck than into the divisions of the smart type of horse box where they have to turn and move sideways as soon as they are up the ramp.

Give the horse as much space to go up into as possible. A rear ramp is easier than a side ramp because the horse can walk straight ahead. Lorry ramps tend to be steeper than trailer ramps so try to drop the ramp on to a bank. It is easier to load a horse, and less dangerous, if the lorry ramp has its own gates. If it has no gates, use movable ones, preferably covered with horse rugs so that they look solid. The horse is also then less likely to get a leg through.

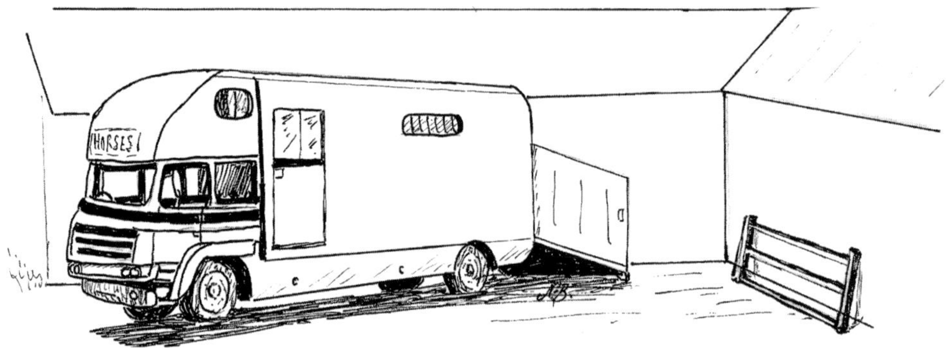

Back the lorry into a corner and have a gate ready to place across the gap.

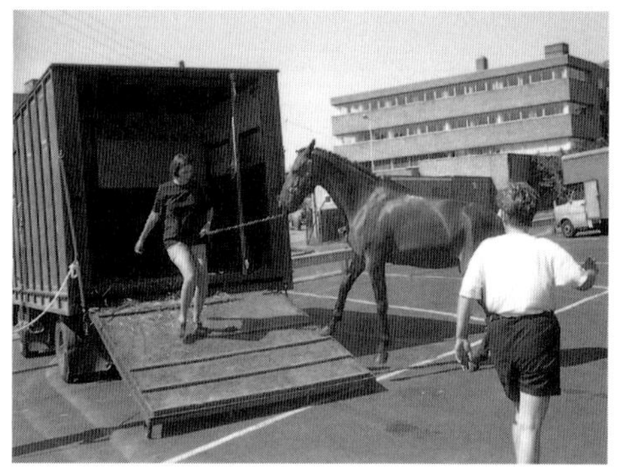

The wrong way to load a horse.

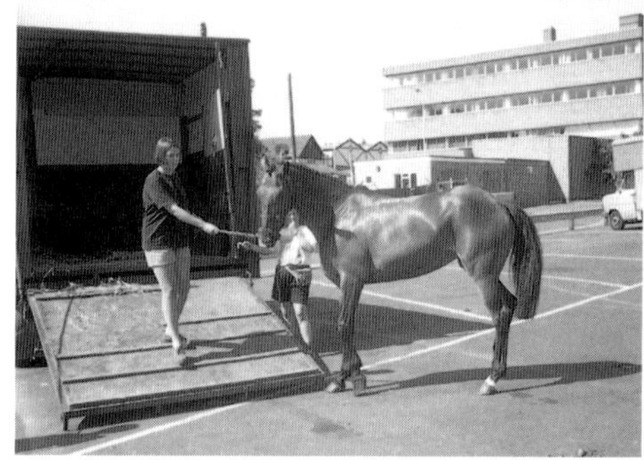

Still wrong.

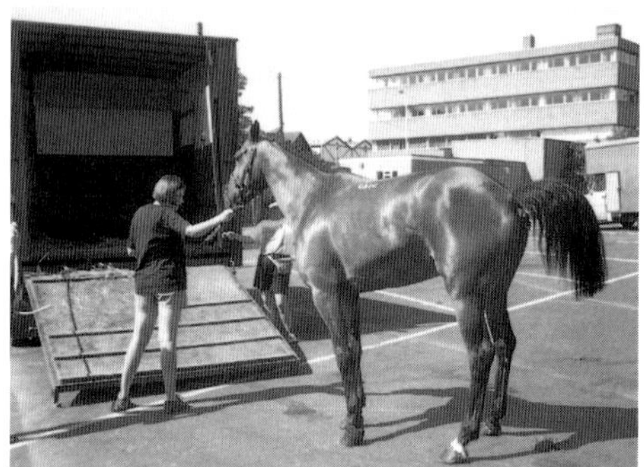

A slightly better attempt but the leader is still looking at the horse and they are trying to put it into a small back section where it will have to turn sideways as soon as it is up the ramp. It would be better to open up the division and give the horse as much space as possible to walk into.

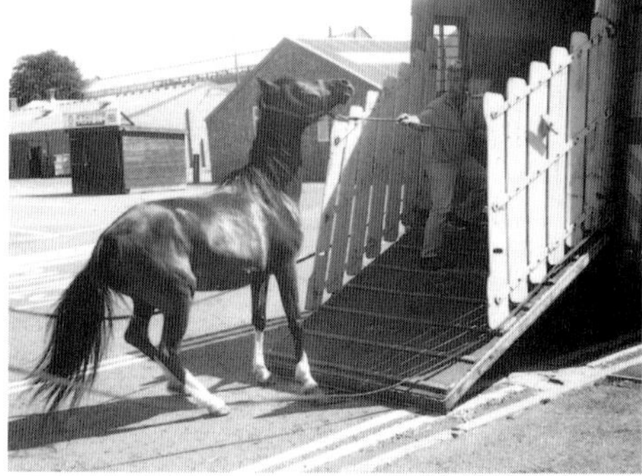

Facing a horse and pulling hard on the headcollar makes the horse run back with its head in the air.

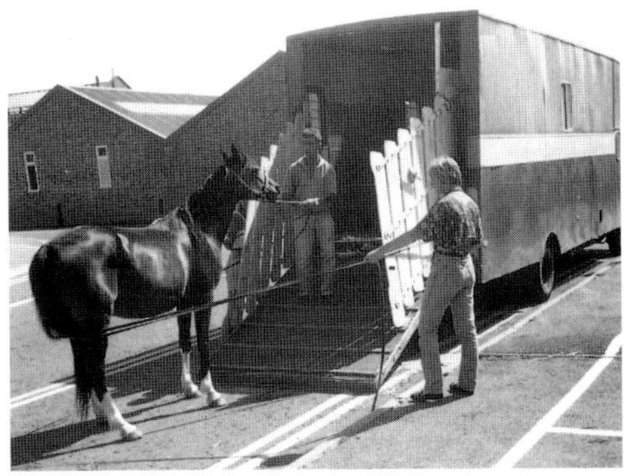

There are now two helpers with a lunge rein behind the horse but the leader is still standing in the centre of the ramp, facing the horse and looking it in the eye.

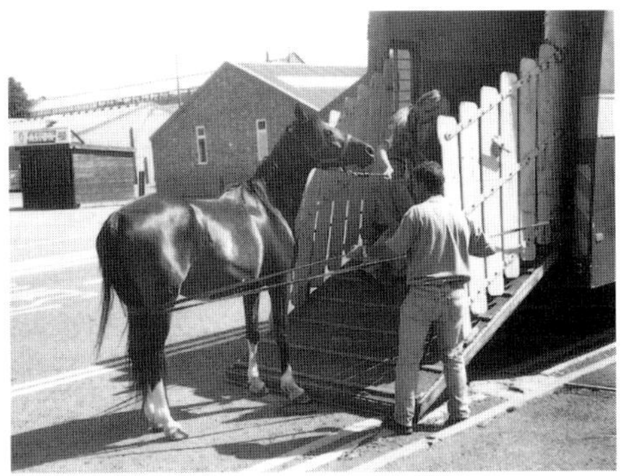

The leader is to one side of the ramp and is not looking at the horse. This time it walked up the ramp and into the lorry.

- At a show or horse sale you may be able to persuade two other lorries to park one on each side of your ramp, so forming a passageway.
- If there are two lorries, both with gates for their ramps, you can back one up towards the rear of the other until the ramps just overlap when dropped. Close both gates on one side of each lorry to form a barrier as they meet. Open the two other gates wide to form a passageway leading into the 'V' where both ramps meet. Lead the horse into this 'V' and close the gates behind it. Wait until the horse has realised that it is completely enclosed, then try to tempt it with food up the ramp of one lorry. If necessary, encourage it from behind. Most of the methods mentioned under loading into a trailer (pages 182–7) can also be used when loading into a lorry.

Loading single-handed

Some horse are only difficult to load if they know you are alone. If another person approaches from their rear, they will immediately walk up the ramp. This is a maddening problem that we all encounter.

Various methods can be tried.

- Attach a lunge line to the back of the trailer or lorry on the far side and lay the line on the ground to form a loop as far back from the ramp as possible. Place it so that when you lead the horse forward you can bend down and pick up the spare end as soon as the horse's hind legs have stepped over it. Keep the lunge line taut above the horse's hocks and use it to encourage the horse to go forward up the ramp. Keep the tension on the lunge line while you slip out of the groom's door (trailer only) to put the ramp up as quickly as you can. With a lorry, keep the tension on the lunge line until you have put a division across to keep the horse in.

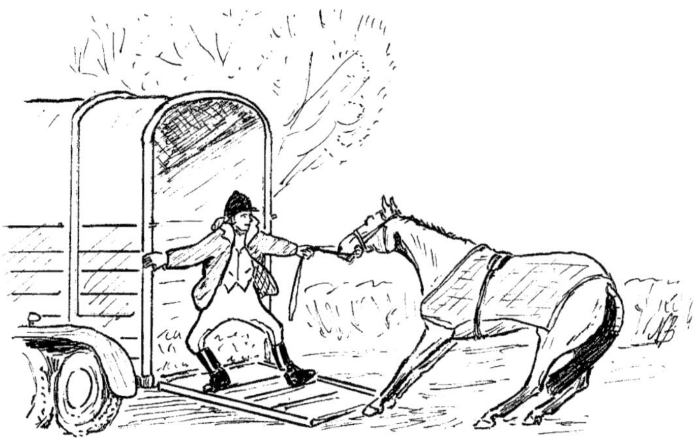

How not to load single handed.

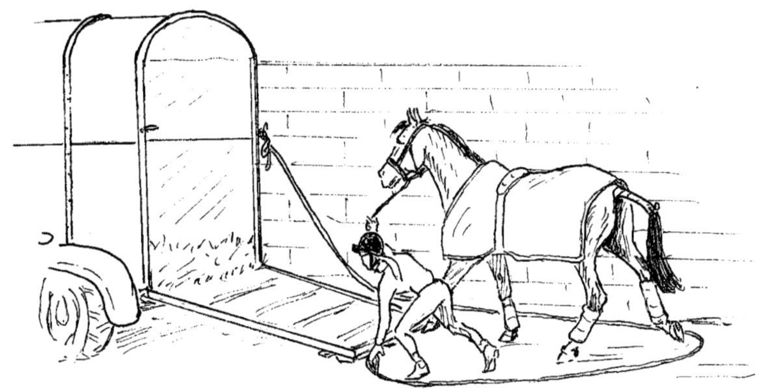

Loading successfully single handed: as the horse walks over the lunge line the leader picks up the spare end . . .

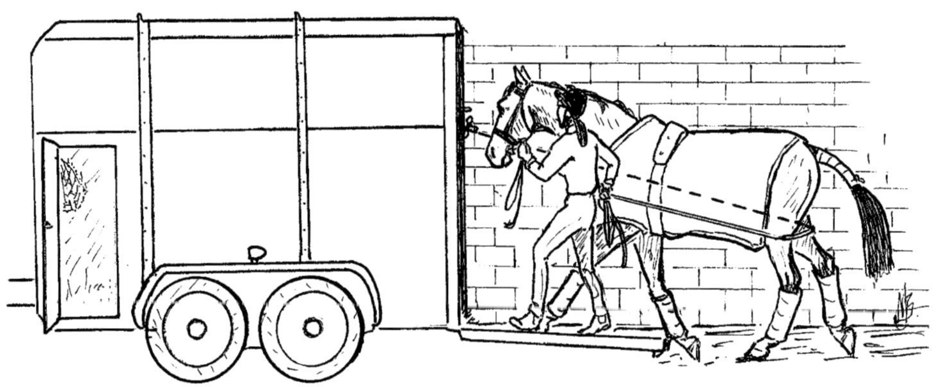

. . . then keeps the line taut above the horse's hocks to encourage it in.

If you know your horse will *never* run back once it is in, you can quickly attach the clip of an already tied-up rope to the headcollar before hurrying round to put the ramp up. However, most horses which are tricky to load will run back and if a horse which is tied up tries to run back when the trailer ramp is down, it is likely to break the headcollar or rope, throw itself down or get a hind leg over the side of the ramp and hurt itself. All of these events will make it even more difficult to load next time.

If the horse is tied far enough forward in a lorry, as long as the headcollar or rope does not break it is less likely to hurt itself. In lorries with divisions it is sometimes possible to pull the division across after the horse, with a rope, as you go in.

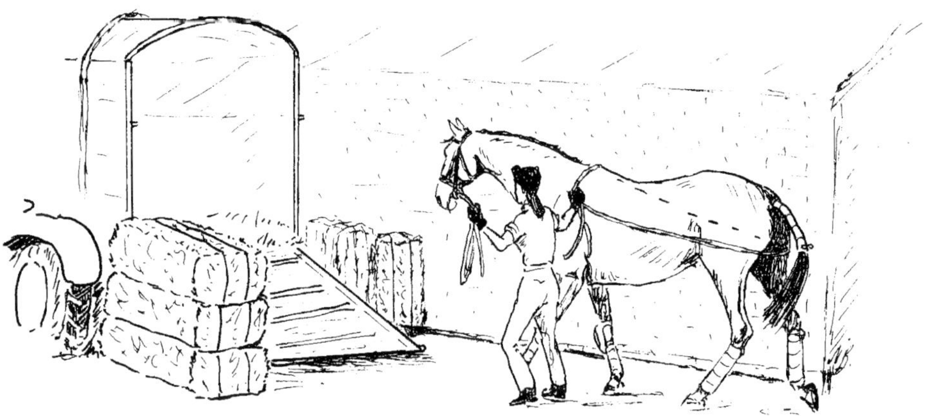

Place a lunge rein or rope round the horse's hindquarters. A little pull on this may encourage the horse to go forwards and load.

- Use a lunge line round the horse's quarters, threaded through the end loop near the withers and on through the headcollar as on page 184.
- Attach the lunge line to the horse's headcollar then take the line forward into the trailer, out through the groom's door and back to your hand. You can then use the lunge line to keep the horse straight while encouraging it in from behind. This method has the great advantage that, as you are driving the horse in from behind, you are in the right position to put the ramp up as soon as the horse is in. The lunge line prevents it from turning round so you can tie it up after the ramp is up.
- If your horse is used to being driven in long reins and has learnt to be obedient, long-rein it up the ramp. Again, you are behind it to put the ramp up. Obviously, this method will be much easier if the ramp has gates or if you form some sort of passageway to help to keep the horse straight.

With time, if the vehicle is driven by someone careful and thoughtful, so that the horse does not find it difficult to keep its balance and the process of

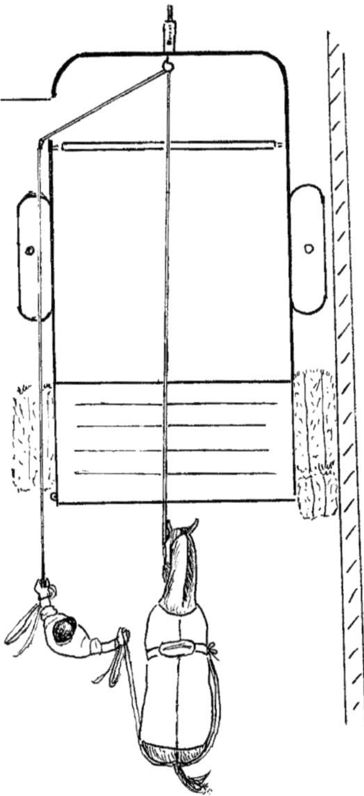

Another way to load single handed. Note the bale of straw in the gap by the wall.

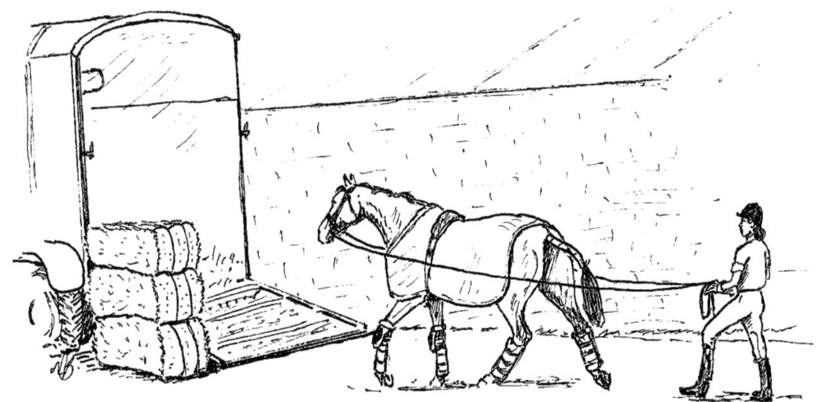

Long-reining a horse into a trailer.

loading is as calm and unstressful as possible, it should become easier to load. *One* journey with a thoughtless driver is all that it takes to make a previously good horse bad to load. One bad experience when loading can also have the same result. Try to reward the horse with food every time as soon as it is in so that it associates loading with something pleasant to look forward to. Gradually decrease the number of 'aids' you need to load the horse.

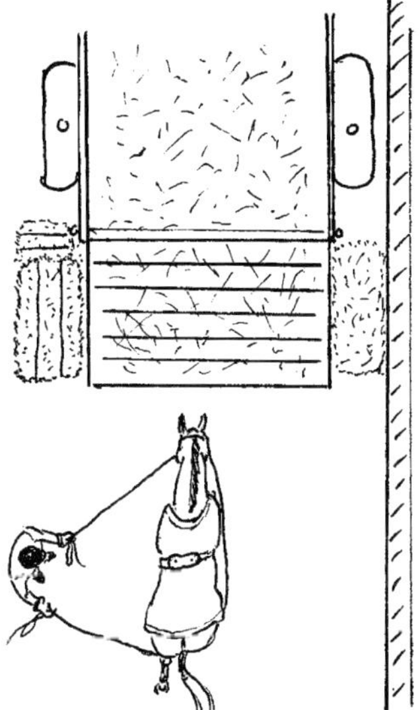

Another method of long-reining into a trailer.

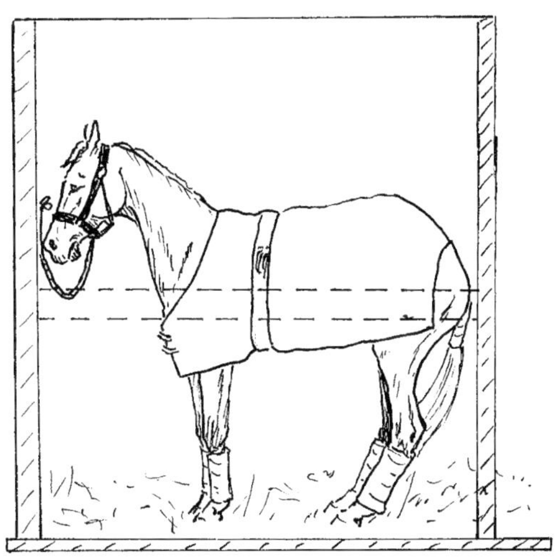

This horse box is too narrow. The horse is forced to stand with its back up and its hind legs right underneath it. This is very uncomfortable for the horse which is also likely to slip and go down behind.

You will not succeed in loading horses if you are in a 'flap', in a bad temper or in a tearing hurry. Nor will you succeed if you are frightened of the horse.

Be calm, quiet and confident. Plan and prepare what you intend to do well beforehand. If you think you may have trouble without an assistant, don't try to load the horse alone, fail, have to put the horse back in the stable then go to find an assistant and have to start all over again. That is a bad lesson. The

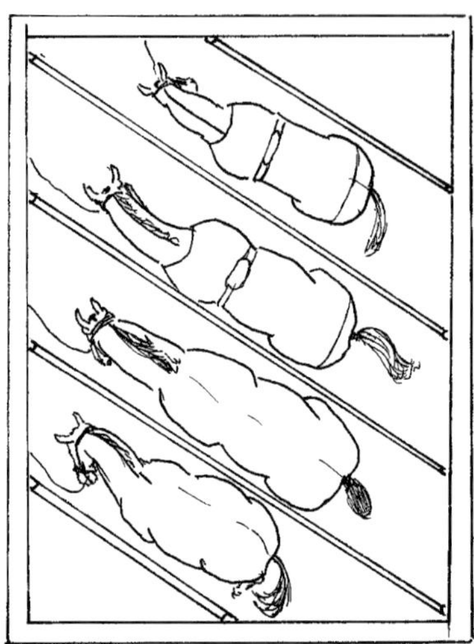

The herring-bone arrangement of the divisions gives the horses more length and they find it easier to keep their balance than when travelling sideways across the vehicle.

horse must learn that it has to go in first time.

If you have this problem in a horse box, again it may have been caused by tying the horse up too short. In this case, travel it loose in half the box or even the whole box.

The problem could also have been caused by travelling the horse in a division running straight across a box which is too short for the horse, thus forcing it to stand with its head tucked in and its back arched. This will cause the hind legs to slip forward under the body. It might only be necessary to give the horse more length by arranging the divisions in a herring-bone pattern or by travelling the horse facing forwards or backwards to cure the problem. Some horses do not like to travel facing backwards so a change of direction may be all that a horse which is having problems in travelling may need.

It is very uncomfortable for a big horse to be forced to stand straight across a lorry with its back arched and its head tucked in so that it can fit. Don't do it.

Unloading from a lorry with divisions

1 Drop the ramp.
2 Untie the horse.
3 Open the division.
4 Lead the horse forward down the centre of the ramp, walking to one side, not in front of the horse.
5 If several horses are all coming out at the same time, untie all the horses at once, provided you have enough helpers. The first horse down the ramp must wait within sight of the second horse to come down and so on, then they are less likely to rush out.

9 RIDING

RIDING AND LEADING

First teach the led horse to trot out willingly in hand (see page 53) and to answer to your voice.

Choose a horse to ride which will not attempt to bite or kick the led horse or it will never learn to keep up level and go happily without pulling back or pulling away in fright.

If possible choose a horse that the led horse knows.

Putting your reins in a bridge

Ride with your own reins in a 'bridge' in your right hand. The left rein should come into your right hand under your index finger and lie across your palm; the right rein should come into your hand under your little finger and lie across your palm over the left rein. Your thumb holds both reins in position and stops them slipping and becoming longer. When you want to turn left, you carry your hand slightly to the right to take the pressure off the right side of your horse's mouth. You then turn your thumb and index finger towards you, bending your wrist so that you put pressure on the left side of your horse's mouth to ask it to turn left. To turn right, carry your hand slightly to the left and use your little finger to turn.

There are several different ways of controlling the led horse but if you are going on the roads it should always wear a bridle, knee boots and brushing boots.

- You can choose to take the reins over the horse's head and lead it in the normal way as you would in hand.
- You can also hold the reins in a 'bridge' so that you can guide the horse more accurately and keep its head straight.
- You can pass the left rein through the right-hand ring of the bit so that this rein lies across the chin (where a curb chain would go). This does keep both reins together more but if the horse pulls away there will now be a severe 'nutcracker' action on the bottom jaw. This is sufficient to make a sensitive horse rear up if it happens suddenly.
- You can remove the normal bridle reins and replace them with a chain or

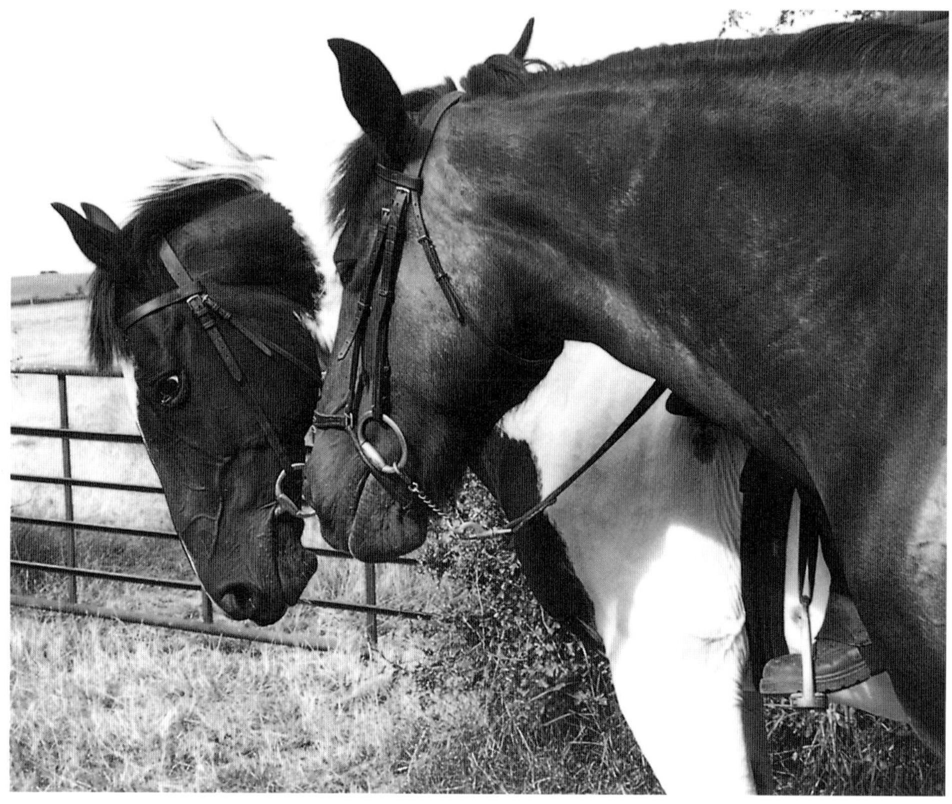

A chain attached to the snaffle bit rings and the lead rein attached to the chain by a central ring.

strap which attaches to each bit ring and has a centre lead ring or D to which a rope or lead rein can be fixed. The advantages are that you have only one rein to hold and the bit cannot be pulled through the mouth as it can with two normal reins if you put all your pull on the rein nearer to you. Also, if the horse gets loose, it will not have the loop of a pair of normal reins to get its feet caught up in.

If your led horse pulls back and just will not keep up, ask an assistant to ride out with you carrying a long whip. Each time you ask the horse to go forward with the reins, get the assistant to give it a sharp flick with the whip.

If you have no help, you can try the method of a rope or rein round the hindquarters suggested to encourage a horse to go forward in hand (see page 193) or attach a crupper on the led horse and tweak this when it won't trot. The pull under its tail may encourage it forward. NB: try out both methods in the stable or a *manège* first for safety!

If your led horse is going to be ridden on arrival at your destination, you can still use the lead attachment. Make its normal reins safe either by putting them behind and under the run-up stirrup irons and leathers (run up so that they

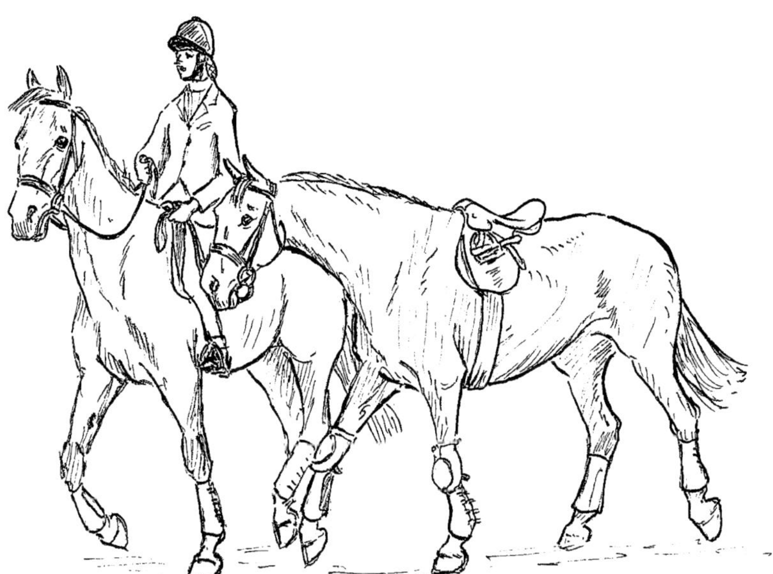

Ride and lead.

cannot come loose, as you would for lungeing, as explained below) or by twisting them and passing the throatlash through one loop (see page 86).

If your led horse is in a double bridle or any bridle with double reins, make the curb rein safe, as explained above, and lead from the bradoon rein only.

Make your stirrup irons safe by running them up in the normal way then wrapping the loop round and in and out of the iron, then passing the end of the leather through the small loop which is left (see page 86).

The led horse should be on your left so that you are between it and the traffic.

On the roads look and listen, plan ahead what you are going to do and give clear hand signals.

Do not ride one horse and lead two horses on the roads. You could not possibly control them if one got upset or anything unexpected happened.

NAPPING

You have had your nice new horse for three days and suddenly it refuses to leave the stable yard, half-rears and whips round, or else it does the same thing a few hundred yards from home. Unless the horse is exceptionally nappy, the problem will not show up at first in a new environment. It is essential that a nappy horse is ridden by a capable, determined, experienced rider. It must be turned in the direction that the rider wants it to go and, immediately it is facing the right way, hit hard and ridden forward with strong legs and hands which *allow* it to go forward if it will.

Horses can be made to nap by riders who use their legs when also hanging on tightly to the reins. The rider's legs say 'go forward' but their hands say 'stop' and the horse does not know where to go or what to do. Nervous riders often do this unconsciously and do not realise that they are causing at least half the problem.

If you hit a horse which is napping, it may shoot forward. It is essential that your body stays in balance with the horse's sudden forward movement and that your hands allow the horse to go forward when hit.

When a horse naps, half-rears and whips round, the rider usually wishes that they had three hands – two to keep it straight, facing the way they want it to go, and one free one to hit it!

In this situation you have at least four options.

1 Try to keep the horse straight, hit it and win the battle yourself (but only if you are a strong, confident rider).

2 Ride with someone else. Get them to go in front out of the stable yard and past the point where the horse usually naps, then take the lead yourself. Progress to going out side by side, then go very slightly in front yourself. Be ready to hit the horse hard, use your legs strongly and growl at it if it so much as hesitates.

3 Get someone very experienced to long-rein the horse out of the yard several times in one session. You or they then ride the same route with someone with a long whip walking behind to encourage the horse forward if necessary.

4 Even a capable rider may need a back-up person on foot when riding a nappy horse. At first, this person should be within the range of vision of the horse, carrying a long whip. The rider can try to keep the horse straight and the helper can hit it if necessary. (The helper must be experienced enough to know how, when and where to hit the horse and must not be frightened.) Next, ask the helper to stay out of sight but to be ready to leap out behind the horse and hit it if it hesitates when asked to go forward.

It is no good just hanging on to the reins and hitting and kicking. The horse must feel that you are not going to allow it to turn round but that you *are* going to allow it to go forward. A nervous or inexperienced rider will not be able to do this and the situation will only get worse. It is no good sending the horse away to be 'straightened out'. It will behave perfectly with an experienced, determined rider but it will revert to its old tricks very soon after coming back to a nervous or inexperienced rider.

A horse which throws its head up and half-rears may be more controllable in a running martingale. A Market Harborough (see page 266) should make it even easier to control.

If your horse suddenly stops, head up, heart beating wildly, it may have seen or heard something in the hedge that it is genuinely frightened of. If the horse does not usually behave in this way, do not immediately start kicking and hitting it because it may fight against you in terror at the thought of having to go nearer to the 'horror'. You may, in fact, teach the horse to nap, rear and whip round in this way. If you knew that there was an unexploded bomb at the side of the track in front of you, wouldn't you fight like mad with anyone who tried to make you go towards it? This is exactly the situation in which you are putting your horse. As long as it will stand quietly facing the way you want to go, give it a few seconds to assess the situation. The animal or bird in the hedge may move; the log or flapping plastic may not seem so terrifying. If the horse relaxes and begins to look forward along the track you wish it to take, ask it to proceed, using legs, voice and, if necessary, stick.

Allow the horse to give the frightening place a wide berth as long as it keeps going forward. Pass and repass the place, allowing the horse to go up and sniff the frightening object if it wants to but never, under any circumstances, try to force it to go up to the object. Dismount and walk in front of the horse to give it confidence, go up to the object yourself and allow the horse to follow you and then look and sniff. Do be aware, however, that you have less control of a frightened horse from the ground and if it rears, runs back or whips round, it may pull you off your feet.

If a horse naps about leaving the stable yard or within a few hundred yards of the stables and you are alone and cannot win on its back, you can also dismount and lead it for several hundred yards before mounting and asking it to proceed. Only dismount as a last resort but it is better to get the horse to do as you ask when led than put it back in the stable having never left the yard.

Some horses will nap when you pass a field in which horses are turned out; some will nap when you come to a choice of turnings towards home or away from home. A strong, experienced, capable rider who is not nervous may overcome these problems. The horse will realise that the rider is boss and will make things uncomfortable for the horse if it disobeys. A weak, nervous rider is likely to continue to have problems with a nappy horse.

Napping when asked to jump

This form of napping is usually caused by a frightening or uncomfortable experience in the past. It is no good hitting the horse. You cannot *make* a horse jump. It must want to jump and, ideally, learn to enjoy it. Go back to the very beginning of jumping. Put poles on the ground and wander about on foot in a very relaxed way, allowing the horse to follow you over them. Next, ride your horse, using a calm, sensible horse to give it a lead, and walk round, beside, then over the poles, first following the other horse, then taking the lead. Have the mildest, kindest-possible bit in the horse's mouth and ride it on a long rein. You will hope to begin to feel that it wants to go straight and forward over the pole. You want it to look straight ahead beyond the pole, not to one side or the other trying to find a way of avoiding a jump as it did before.

Proceed very gradually in rising trot over poles on the ground then over cross poles and and very small fences. Trot through a wide gap between the two sections of a wall, brush fence, barrels or fillers to let the horse know that there is a safe way through and to give it confidence. Sit forward in balance with the horse so that if it does shoot through the gap you will go with it and not pull its mouth. Only when it is going forward steadily and confidently through the gaps should you attempt to jump the wall, brush fence, barrels or fillers pushed together. You need someone on the ground to make the alterations to the fences so that you do not have to keep getting off the horse.

As long as the horse wants to jump, goes calmly and willingly forward and looks ahead beyond the jump, you know you are working in the right way. If the horse starts to lose confidence and is hesitant about going forward, you have gone too fast too soon. Go back a step or so, make it easier for the horse and progress more slowly.

When a horse has lost confidence about jumping it *must* be ridden by a confident, capable rider who can sit quietly in balance with the horse and will never, under any circumstances, pull its mouth.

Rubbing the rider's leg against a wall or fence

Some horses and ponies have learnt that they can get their own way if they put the rider in a difficult position such as going very close to a wall or fence and leaning on it so that the rider's leg will be trapped unless they move it quickly. With one leg out of action and the rider now in a precarious position, the animal can take advantage and go where it wants to.

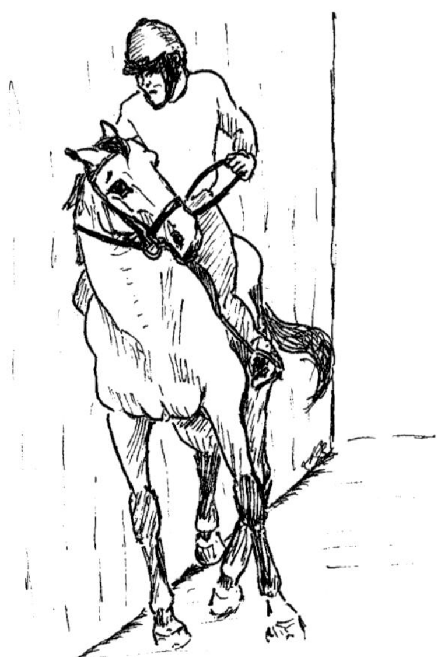

Using the left rein makes the horse lean on you even more.

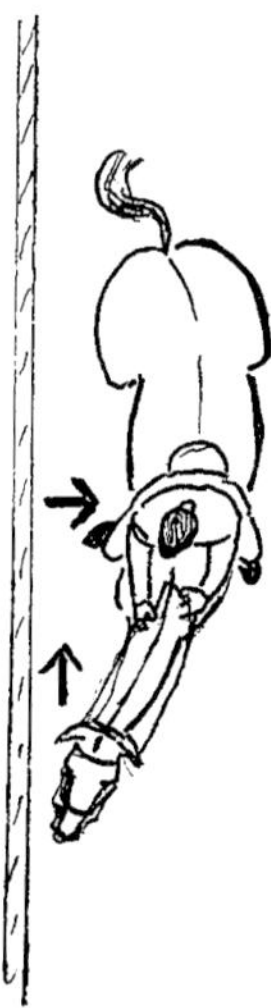

Use the right rein and right leg to move the horse's body away from the wall.

The first time it happens, you are likely to be taken by surprise and your instinct will be to turn the horse's head away from the wall. Unfortunately, this action puts the horse in an even better rubbing position. Use the rein and leg nearer to the wall so that the horse's head is towards the wall. If necessary, circle and ride forward again. In my experience most horses or ponies (and it is mostly ponies who are intelligent enough to think of this trick) always rub on the same side, so it is easier to correct.

OPENING AND SHUTTING GATES

If your horse runs back and seems frightened when you approach a gate to open it, someone has probably allowed a gate to bang against the horse or catch its heels as it went through.

Dismount and lead the horse up to the gate, asking it to stand parallel to the gate, tail towards the hinges, as it will have to do when you open a gate when mounted.

Make it stand still while you open the gate really wide. Be very sure that no part of the gate accidentally touches the horse as you lead it through. Turn the horse round, again tail towards the hinges as it must be when you shut a gate when mounted. Carefully manoeuvre the horse backwards and sideways until you have shut the gate. Make it stand still parallel to the gate after it is shut and wait there for a few seconds.

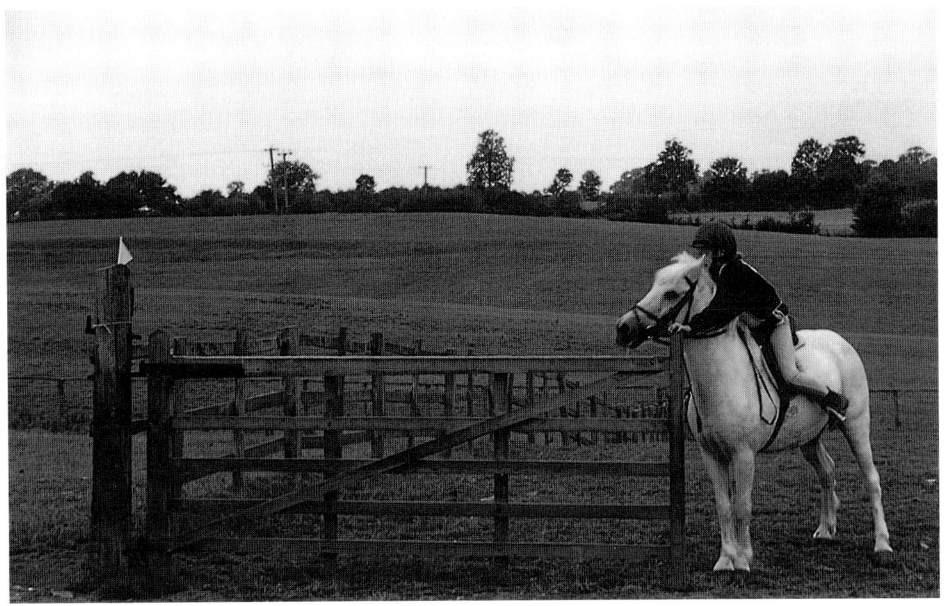

The wrong way to open a gate. The pony is incorrectly positioned and the rider is using the wrong hand and getting into a mess.

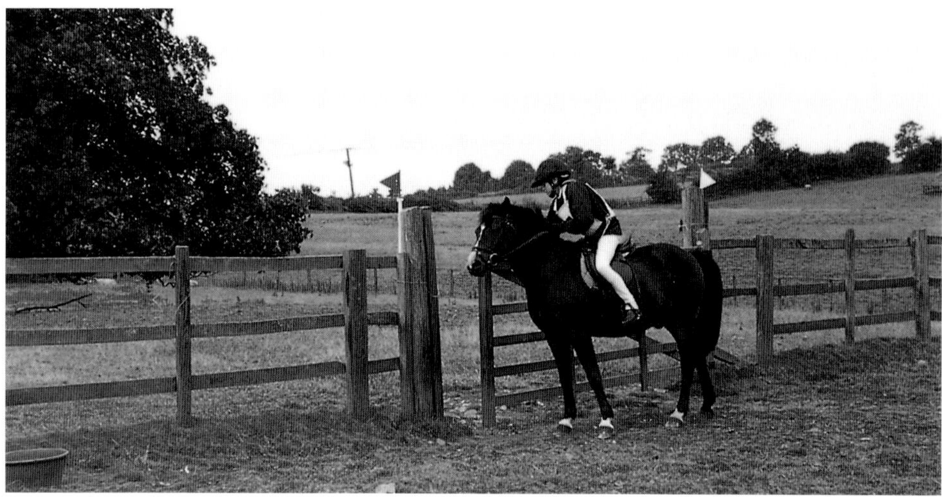

This pony is parallel to the gate with its tail towards the hinges. The rider has both reins in her left hand and is using her right hand to open the gate.

When it has ceased to get agitated when you open and shut a gate dismounted, try to do it mounted. Choose a very easy gate which opens away from you. With the horse standing parallel to the gate, tail towards the hinges, use your hand nearer the gate to open it. Both reins and your whip should be in the other hand. Make sure that you do not accidentally pull on the reins as you bend down to open the gate. Be very calm. Do not get cross with your horse if it moves. Talk to it and reassure it. Shutting the gate is more difficult so, at first, get someone else to shut the gate or, if you are alone, dismount and shut it.

Gates which open towards you are potentially dangerous as if the horse tries to rush through before you have got the gate open wide enough, the gate will trap and frighten it. You may also get your leg caught and, if the horse then dashes through, you may be pulled off. Do not attempt to open a gate of this description until you and your horse are very confident and calm and you have very accurate control of the horse.

Never go through a gate and try to pull it closed behind you as you pass through. The gate will bang the horse's hind legs and it may even get a foot caught under the gate.

Always turn your horse's tail towards the hinges and open and shut a gate with the hand nearer to the gate.

Be aware that reins and martingales can very easily get caught up on gates.

If someone else has opened a gate for you, always put both reins into the hand further from the gate and put the hand nearer the gate out ready to prevent the gate from banging against your horse if the gate starts to swing to.

If the gate will not stay open, hold it ready for the next person to catch when several people are going through one at a time.

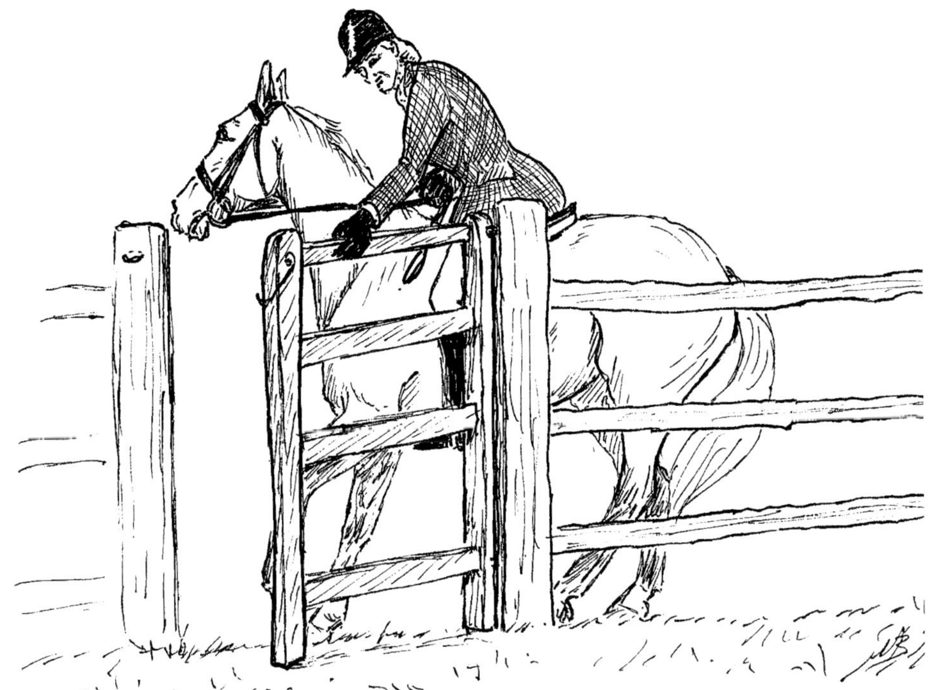

Shutting a gate.

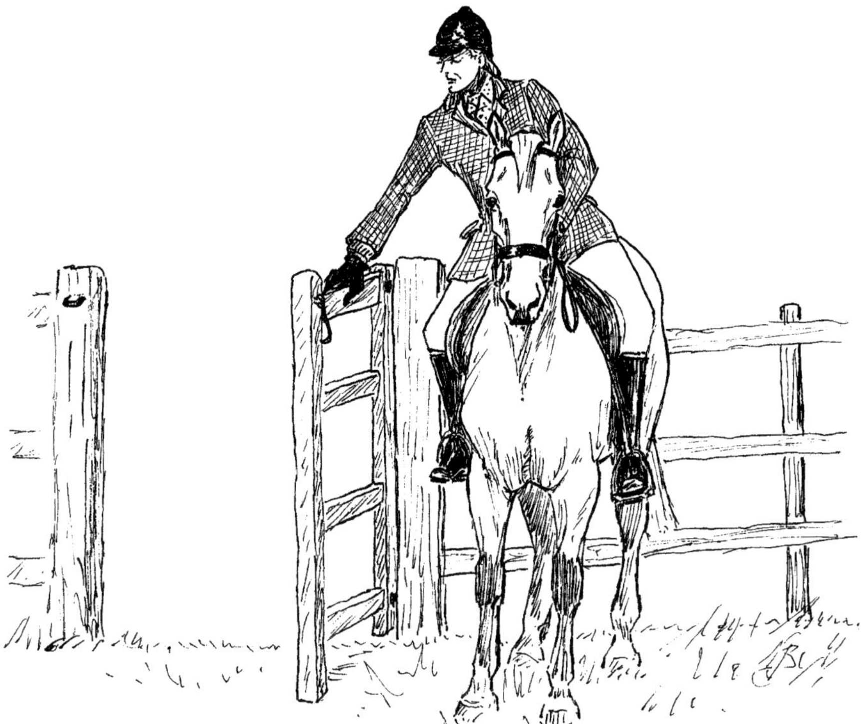

Opening a gate that opens towards the horse and rider.

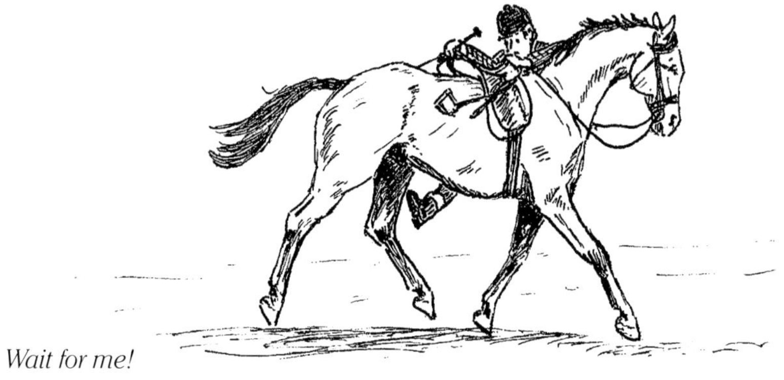

Wait for me!

MOUNTING

Some horses will not stand while you mount simply because they have never been made to do so. If possible, always use a mounting block. It is better for the horse's back than mounting from the ground when all your weight makes the saddle press on the off side of the horse's spine each time. You can also get on more quickly from a mounting block, which makes it easier to control the horse and to insist that it stands still while you mount and for several seconds afterwards so that you can adjust stirrups or girths.

Some horses dislike being mounted for the following reasons.

- The rider sticks their toe into the horse just behind the elbow which is a very sensitive area.
- The rider overshortens the reins and has a tight hold on the horse so that it goes backwards.
- The rider has one rein shorter than the other, which makes the horse turn towards or away from the rider.
- The rider comes down heavily in the saddle and the horse anticipates the discomfort.
- The horse has a bone or muscle problem in its back. (See Back Problems, page 118.)
- The saddle is pressing down on the top of the horse's withers and is hurting it.
- The saddle is pinching and pressing inwards on each side of the withers and hurting.
- The back of the saddle is pressing down on the horse's spine and it is anticipating the discomfort.
- The horse anticipates a wild, exciting ride and is impatient to be off.

A horse which has always stood quietly for you to mount in the past is probably finding that the saddle hurts, so check the saddle fitting very carefully. If it is necessary to have someone to hold the horse when you

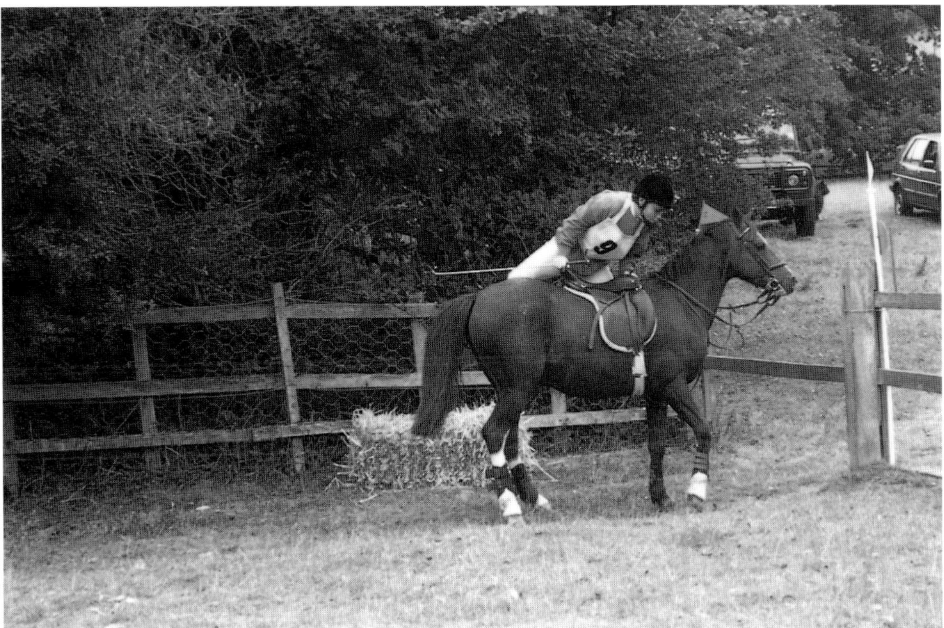

Mounting dangerously with the reins in loops and a long whip in the right hand.

mount, ask them to hold the back of the noseband. They will then not affect your contact on the reins. Progress so that this person soon simply stands by the horse and then only nearby in case they are needed.

Dismounting

Teach your horse to halt and stand still. Do not dismount immediately when the horse halts. After you dismount, make the horse stand still for a few seconds.

- If a horse which has always stood still for you to dismount in the past suddenly starts to shoot forward or backwards as you lean forward preparatory to dismounting, it is almost certainly feeling discomfort from the front of the saddle pressing down on its withers. This is because, as you lean forward, more of your weight is put on the front of the saddle.
- If a horse which has always stood quietly and happily for you to dismount in the past suddenly starts to throw its head up and perhaps lay its ears back as you lean forward preparatory to dismounting, it is almost certainly feeling painful pressing or pinching from the saddle. In all cases, check the saddle carefully and also check the horse's spine in the area in front, under and behind the front arch of the saddle and the area below and to each side of the withers to see if it is painful. Change the saddle or get it restuffed. If the horse's back is painful, do not put the saddle on it for a few days. Make sure the pain has gone before you use a saddle again.

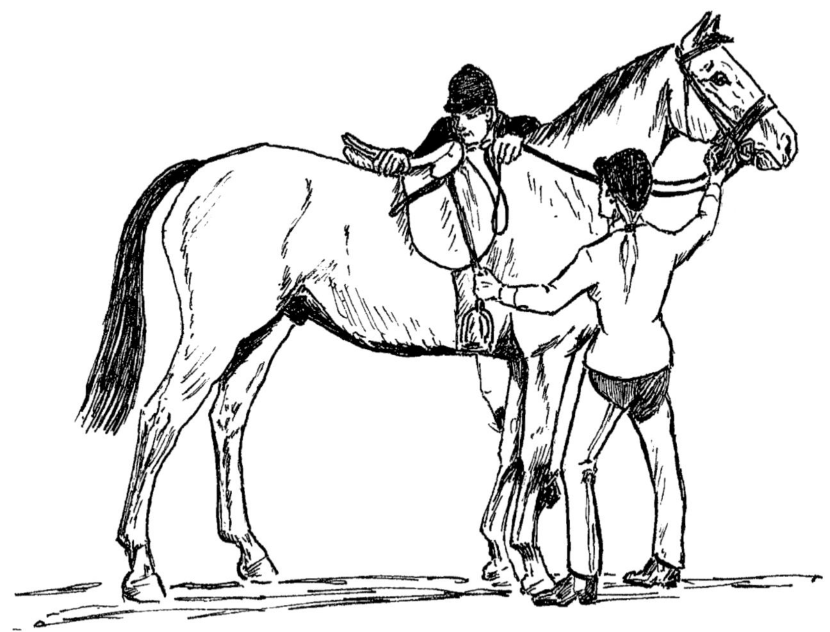

Mounting with an assistant holding the noseband and stirrup.

COLD BACK

When you mount and put your weight in the saddle, does your horse crouch right down behind and perhaps walk along for several minutes in this position? These are the symptoms of a 'cold back'.

Use a thick, fleecy numnah. Make sure the saddle fits comfortably (test it without a numnah). Tie the horse up and put the saddle on fifteen minutes before you intend to ride. Mount from a mounting block. Do not sit in the saddle; stand in your stirrups and keep your weight well forward out of the saddle. Ride in this position for several minutes then lower your weight gently into the saddle. The horse will probably be perfectly all right now but if it does crouch down, keep your weight out of the saddle for a little longer, then try again.

Some horses just do behave in this way. Nothing appears to be wrong with them and as long as you keep your weight out of the saddle to start with, there is no problem. Check the horse's spine towards the back of the saddle to see if it is painful. Make sure the saddle fits correctly and is well clear of the spine and with a channel between the stuffing that is wide enough to ensure the spine is not pinched.

Some animals which live out may crouch down when you mount if their backs are cold and wet after rain.

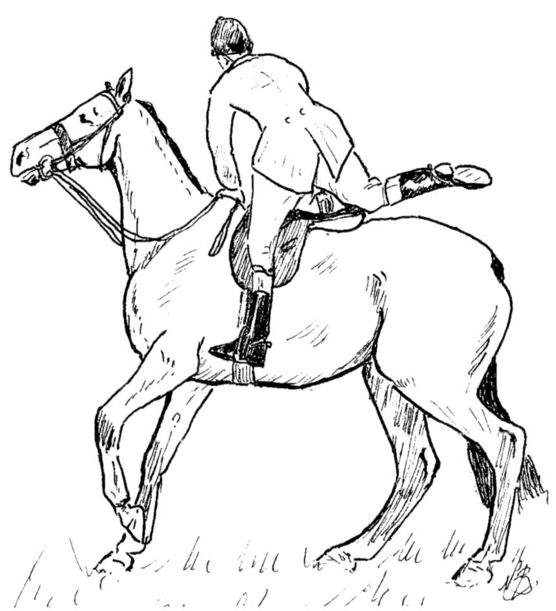

As the rider mounts, the horse's back goes down and the horse crouches as the rider's weight is felt.

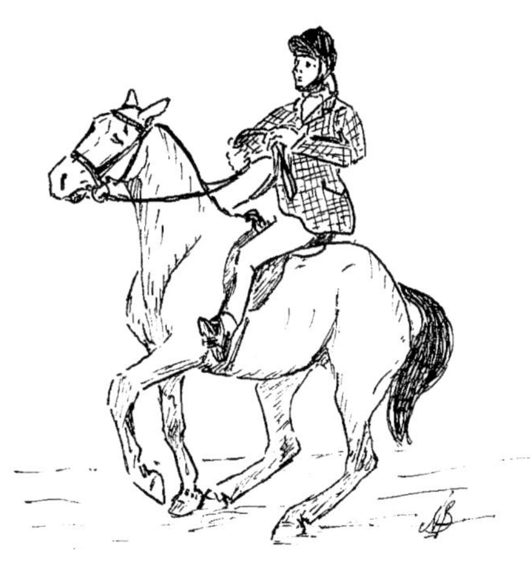

The wrong way to sit after mounting a cold-backed horse.

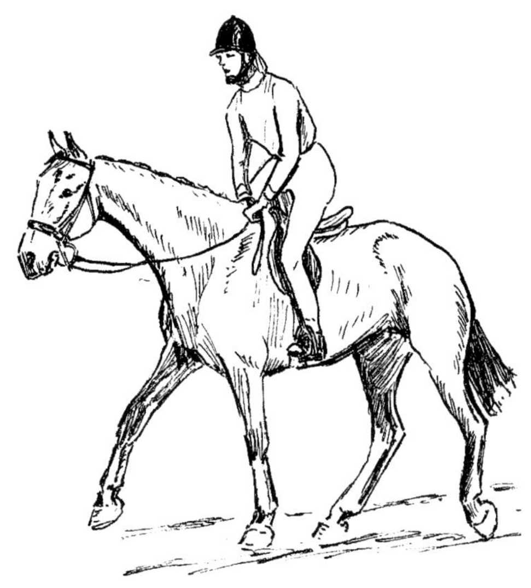

Sitting forward after mounting.

JOGGING

This annoying and tiring habit is often found in a tense, excitable horse. It just cannot relax, lower its head and swing along in an easy walk. Gently steady the horse to a walk and, as soon as it walks, ease the reins and give it as long a rein as possible. The second it begins to jog, steady it to a walk and release the reins. Sit lightly in the saddle. Use your voice to calm the horse, repeating 'W–a–l–k' in a slow, deep voice. If the horse only jogs during the last mile or so of the approach to home, or if it jogs as soon as it thinks it is now on the way home, dismount and lead the animal. Many horses will immediately relax without a rider on their back. If it has walked calmly for five or ten minutes when led, remount very gently and quietly, keep your weight a little forward so that you are sitting light in the saddle and leave the horse's head alone, giving it as long a rein as possible.

If you are riding in company, your jogging horse is unlikely to walk unless it is in the lead, so ask any companions to keep their animals a horse's length behind yours. A young horse must be treated gently and calmly. An older horse may respond to the discomfort of a sharp jerk in the mouth every time it begins to jog, immediately followed by a loose rein. This may have to be repeated several times before the horse associates the discomfort with jogging. Use the word 'Walk' at the same time. This seemingly disgraceful advice really does work wonders with some horses which will soon respond by walking as soon as they feel you begin to move your hands preparatory to jerking their mouths. Soon they will respond to the word 'Walk' alone. Obviously, some horses will become tenser, more worried and jog more if their mouths are jerked, in which case you should cease to use this method.

Some horses respond to a pull on a neck strap to steady them to walk.

Another possibility is a second rein attached to the side rings of a drop noseband. Use this extra rein to steady the jogging horse instead of the bit rein.

Some horses will walk if you take a piece of skin near their shoulder blade between your finger and thumb and pinch and really twist the skin every time they jog.

If the horse is ridden alone and jogs the second the ride is beyond the halfway mark and it knows it is now travelling towards home, refrain from ever trotting or cantering towards home so that there is less to get excited about. Never turn in your tracks so that one minute you are going away from home and the next going towards home as this often excites horses. You can usually find something to ride a loop or circle round and so avoid a direct turn. Turning round in your tracks can encourage a horse to nap and argue with you when it wants to go home and you want it to go on further.

Try all of these methods and see which works best for your horse. To break the habit, for several weeks try to avoid the situations which you know are most likely to cause the horse to jog.

Even a calm, sensible horse will learn to jog to keep up if its companions on a ride are bigger than it, longer striding or simply have a naturally faster walk.

Lengthening the stride in walk

It is possible to improve the length of the walk stride in most horses. Ride the horse out alone so that it will not be tempted to jog to catch up with another horse. Encourage it to lower its head and lengthen its neck by giving it a long rein. Use your legs alternately, using your right leg as the horse's off (right) foreleg begins to come off the ground and your left leg as the horse's near (left) foreleg begins to come up off the ground. Lengthening the horse's neck and lowering its head will encourage it to take a longer, lower stride. Using your alternate legs as each stride begins will encourage the horse to step forward further, using a longer stride. It will learn to use its shoulders freely and swing along. The horse must never be allowed to slop along when you are riding at walk. It must be constantly ridden forward at an active walk. It is hard work for the rider who must persevere, sometimes for several weeks, before the results of their efforts will begin to show.

A tense horse must first learn to lengthen in a long, low outline before it is asked to lengthen on the bit.

SMELLS

Horses are very sensitive to the faintest odour and may react completely out of character on occasions if they do not like a smell. They may be frightened by, and try to get away from, a smell on a person approaching them by running back if tied up in a stable or by whipping round and even threatening to kick out if loose in one. They may become wide eyed, snort, breathe rapidly and carry their heads high. If in a field, they may gallop off as soon as the smell reaches their nostrils and not dare to approach you again.

If other animals, such as pigs, goats, cattle or sheep, have been in a horse box or trailer, a horse that is normally perfectly good to load may snort and fuss and absolutely refuse to go in. Do not chastise a horse in these circumstances or you may make it permanently difficult to load. Clean the box out really well. Try to disguise the smell, perhaps with disinfectant, or put some of the horse's own dirty bedding and droppings on the ramp and in the vehicle. Some horses will refuse under any circumstances to go into or even past a vehicle which smells even faintly of pigs.

Many horses will be frightened of even a faint smell of blood on your clothes or hands.

Some horses do not like the smell of perfume and have been known to become aggressive if they smell it. If you do not normally wear scent when dealing with your horse and do one day wear some, the horse may react quite differently to your presence.

Horses can be frightened of a smoky smell and be loath to pass such a place. The faintest odour of pigs can produce really violent napping when hacking out. The horse is often genuinely terrified and if you are alone it is often best to choose another route. If the smell of pigs has terrified the horse and it then sees them grunting and gambolling about, it may panic and become completely uncontrollable. If you did get off to try to lead the horse past, it is unlikely that you would be able to keep hold of it.

Vets and blacksmiths have special smells and many horses snort and back off as soon as they enter the stable.

Putting a little Vick in each of the horse's nostrils can mask the smells it dislikes. However, the Vick must be applied before the horse catches a whiff of the smell it dislikes or which frightens it.

SHYING

Horses shy from fear and also from sheer naughtiness.

Some horses are more frightened of sounds, for instance a bird scratching under a hedge or a gun going off. Others are frightened by strange sights, such as a log or a piece of plastic.

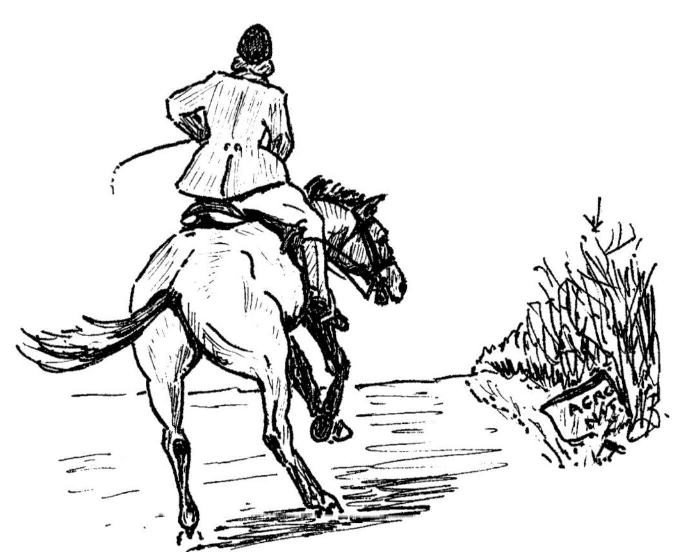

When this horse shied the rider pulled on the right rein, sending the horse out into the road where a car might well be approaching.

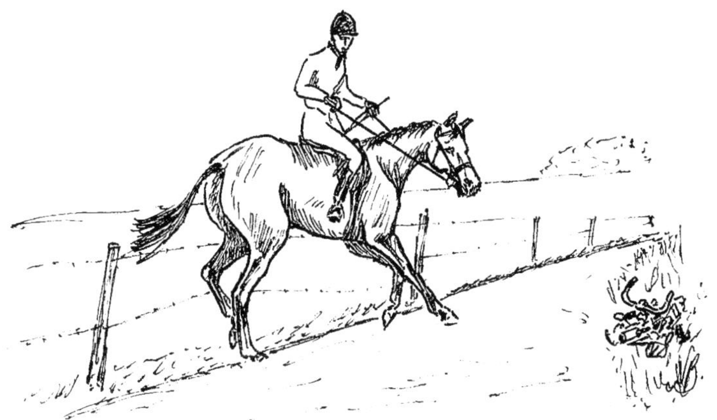

Because the rider used the rein nearer to the 'spook' to try to control the shying horse, the horse is going to run into the wire which it is unaware of.

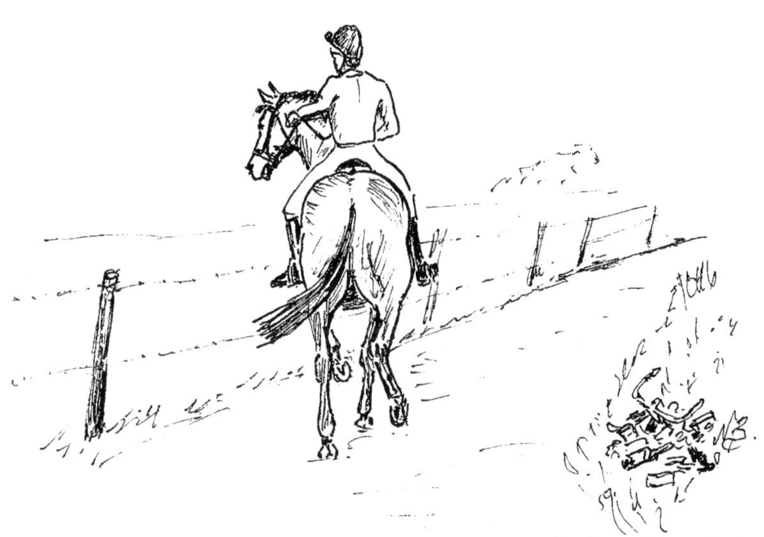

This rider uses her left rein and right leg. The horse goes past the 'spook' and also sees the wire.

A frightened horse will raise its head, eyes popping, and you may feel its heart beating hard and fast. It will probably shoot sideways still looking towards the frightening object. Its whole mind will be on the scary 'demon' so it may well be oblivious of anything else going on around it. It is for this reason that a horse which shies badly is very dangerous to ride out on the road as it will shy out into the road even when a big lorry is coming.

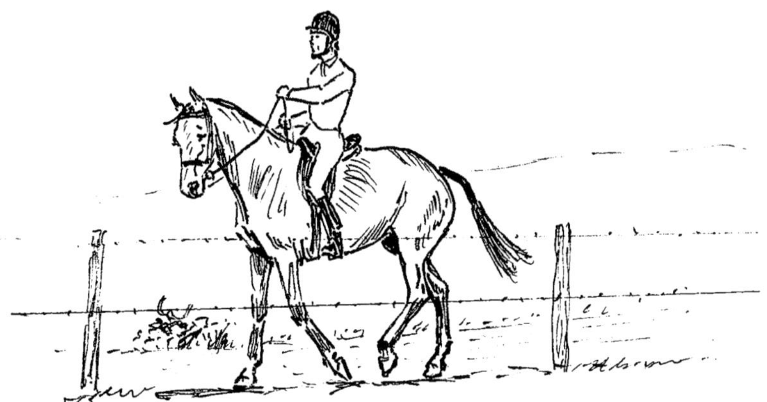

When viewed from the other side we can see that the rider's left hand is raised and the left rein is being used strongly against the horse's neck which prevents it from bulging out through its left shoulder and shying into the wire. The right leg is used strongly to control the hindquarters. Even if there is no road or dangerous hazard on the left, this is the correct and most effective way to ride a horse past a scary object on its right.

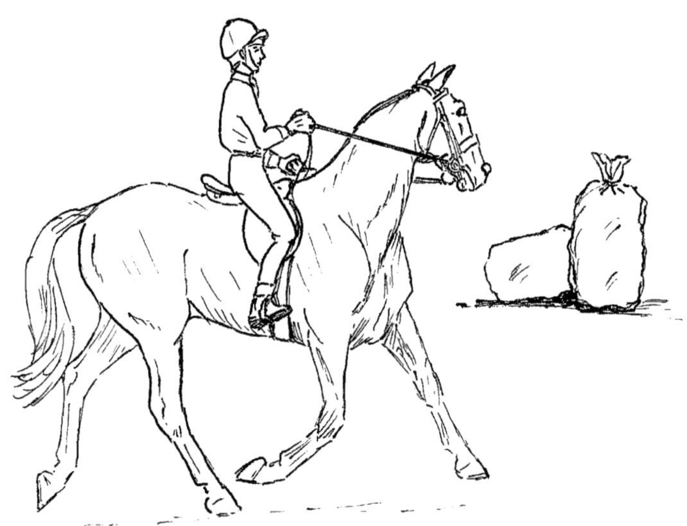

This 'spook' is on the other side of the road so the rider uses her right rein held high to control the neck and right shoulder while the right leg keeps the horse going forward.

Overshortening the reins

You can make a horse shy by overshortening and overtightening the reins as you approach anything that you think your horse might shy at. The horse feels your fear and apprehension via the reins and your tense body and thinks. 'My rider is frightened; perhaps I ought to be too'.

While riding out, your horse may raise its head and prick its ears, looking intently at something it is not sure of. As soon as you begin to feel or see this happening, ride the horse forward with firm, confident legs. The horse must feel your hands allowing it to go forward and your legs asking it to do so. If it shies sideways away from a frightening object on its right use the left rein to bend its head away, thus helping to control its left shoulder and prevent it from shooting sideways with its left shoulder bulging out. Use your left leg behind the girth to control its quarters. Your right leg asks the horse to go forward and your right rein allows it to go forward. Sit upright and ride the horse forward with your seat and back. Allow the horse to pass the object on a track a little way from it if necessary.

The priority is to keep the horse going forward without arguing, not to get it to pass as close as possible after an argument. Pass and repass the object until the horse is close enough to have a look or a sniff if it wants to. Never, ever try to ride a horse directly at something it is frightened of as it may, through fright, learn to take strong evasive action it has never used before, such as whipping round or rearing.

Never use the rein nearer to a frightening object to try to control a shying horse. First, it will think you want it to go up to the 'horror' so it will only shy even more. Second, you will be allowing the outside shoulder to bulge out and carry the horse sideways in the direction it wants to go.

Some horses will shy from sheer naughtiness and a large leaf bent the wrong way is sufficient excuse. If you are approaching something which you know your horse will shy at from naughtiness, reverse your whip, holding it in the hand further away from the 'spook'. Hold the whip at your horse's eye level and move the end up and down beside the horse's eye while riding it forward strongly with your legs. It can then see the whip which you are using as a warning to discourage it from misbehaving and shying out of naughtiness. Weak or nervous riders do teach horses to shy out of devilment and such horses may even deliberately try to unseat their rider by a sudden shy. A reversed whip and firm forward riding can cure this habit in time.

Do not reverse your whip on a genuinely frightened horse. It needs to gain confidence – not to be threatened.

ROLLING WHEN RIDDEN

Woolly-coated animals will roll when they are hot and sweaty, often flopping down with little warning. Some young horses will try to roll when they first feel hot and uncomfortable under the saddle.

Horses, particularly ponies, will roll when they come on to a sandy surface or wood chips in an indoor or outdoor school. In such situations, the second the animal drops its head and looks at the ground you must suspect that it is going to roll and ride it forward really strongly, using a stick if necessary. After looking down, the next stage is bending one foreleg and, in a second, it has gone down! Get off immediately, shout, jab on the reins, hit it, *anything*, to stop it rolling over on your saddle and breaking the tree!

When you remount, be careful as the desire to roll will still be there.

If your horse stops and paws the water as you are crossing a stream, it is not testing the depth nor telling you that it wants a drink – it is probably about to roll so if you don't want to get wet you should use your legs and stick quickly!

WHIPPING ROUND

This habit is often accompanied by the habit of dropping a shoulder (see page 217) to get the rider off. Many horses start off by whipping round because they are genuinely frightened of something. Perhaps their rider then falls off or becomes unbalanced and loses control of the horse which quickly learns that this is an effective way of getting rid of its rider or of taking charge itself. The horse soon begins to look for any excuse to whip round – a different-coloured patch of grass, leaves moving – things which no horse would really be frightened by. The next stage is to whip round at nothing with the sole intention of getting the rider off or taking charge.

The rider with whom the horse has learnt to misbehave will not be able to cure it because the horse has no respect for them – it knows that it is boss. A strong, experienced, capable rider who is not in the least nervous must ride the horse every day. The rider must sit deep in the saddle, heels well down, legs in contact with the horse's sides. They must use their seat, back and legs to ride the horse forwards. Their hands must have enough contact on the reins to keep the horse straight but not so much that the horse feels the rider is stopping it going forward. (Nervous riders tend to tighten their reins and clutch, which makes most horses misbehave.)

The rider must be one hundred per cent attentive all the time and the very second that they feel the horse *begin* to think of whipping round, they must ride it forward very strongly. The most important thing is to prevent the horse from turning round and to do this it is necessary to have one hand on each rein so that it is impossible to hit the horse at that exact moment. If the horse always whips round in the same direction (as some do) it may be possible to use a long whip on the hindquarters while still holding both reins. If the horse always whips round to the left so that its quarters go to the right, the whip should be carried in the right hand and used on the off (right) side of the horse's hindquarters.

Another method to try if the horse always whips round to the left, is to carry a long whip upside down in the left hand so that the end of the whip lies along the left side of the horse's neck fairly near its left eye. The horse is conscious of the whip there and if, as it *begins* to think of whipping round, the whip is waggled up and down and the horse is driven forward strongly, it may change its mind.

If the horse does succeed in whipping round, turn it to face the desired direction and quickly give it two or three really hard whacks while sitting well down in the saddle and riding it forward very strongly. It is essential to stay on the horse, really boss it and punish it instantly for misbehaving. It must know why it is being hit.

Most animals will revert to this habit once more if they are ridden by a nervous or inexperienced rider.

DROPPING A SHOULDER

This nasty habit is used by animals which have learnt that it is a very effective way of depositing their rider on the ground! They shoot sideways, say, to the right, to unbalance their rider, then suddenly drop their left shoulder to tip the rider off. They may whip round or buck to unbalance the rider before dropping their shoulder just to finish them off. They may also run out at a jump and do it.

Some horses always do this in the same direction which is a slight help because you know what to expect and can be ready for it.

It is absolutely essential that a horse which drops its shoulder is ridden by a strong, determined rider with a very firm seat. The habit can be broken but the feel of a wobbly or unconfident rider will almost certainly make the horse revert to the habit.

BUCKING

Why does your horse buck?● Is it excitement or sheer joy of life?
● Is it trying to get you off because it dislikes being ridden?
● Is its saddle uncomfortable, making its back sore, bruised or pinched?
● Has it got a back problem? (See page 118.)
● Has it learnt that if it bucks the rider comes off and it is free?
● Is it overfed or underexercised?
● Is it young, perhaps recently broken, and bucking at the unusual feel of a tight girth?

If your horse is bucking you off, you need expert help immediately from someone who can answer some of these questions. Once the cause is known, various remedies can be tried.
● Young horses may need lungeing before they are ridden so that they can get rid of any bucks at the girth before you get on. Even with a quiet young horse that is kept out, if you have not been able to ride it for a week it is sensible to lunge it before riding it.

- Too much hard food for the amount of work being done, or for the rider's own ability, causes many problems. If the horse is normally stabled all the time, if possible turn it out every day before riding it. Feed nothing but good quality hay, which is quite sufficient for most horses that are just hacking. When the horse has calmed down, you can begin to give it a little hard food if necessary.
- A horse which is quite deliberately bucking its rider off must be ridden by an experienced rider capable of staying on it and controlling it accurately. If you are an inexperienced rider and 'clutchy', the horse will know. It is likely to behave well with an experienced, capable rider but to buck again if it feels you wobble or clutch.
- If a sore, bruised or pinched back is the cause, the horse must be given time to recover before putting on a well-fitting saddle which has been checked by an experienced person. At first the horse should be ridden by a capable rider because it may think that the saddle is still going to hurt and buck in anticipation.

When riding a bucking horse, try to keep its head up. Holding your reins in a bridge (see Diving, page 225) may help to prevent you from falling forwards as the 'bridge' on the horse's neck will stop your hands from sliding down each side of its neck.

Keep the horse going forward, then it will find it more difficult to do large bucks. Alternatively, turn the horse short on a tight circle. Keep your heels down and your head up.

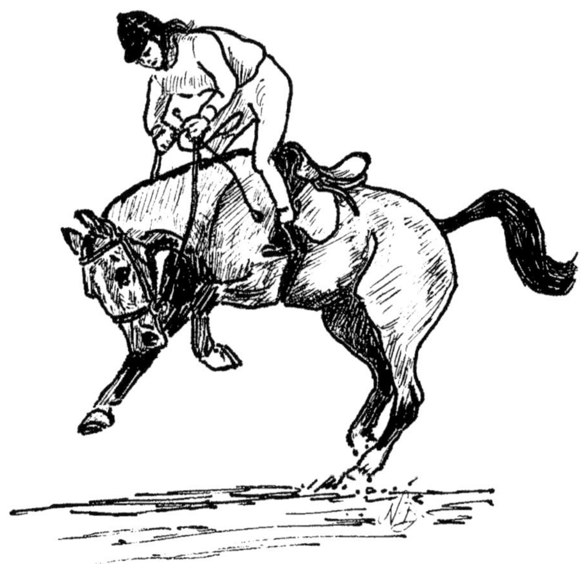

This rider is about to be bucked off.

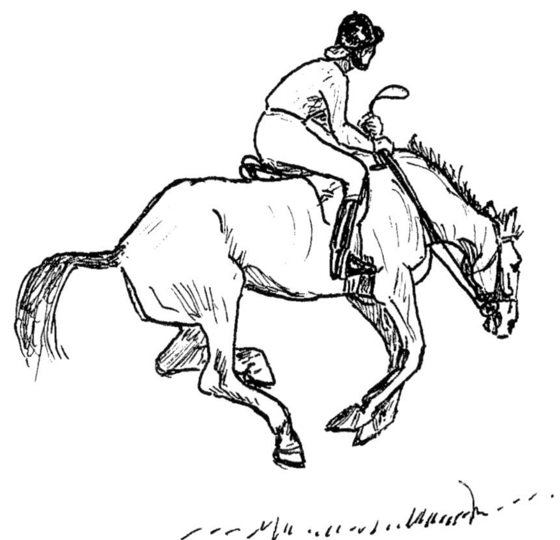

This rider is holding a neck strap and sitting in balance with the horse. Her chances of staying on are much better.

Many people will advise you to hit the horse hard as soon as it starts to buck but that is easier said than done!

Sour and ungenerous animals will buck when they do not answer to the leg when asked to increase pace and a stick is used. They hump their backs, swish their tails and sometimes stop dead or turn sideways when hit. Using a stick makes this type of animal worse and what started as resentful humping of the back can become a series of very large bucks intended to dislodge the rider.

Sometimes horses who react to being hit in this way will go forward when the rider wears blunt spurs. Sometimes just the use of the voice and making every ride enjoyable and interesting for the horse can change its attitude to life. This is particularly true of some riding school horses which have become so bored by going round and round with different beginners that they have lost all interest in life.

Ponies which buck and are too small for an adult to ride can sometimes be controlled by two pieces of cord which run from the D at each side of the front of the saddle to the pony's crest where they are knotted (to prevent them opening up when the pony tries to put its head down) through the brow band loops and on to the bit rings. The cords should be adjusted so that they do not affect the pony's normal head carriage and only come into action if the pony tries to put its head down. They can also be used as grass reins to prevent the pony from diving its head down to graze. (See page 88.)

Many young horses are frightened by the feel of mud, soil or gravel being thrown up against their tummies by their own feet or the feet of nearby horses and can leap and buck in a truly alarming way. Some older horses never accept this feeling and will always buck in that situation.

It is not easy to arrange a situation whereby the horse can be gradually accustomed to this, although riding in a very waterlogged outdoor *manège* can help. A bad fright early in life often triggers longlasting memories.

Fly bucking

This habit is often caused by an overexcited horse being held back too strongly by the rider. The horse leaps forward with all four feet off the ground as if it is jumping a fence which is not there. It will often throw its head up and leap almost in one movement. To make a really big leap it must take off evenly from both hind feet.

Possible ways of preventing fly bucking include:

- Using as mild a bit as possible.
- Not taking the horse among others which are tearing about.
- Riding only with a knowledgeable person who is on a quiet, sensible horse.
- If you feel the horse's muscles tensing up under you preparatory to fly bucking, ride the horse forward on to a small circle but be aware that as your circle comes round in the direction in which the horse wants to go, it may leap forward again.
- As soon as the horse lands from a fly buck, circle it and be ready to make another circle if necessary. By turning the horse you are making it more difficult for it to make an enormous leap by taking off from both hind legs equally as it will have more weight on one hind leg when travelling in a circle.
- Put on a running martingale (see page 100) or a Market Harborough (see page 266) to help to prevent the horse's head going up preparatory to leaping.
- Play with the bit with your fingers. Try not to hold the horse back strongly with both hands. Most people instinctively do this when they feel a horse tense up but it really does make the situation worse. Instead, play with one rein, try to get the horse's head round to one side so that you put it slightly off balance, and ride it forward with your legs. The feeling that the rider is trying to stop it going forward makes an excitable horse fly buck. Try to let the horse feel that you will allow it to go forward but at *your* choice of gait. Keep your weight forward so that you are going with the horse. To stay with it if it really leaps, you are going to have to sit as you would at the take off for a large fence.

Some horses get so overexcited that they will do enormous fly bucks forward without thinking about where they are going to land. This is a very dangerous situation because they can crash into trees, get tangled up in a wire fence, land on top of other people and horses or leap out in front of traffic. If you get into this situation, dismount and lead the horse away, if possible with another quiet horse for company. In a few minutes, away from the excitement, it may calm down enough for you to remount and ride it quietly home. Do not put yourself or the horse in this dangerous situation again. Get an expert to ride and school the horse. Most horses will grow out of this sort of behaviour but a few will persist in certain situations, such as when queuing for a jump out hunting.

Exploding at the girth

All their lives some horses will react adversely to the feel of a girth. They may stand absolutely frozen rigid when you first do up the girth in the stable, then suddenly explode in leaping bronco bucks. They may stand shaking with fright afterwards or may be perfectly relaxed and cause no more trouble that day, only to repeat the performance next day.

Some horses are perfectly all right until you are on their backs, when they freeze rigid and, when asked to move forward, leap forward in a series of bronco bucks.

If, for any reason, you have not ridden your young horse for several weeks (or in some cases even days) it may be necessary to treat the horse as if it has never had a girth on before.

1 Do up the girth loosely.

2 Circle the horse in both directions in the stable.

3 Tighten the girth one hole. Circle the horse again.

4 Lunge the horse on both reins, if possible including canter because it is at this gait that the horse will feel the constriction of the girth most and be more likely to buck.

5 Get on the horse immediately it has been lunged. If you retighten the girth before mounting, circle the horse in both directions.

6 Using a girth with elastic inserts and always circling the horse in both directions before you mount can cure this problem.

7 Many older horses which have been out of work for some months also have to be restarted as if they were youngsters.

HANGING

When you are trying to ride in a straight line when schooling or out on a hack, many horses will 'hang' towards home or towards other horses. Their tummies and one shoulder bulge out towards the direction in which they want to go. They are looking, say, to the right, away from the direction in which they want to go but moving forward and sideways to the left towards this direction. Most riders' instinct is to use even more right rein, in which case the horse will only increase its sideways movement. Both reins and legs must be used to check

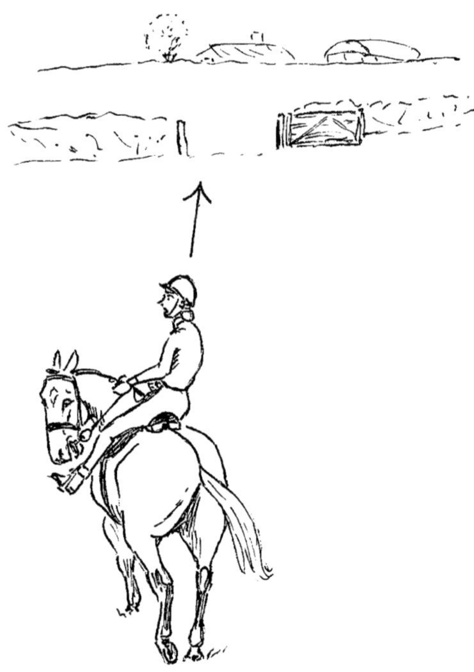

This horse is running sideways. The rider is using her left rein only and no leg at all. The horse is bulging out through its right shoulder and continues going towards home.

the horse, then the left rein must be used to keep the neck straight and the left leg to prevent the left shoulder and the tummy from bulging out. It is helpful to carry your stick in the left hand and hold it vertical so that you can tap, tap, tap the horse on the left shoulder if necessary to help to prevent it from bulging out. Again, think ahead and position the horse so that you can prevent it from 'hanging' before it starts to think about doing so.

RUNNING SIDEWAYS

The same method can be used to prevent a horse from running sideways. The horse may gather itself and run sideways at speed in the direction in which it wants to go while still looking in the opposite direction. The first thing you must do is slow the horse right down to a halt before you try to correct the direction in which it is going. If it shoots sideways to the left, but is looking to the right, use mainly your left rein and left leg, quite strongly if necessary, to bring it quite sharply to a halt. As you do so, sit down in the saddle and put your weight back. Both legs, but your left leg more strongly, must ride the horse forward into your 'holding' hands to control and correct it as the horse has learnt that by bulging its shoulder towards the direction in which it wants to go,

| Home |

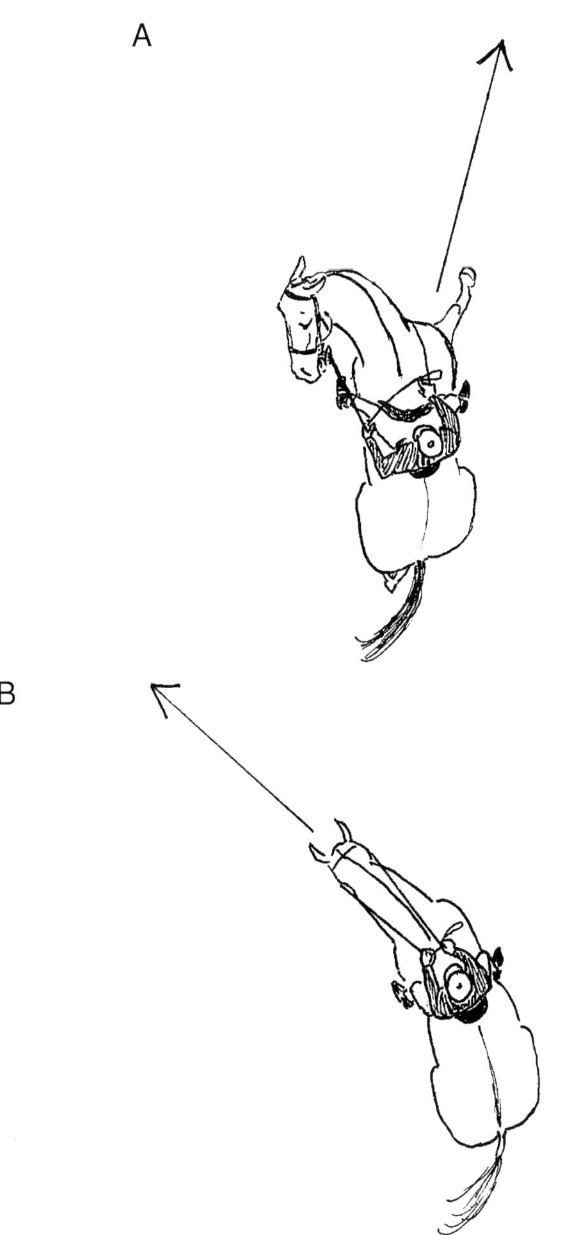

Rider A is using the left rein only and cannot stop the horse running sideways. Rider B is using the right rein to control the right shoulder and her right leg to bring the horse over to the left. A little left rein only is needed to guide the horse.

it can escape the rider's control. Preventing the outside shoulder from escaping is all important. The outside rein and leg must do this. To control the bulging left shoulder it may be necessary to ride the horse so that its head and neck are turned slightly left as a correction.

The faster you are going, the more control the horse has. The slower you go, the more control you have, so, first of all, slow down to halt if necessary, using the rein on the same side as the bulging shoulder to do so.

Lifting up the hand and rein trying to control the bulging shoulder and bent neck make them more effective.

Running sideways in company

An excited horse will run sideways if overrestricted by the rider's hands. This is particularly true if the rider is taking a strong, steady pull, literally trying to hold the horse back.

When the horse runs sideways, say, to the right, the rider invariably tries to control the horse by using the left rein. This bends the horse's head to the left, allowing the right shoulder to bulge out and continue the sideways run to the right. When the horse's head is bent left, its near (left) hind leg steps under and across to the right enabling it to push its body forcefully to the right. The horse is able to continue going sideways fast to the right and the rider has little or no control and can often be heard saying, 'I am frightfully sorry, I am frightfully sorry' as they bump into horses or mow people down like ninepins.

Prevention is better than cure. Steady the horse, using your fingers to squeeze the reins – steady, steady, steady in a rhythm with its stride. Allow it to go forward with the other horses but at a steady pace. If you try to hold the horse back strongly with a continuous pull on the reins, it will try to go sideways in exasperation. As soon as you begin to feel the change of balance and movement of muscle telling you that the horse is about to try to run sideways, say, to the right, push your hands forward a fraction to encourage it to continue going forward and ride it forward with your legs. Then feel, feel, feel on your right rein to ask the horse to bend its head slightly to the right. This will prevent its right shoulder from bulging out and carrying the horse to the right. Raise your hand slightly as you use your right rein and allow the rein to press on the right side of the horse's neck. This will help you to keep the right bend and control the right shoulder. Sit down in the saddle and ride your horse forward strongly with your seat, back and legs. Have your right leg behind the girth and use it to keep your horse's hindquarters following in the same track as its forehand, going forward and straight. This will help to prevent the horse from stepping under and across with its near hind leg and so pushing its body to the right.

Tactful co-ordination of hands, legs and seat is needed to control an excitable horse. You must have a steadying but allowing hand and both legs on its sides to keep it going forwards at the speed you want.

DIVING THE HEAD DOWN

Horses which suddenly and violently dive their heads down are very tiring to ride and can injure the rider's shoulder muscles. Some horses do it from excitement, others have learnt that they might gain an inch or two of rein or even snatch the reins out of your hands by this method and so get their own way.

Holding the reins in a bridge in both hands may help because the horse is then pulling against its own neck and not your shoulders. The left rein comes into your hand by the little finger, goes across your palm and out by your index finger, leaving a 7–10 cm (3–4 in) gap of leather before it enters your right hand by your index finger, goes across your palm and out by your little finger.

The right rein comes across your right hand and then your left hand in the same way. The reins lie on top of each other with a 7–10 cm (3–4 in) gap of reins between your hands.

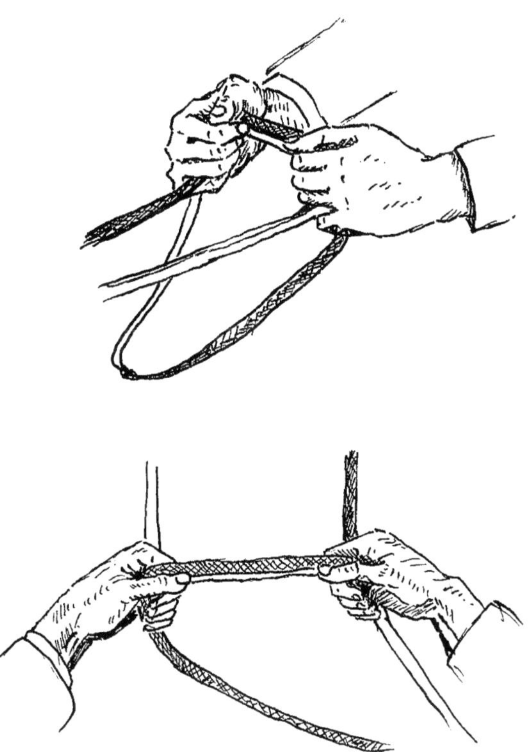

Bridging the reins will help to prevent a horse from diving its head down. It also gives the rider greater security on a horse that bucks as the bridge will prevent the rider's hands from parting on each side of the horse's neck.

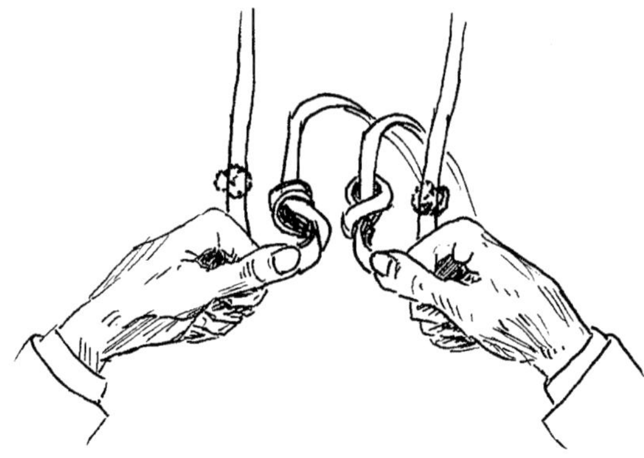

Knots in the reins will prevent them from slipping through your hands on a wet day or if the horse is pulling. Normally the knots should lie between your little finger and the bit but when you shorten the reins the knots come back near to your thumbs to give you control.

If your horse is just strong and excited to start with when hunting or going across country, knots in your reins can prevent them from being pulled through your hands. The knots should be a hand's width forward from where you normally hold your reins. To have more control, shorten your reins by putting your hands just beyond the knots so that your index finger and thumb are against the knot. It is now not nearly so easy for the horse to drag the reins through your hands.

A gag snaffle bit's upward action can help to prevent a horse from diving its head down. A gag bit should always be used with two reins so that the gag action can be used when necessary and not all the time.

If your horse is normally ridden in a Pelham bit or a snaffle, you can make a neat gag-action running-rein by undoing the centre buckle of an extra rein and joining the stud billets from each end (usually attached to the bit) to each other. Lay this join on top of the bridle at the poll. Pass each end of the rein through the brow band loops, down by the cheeks of the bridle and through the largest ring of the bit from outside to inside then up on to the top of the horse's crest where the buckle can be done up again.

You can slip both hands into this 'emergency rein' while still holding your normal reins. It is a great help on a horse which leans on you, tries to pull you forward out of the saddle and dives its head down when going downhill. It is not there to be used all the time, just when needed.

Some horses will dive their heads down from pain or discomfort. Possible causes of this include:

● The cavesson noseband is too low so that when you feel on the reins the bit rises in the mouth and the lips are trapped between the bit and the noseband. This problem is quite common and often goes unnoticed

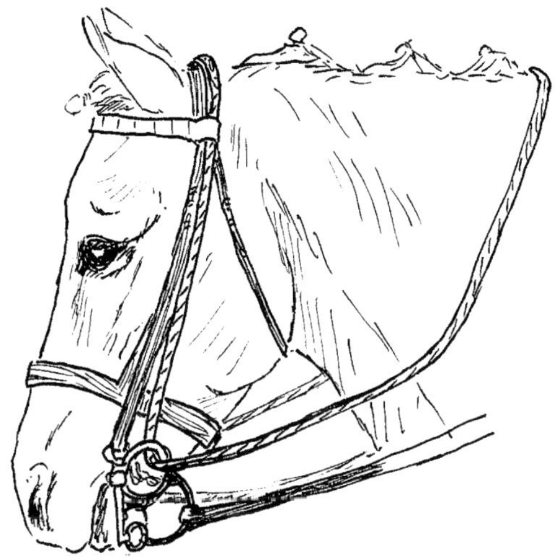

A rein as a gag for emergency use with a Pelham.

because when the reins are not being used there is a gap between the bit and the noseband and all appears to be well. The severe pinching only happens when the reins are used to steady the horse. (See page 79.)

- The bit is worn at the joints and is pinching or cutting the corners of the mouth. There are painful splits in the corners of the mouth.
- The horse has sharp teeth which are cutting the insides of its cheeks. (A horse's teeth should be checked at least once a year.)

Some temperamental horses will always reach and dive when put in an exciting situation but many can be cured by calm, steady schooling. A rider with the knowledge of how to make it uncomfortable for the horse by letting it jerk against its own neck, or by not giving with their hands when it dives will have a gentle, sympathetic, allowing hand when the horse is going kindly. With perseverance, the horse may learn from this method.

RUNNING BACK WHEN RIDDEN

This habit is very often started by nervous riders overshortening their reins and literally hanging on to the horse's head. The rider urges the horse forward with their legs but their hands do not allow so that the horse feels it can't go forward because the rider's hands are holding the reins short and tight. The horse feels it cannot go forward so it goes backwards. It soon learns to use this action as an evasion whenever it sees something it is slightly frightened of or if it does not want to go in a certain direction. Sadly, very many good horses have been spoilt in this way.

If you have this problem, get help as soon as it begins to occur. Get an experienced, determined but sympathetic (*not* rough) rider on the horse, someone who will ride the horse forward with their legs and use a whip behind their leg if necessary (not on the shoulder because they want the horse to go straight forward, not sideways). Above all, they *must* have allowing hands so that the horse feels it can go forwards when asked. If the rider uses a whip, they must be ready in their upper body to go forward with the horse if it shoots forward in response to the whip and must also be ready to push their hands forward so that there is no possibility of the horse having its mouth pulled if it overreacts to the request to go forward by shooting forward suddenly.

When the horse is responding well to the experienced rider, immediately get on it yourself, ride it forward strongly and, above all, allow it to go forward. At first, have someone on foot or on another horse to go with you to give you confidence and assistance if necessary. Always let your horse feel that your hands are allowing it to go forward.

Overshortening and overtightening the reins

This instinctive reaction by nervous or inexperienced riders causes many problems and spoils many good horses.

When riding out on the roads some riders, on seeing or hearing a lorry approaching, immediately overshorten their reins and hang on to their horse's heads while tensing their own bodies and leaning forward. This at once makes the horse think, 'My rider is all tensed up and holding me tightly. This thing approaching must be dangerous. I can feel via the reins and their body contact that they are frightened of it. I had better take evasive action'. The horse may shoot forward, sideways or backwards, or whip round according to the direction from which the lorry is approaching. This horse will very quickly become bad in traffic, anticipating its rider's nervousness.

If you are nervous of riding in traffic, do not ride out alone. Make yourself breathe deeply and slowly and sit in a calm, relaxed way. Do not shorten up your reins or tighten your feel on them. Hum or sing quietly. Talk to the horse quietly and calmly to give it confidence by letting it feel that you are not frightened of traffic. If things do not improve, let someone more confident ride your horse in traffic but go with them yourself on a very quiet horse to regain your own confidence and watch your horse also gaining confidence from a different rider. Only when you and your horse are confident again should you begin to ride it in traffic yourself. Have someone on a quiet horse with you until you and your horse trust each other.

REARING

There are many reasons why horse rear.
- Through pain caused by:
  – a heavy-handed rider;
  – a bit that is too severe;
  – a sore mouth or gums;
  – a painful, unhappy experience when jumping.
- Through fright caused by:
  – fear of something they have seen or heard in front of them;
  – fear of going out alone;
  – fear of deep mud, water, a narrow gap, waving branches, flapping plastic.
- Through nappiness shown by:
  – not wanting to leave other horses or the stable yard;
  – when out on a ride, not wanting to turn away from home or to pass other horses ridden or grazing in a field.

First you must try to work out the cause. If in doubt, ask an experienced person for help and advice.

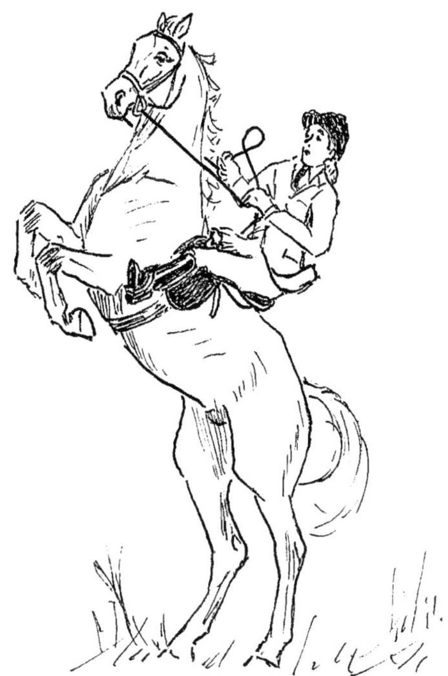

The rider is out of balance and hanging on by the reins. She could pull the horse over backwards.

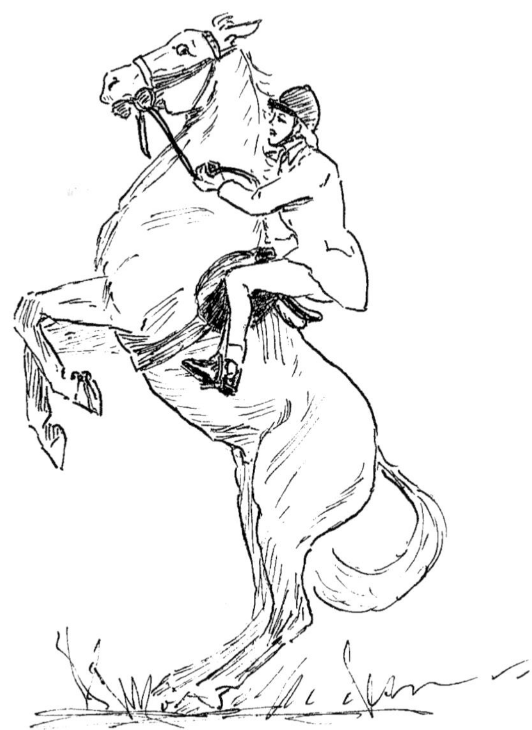

This rider is in balance but is holding the reins too tightly so the horse is unable to stretch its head and neck forward to bring its forelegs down easily. Its hind legs are so far forwards under it that it may fall over backwards or sideways.

If a horse has been rearing and napping with a rider and getting away with it, it is almost essential to change the rider. A strong, capable, experienced rider, not nervous and with sympathetic hands, is needed to improve a rearing horse. If the horse rears dangerously high, the safest way of trying to cure it will be to get a really capable, experienced person who is not nervous to long-rein the horse in the area where it has been rearing. This person must use a cross, 'growly' voice and also the whip if the horse misbehaves. An experienced assistant may be necessary.

If the horse is genuinely nervous and panicky, snorting and shaking before rearing, lead it, following another very quiet horse, first past, then right up to, anything frightening. Then allow your horse to go right up and sniff anything frightening. It is no good hitting a really frightened horse or trying to make it pass or go up to something that it is genuinely afraid of. This will only make it fight and rear in terror. A horse can learn to rear if the rider tries to force it to pass or go up to something it is genuinely terrified of. Wouldn't you fight to get away if someone tried to make you go up to something you thought was going to attack you?

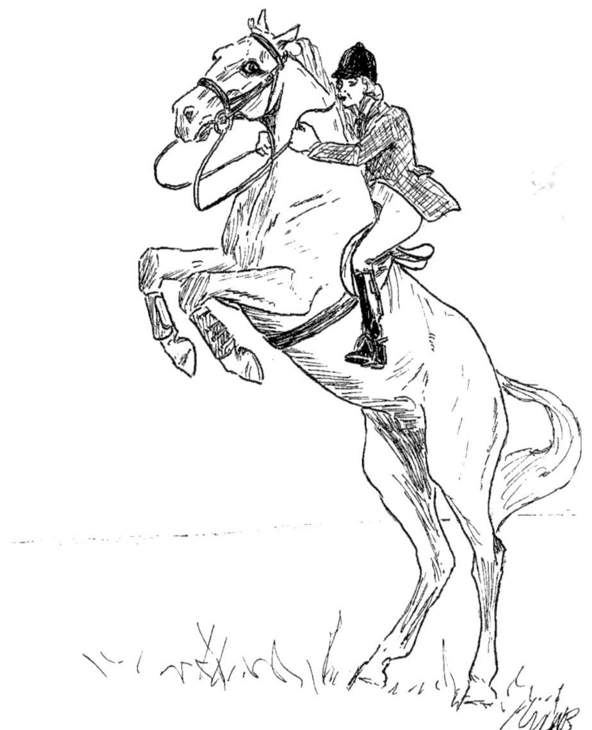

This rider is in balance and is giving the horse a completely loose rein so that it can stretch its head and neck forwards and come down safely on to its forelegs.

Be patient with a nervous horse but, once it has explored the frightening place or object and passed it calmly in both directions, then be very firm if it starts to misbehave again.

A horse that is inclined to rear must feel that your hands will allow it to go forward and will not pull on or jab its mouth.

You must use the mildest possible bit, such as a rubber, nylon or thickish metal snaffle with no worn joints or sharp edges. Make sure that neither the bars of the horse's mouth nor the corners of its lips are sore. A martingale (see page 268) or a Market Harborough (see page 266) will definitely help to discourage the horse from rearing.

Ride the horse forward strongly with your seat and legs before it starts to think of rearing.

If the horse does go up, the most important thing of all is not to pull on the reins or to try to stay on by holding on tightly to the reins. If you do this you can very easily pull the horse over backwards on top of you. Very few horses will go over backwards voluntarily when rearing. They are almost always pulled over by the rider. Sit forward, get your arms round the horse's neck and your head against its neck and to one side of it. Allow your feet to come back under you. Sit still.

To rear, a horse must balance on both hind legs so using one rein out to the side to turn the horse's head and thus unbalance it can make it more difficult for the horse to start to rear. There must be no backward pull.

If the horse just does several quick, small, 'threatening' rears, pummelling it on the top of the head and between the ears with your fists while using a cross, 'growly' voice and riding it forward strongly can surprise it and change its mind. Many horses which are old hands at rearing will try a rider out to see what they can get away with. Be firm and determined as soon as the horse begins to think of misbehaving but, above all, let the horse feel that your hands, though guiding it, will allow it to go forward.

Shortening or tightening your reins at the slightest sign of trouble causes more problems with horses than almost anything else.

When the horse will go forward without offering to rear, an experienced, capable rider may ride the horse along the same route with the person who has been long-reining it following behind carrying a long whip. If the horse tries to slow down or even thinks of stopping preparatory to rearing, the person walking behind must instantly use the same cross, 'growly' voice they used when the horse misbehaved on the long reins and also wave the whip so that the horse can see it.

Some horses will rear in company if they are asked to take the lead but most will only rear if they are asked to leave other horses or pass other horses going in the opposite direction on a ride. Refusing to leave the stable yard is probably the most usual place to have a rearing problem. When out on a ride, choosing a turning leading away from home when the horse wants to take the one towards home can make a horse rear to get its own way. If you know there is a certain place where you always have trouble, ask an experienced, capable person, who has dealt with this problem successfully many times before, to hide at that place. When the horse begins to argue, they must leap out behind the horse, using a cross, 'growly' voice and waving a whip or rustling a plastic bag, anything to get the horse to go forward and keep it going forward.

The horse may learn to respect and obey a capable rider but a nappy horse will invariably revert to the habit with a nervous, 'clutchy' rider. For this reason, if you are the slightest bit nervous it is better to get rid of a horse that rears.

RIDING IN TRAFFIC

A bad fright received by a young horse is never forgotten. Once I was riding a home-bred four year old through a small village when a boy came up behind us and went past on a motorbike. The mare was not at all worried by this. A few minutes later, however, the boy came back round a bend towards us going absolutely flat out. He skidded and came off the bike which skated noisily towards us on its side, engine running, sparks flying. My mare was absolutely terrified and never again heard a motorbike engine without being frightened.

Another time, when I was riding a young horse along a small lane just after heavy rain which had left lots of deep puddles, a police car approached very fast from behind. I signalled to it clearly and correctly to slow down. The driver took not the slightest notice and tore through a deep puddle, the car tyres flinging what seemed like a bucketful of water at the horse's legs. The horse leapt up in the air and down into the ditch. It was some time before I could convince it that all cars would not throw water at it in passing!

These stories illustrate how important it is to try to avoid frightening incidents when a young horse is first taken near traffic.

Avoid narrow lanes without verges where a horse can feel trapped if a large vehicle comes along. The horse may try to turn round in a panic and may then actually be touched or even bumped by the moving vehicle. This is something it may never forget. Tractors, motorbikes, bicycles and prams can cause problems, especially as cyclists and pram pushers are usually totally unaware that they are frightening to a horse.

If you have been offered a horse for sale which is known to be bad in traffic, I do not think it is worth having it even if it is cheap. The traffic nowadays is so fast on small narrow roads that these are almost more dangerous than the big, wide main roads.

If an older horse is found to be bad in traffic there is often some specific situation that it takes exception to. Something frightening has happened in its past and it has never forgotten and probably never will. The 'monster' could have been a very rattly trailer, or a pick-up truck with dogs in the back which suddenly all leapt up barking as they drew level with the horse. Perhaps it was a flapping plastic sheet, or the air brakes of a heavy lorry which braked when level with the horse.

When you ride such a horse in traffic, a calm, traffic-proof companion and a rider who does *not* tense up or shorten their reins, or take a firm hold of the horse's head as soon as they see a lorry coming, are essential.

Horses are great copy-cats. If one shies the others near it will do so too. If the rider gives clear signs of nervousness by shortening their reins and tensing up, the horse will be aware of this and think, 'Well, if they are frightened of this lorry it must be dangerous. I think I am going to be frightened of it also'. A nervous rider makes their horse nervous also. In no time at all horse and rider are both preparing themselves to be frightened whenever anything out of the ordinary approaches. This is a vicious circle – as the horse becomes more frightened, the rider shortens the reins and clutches even more, so soon the horse starts to whip round as the vehicle approaches. The rider's tight rein clearly indicates to the horse that it might be dangerous to go forward – so it doesn't.

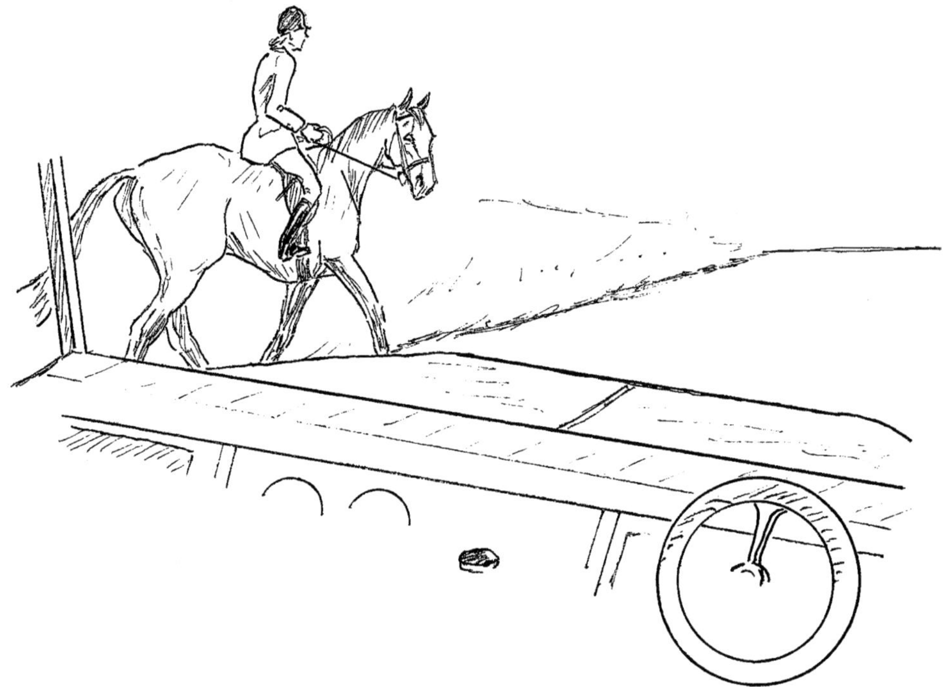

The horse sees the vehicle with its right eye. The rider's right leg keeps the horse's hindquarters out towards the hedge, well clear of the vehicle.

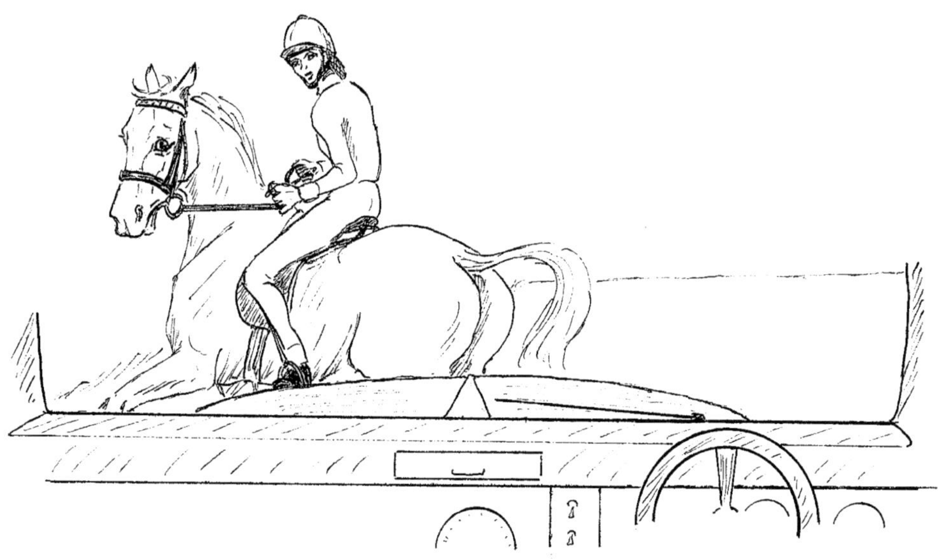

The rider has used the left rein and the horse is looking at the vehicle with its left eye. The hindquarters have swung out into the road where they may easily be hit by the vehicle.

By now there is a real problem. A calm, confident rider who will, if possible, take the horse out in only light traffic on a road with wide verges is necessary. The rider must sit in a relaxed heap, leave the reins alone, not moving their hands at all as traffic approaches but just using their legs to ride the horse forward. They should talk to the horse quietly all the time and, whatever it does, try not to grab suddenly at the reins and hang on to its head. If you sit quietly without moving your hands at all, most horses will hesitate and cock an ear back at you, wondering why you are not shortening the reins or tensing up. They may then voluntarily stand quite still while the vehicle passes, then walk on as if nothing has happened. They may also step sideways and go a few steps further away from the traffic as it passes them. The rider must not try to correct this behaviour. It is acceptable under the circumstances. If the horse does try to turn round, the rider must use as gentle rein aids as possible to correct it and always let the horse feel that it has the freedom to go forward. The rider's legs must urge the horse forward, squeezing rhythmically.

A calm horse ridden between the nervous horse and the traffic will help to give it confidence. If the horse is most often frightened of traffic coming towards it, use its companion as a leader. If it is most often frightened of traffic coming up behind it, have the companion at the rear.

When traffic is coming up behind and you are riding correctly on the left-hand side of the road, use a little right rein and right leg to make sure that your horse sees the approaching traffic with its right eye. Horses tend to keep their eye on something that they are frightened of, so if the horse continues to look at the vehicle with its right eye, its hindquarters will stay out towards the left side of the road, away from the vehicle.

If the horse sees the vehicle coming up behind it with its left eye and continues to keep that eye on it, its hindquarters will swing out into the road towards the vehicle and may be hit by it. This is the cause of very many traffic accidents involving horses. As the horse's hindquarters go out to the right into the road, the rider frantically shortens the reins and tries to turn the horse left on to the verge. The horse then actually backs into the traffic and is hit by the vehicle.

If you notice something on your side of the road which a horse might shy at, try to avoid passing the 'spook' just as a vehicle is driving up behind you, in case the horse shies out into the road.

If you see something pretty horrific approaching, try to be near a wide verge, a side turn or a gateway as it draws level but don't tense up and make 'preparations' which the horse will be aware of.

See Shying (page 212) because a horse which shies away from things on the verge out into the road and is so totally unafraid of traffic that it doesn't think about what is approaching and which may hit it is an almost worse danger than a horse that is nervous in traffic.

JIBBING

Jibbing is usually a more passive resistance, whereas napping is an active resistance. Horses which jib either stand woodenly still and refuse to budge, or step slowly backwards. When hit, they will often buck on the spot. The cause is usually not wanting to leave, or turn away from, home, or not wanting to leave other horses. Some horses will jib when hit and are more likely to go forward if ridden gently, asked to go forward and to one side or the other instead of straight ahead, or turned in small circles several times before, once more, being asked to go forward. Do not hold the horse on a tight rein. It must always feel that your hands will *allow* it to go forward.

Sometimes jibbing is simply the result of boredom. For instance, some riding school horses get so fed up with going round and round in endless lessons that they stand still and refuse to move. They have switched off and lost all interest in life. A horse with this temperament is not suitable for riding-school work but many jibbers can be transformed by being hacked out with others and not used in a lesson or schooled in circles for several months, introduced to little natural jumps on a hack, or taken hunting. They will begin to enjoy life and take an interest again. This can be a very rewarding experience for the rider.

If you sit still and wait, sometimes a jibber will decide to go forward. If you sit quietly for some time, then suddenly use voice, legs and stick all at once, the horse may also go forward. You could try turning the horse round and asking it to go backwards in the direction in which you want it to go. After backing for several yards, turn it round and ask it to go forward again. Repeat if necessary.

A well-bred, hotter-blooded type of horse is more likely to nap, offering active resistance. The commoner, colder-blooded type of horse is more likely to use the passive resistance of jibbing.

Occasionally, jibbing can be caused by discomfort from badly fitting saddlery; a breast girth or breast plate that is tight or rubbing; undue pressure or bruising of the back near, or on, the withers, or discomfort in the mouth. Check all of these possibilities.

CONFRONTATIONS

Avoid confrontations unless you are sure that you can win. Each time that a horse or pony gets its own way will build up its self-esteem and lower its opinion of you as a rider. It will play up more and more.

Don't give up but use your brains to think of an easier way of asking the horse to do what you want; a way in which you will win.

Learn to recognise the difference between a horse which is naughty and one which is genuinely frightened of something and needs time and patience, not punishment and forcing. Punishing a horse which is genuinely frightened and trying to force it to go past something scary can often teach it to rear, nap and buck in protest, things it would probably not have tried to do otherwise. Once these habits are learnt they will be used again.

A genuinely frightened horse can have been going quietly in a relaxed manner until it suddenly sees something strange. Its head will come up, its ears will prick, its body will tense, it will shorten its steps and may slow down. Try to keep it going forward while stroking its neck and talking to it. Allow it to deviate from the track close to the frightening object as long as it keeps going forward. If it does come to a stop, allow it to stand still but not to turn round. Give it a minute or two to assess the situation – perhaps it is not as frightening as it first thought and it may relax and walk on. If it does not do so of its own accord, squeeze with your legs to send it forward. Allow a deviation if necessary but going forward is essential. It is far better to pass something on a big curve than have a fight to pass close to it.

A naughty horse may be feeling fresh and lively, head up, ears twitching, perhaps jogging a few steps, just looking for any excuse to shy or whip round even at a large leaf. Ride it forward into a light contact on the reins so that it feels that you are controlling it between your legs and your hands. Riding forward is the most important thing, using your legs, seat and back and letting the horse feel that your hands are allowing it to go forward but will prevent it from turning or whipping round. A well-timed smack may be necessary.

Overtightening of the reins on a fresh, lively horse is the commonest cause of this behaviour which may, under these circumstances, cause the horse to canter sideways, run backwards, whip round or rear.

Having had the confidence to pass a 'monster' once, a genuinely frightened horse may not be frightened of the same thing a second time.

A naughty horse may regularly spook at the same log or bench and use it as an excuse to misbehave. The naughty horse must learn to respect and obey you. The frightened horse must learn to have confidence in you and believe that it will be all right if it obeys you and goes where you ask it to. You have a responsibility to a young and nervous horse. If it is to continue to believe in you, you must not ask too much too soon. Build up its confidence gradually; whether you are hacking out, teaching it to jump or rebuilding its confidence when jumping, don't ask too much too soon.

SENDING YOUR HORSE TO AN EXPERT FOR HELP

If you have had problems with your horse such as napping, whipping round, shying and dropping a shoulder or bucking to get you off, you must realise that it is almost certain to revert to these bad habits when you ride it again. It is essential that you ride your horse in the company of the expert so that they can help and advise you. You must regain your confidence and determination and your horse must learn to respect you and obey you. If possible, also get the expert to ride out with you when you get your horse home because even if you have managed to control it on the expert's ground it is almost sure to 'try it on' again on its home ground where it has previously had success and got its own way.

TURNING DIFFICULTIES

There can be several causes of this problem.

- The horse may have sharp teeth on one side of its mouth. When you use the rein to ask the horse to turn, pressure may be put on its cheek so that it comes in contact with the sharp teeth. The horse may then throw its head up to avoid the pain and be loath to turn in that direction. Get a vet or horse dentist to check and, if necessary, rasp the horse's teeth. As a routine, horses should have their teeth checked at least once a year.
- The horse may have discomfort in its spine – anywhere from its head to its tail. It may turn reluctantly and stiffly as if it is trying not to bend any part of its neck or back. Sometimes you may feel this resistance only when asking the horse to turn in one direction; sometimes it is reluctant to turn in either direction. There may be other signs of discomfort (see Back Problems, page 118). Ask a registered equine chiropractor to check the horse over.
- The horse may simply be stiffer on one side than the other and find it easier to turn in one direction than in the other. This is true of most horses to some extent, unless they have been very well schooled and suppled. (See the suppling exercises on pages 257-9.)
- The horse may have learnt to fall out through the opposite shoulder and to continue to move away from the direction in which you are trying to turn it. This habit is usually caused by riders who try to turn left by using the left rein only, leaving the right rein slack. The horse turns its head and neck left, falls out through its right shoulder and continues to move right in the direction that it wants to go, usually towards home or towards other horses.

When turning a horse, there should not be any more bend in the neck than there is in the rest of the body. To keep this slight, even curve when asking a horse to turn, you must keep a contact on the outside rein because it is this rein which not only controls the pace, but also controls the amount of bend in the neck.

It is a common sight to see riders trying to turn a horse by using one rein only. When the horse's body does not follow its head, they then use that one rein more and more until the horse's head is almost on their knee, yet the horse continues to move in the opposite direction. When you pull a horse's head round to the left (and pull is what many riders do in desperation!), it will step across and under with its near (left) hind leg and push its body over to the right with its right shoulder leading the way.

You must have a contact on the outside rein *before* you start to ask for the turn. If you know you are approaching a place where the horse may argue because it wants to go towards home or towards others, you must begin your preparations before the horse starts to think about what it wants to do. Prevention is far easier than correction, so think ahead. If you have a horse which has learnt to argue, it may be necessary to be quite strong with your outside rein when you are trying to control the amount of bend in the neck. You must, of course, also use your legs very strongly at the same time, using your outside leg on the girth to prevent the horse's shoulder from going sideways in the direction that it wants to go. Use your inside leg behind the girth to ask the horse to move its quarters over so that its forehand will come round in the direction that you want to go.

It can be helpful if when, say, turning left, you take your left hand out and away from the horse's neck and almost lead it round with a feel, feel, feeling action. At the same time, use the right rein quite strongly on the right side of the horse's neck so that you are both controlling the amount of bend and 'neck reining' the horse round the turn. When turning left, carry your stick in your right hand and tap, tap with it on your horse's right shoulder.

You will find it much easier to turn a horse if it has more weight on its hindquarters than on its forehand because it will not then lean on your hands and feel heavy in front. Begin your preparations to turn by using your legs to make your horse step under more with its hind legs, while checking slightly with your hands. This should have the effect of rebalancing the horse by moving its centre of gravity further back. Known as a half-halt (see page 269), this rebalancing is necessary to some degree before all changes of pace, gait or direction.

Suppling exercises (see pages 257-9) will help to correct a turning problem.

Bits

I think it is easier to turn a horse and guide it accurately in a jointed bit than in a straight bar bit because the jointed bit wraps round its lower jaw.

A jointed bit with cheeks, in conjunction with a drop noseband, can be very helpful on a horse which is difficult to turn or guide accurately.

EXCITABLE HORSES

Some horses are naturally more highly strung and excitable than others. Others have become overexcited by the way they have been ridden.

A calm, confident, experienced rider who sits in balance with the horse, has sympathetic hands and uses smooth, gentle aids will get on better with a highly strung, excitable horse and may even make it appear easy to ride. A rough, uncoordinated, unbalanced or nervous, clutchy rider may transform the same horse into a cavorting prancing bag of nerves within seconds of getting on it. It will appear almost unridable while this person is on it.

Sensible horses can become overexcited and difficult to ride if the rider constantly races others, uses sudden, jerky aids, whips the horse round in its tracks and then goes flat out immediately. A horse can be upset by a rider who constantly hits it for no reason that the horse can understand. A too-severe bit can also upset and overexcite a horse.

Ride an excitable horse in the mildest bit possible, perhaps a rubber or nylon snaffle. Some horses prefer a jointed bit to a straight bar, so see which suits your horse. The horse may be even calmer in a mild bitless bridle but try this out first in an enclosed area to be sure you have enough control. Some horses are calmer alone, others are calmer in company. See which situation is best for your horse. Some horses are calmer out on a hack, others settle better when ridden in a small, enclosed area.

Ride your horse wherever it goes most quietly. Ride it in a rhythm and try to have a 'metronome' in your head so that you will notice if the horse's rhythm quickens. Talk or sing to the horse to keep it calm. Think ahead and prepare the horse carefully and gently for every change of gait or direction. As the horse relaxes, it will adopt a lower head carriage, longer, lower stride and quieter, softer hoofbeats. Ride with a very light rein contact and teach the horse to respond to the lightest aids. Using the slightest change of your weight, or your voice, rather than your reins to slow down or turn often helps to keep the horse calm.

Only when your horse will go calmly and in a rhythm in all gaits on a light rein contact can you begin to school it further and ask it to come on the bit and be as obedient and accurate as in a dressage test. If you attempt to school a tense, excitable horse, it is likely to shorten its stride and raise the level of its head carriage. Its hoofbeats will be loud and staccato. Its response to your aids will be quick, jerky and unbalanced. It may lean on the bit and stiffen against your hands.

The problem is often one of mental worry and stress so you must be patient and understanding.

HOLLOW BACK, HEAD IN AIR

The result of this is often the same as head in air, hollow back but the cause can be very different.

If it is hollow back that is leading to head in air, one of the following causes is probable.

- A sore back caused by an ill-fitting saddle putting pressure on the horse's spine. A scalded back caused by excessive movement of an ill-fitting saddle.
- An unbalanced rider sitting too far back in the saddle and causing pressure on the spine. A scalded back caused by the rider sitting over to one side, thus producing excessive sideways movement of the saddle.
- A heavy rider making the horse uncomfortable by sitting very much behind the movement (behind the horse's centre of gravity) too near to the horse's loins (the weakest part of its back). (See Sitting in Balance, below.)
- Damage to the horse's spine or pelvis, which could be painful when ridden. (See Back Problems, page 118.)

A horse which goes hollow-backed because of any of these problems is almost certain also to go 'head in air'. As the back goes hollow and the hind legs are left behind, the head and neck automatically come up. Try it yourself on hands and knees or even sitting in a chair. Hollow your back and you will feel your head and neck come up. Now round your back – you will find raising your neck and head much more difficult.

Ask an experienced person to check the fitting of your saddle, your horse's spine and the muscular area on each side of the spine which carries the saddle. Ask them to watch you riding both from the side and from the back. If there is no obvious cause for your horse's back problem, ask a qualified equine chiropractor to examine your horse.

Sitting in balance with your horse

Use a well-fitting saddle which is comfortable for both the horse and you – one which helps you to sit in balance over the horse's centre of gravity by having its lowest point fairly close to the stirrup bars. A saddle which tilts up in front and slopes down towards the back will encourage your seat to slide back to its lowest point. Your lower leg will then come forward so that you will be sitting behind the movement, behind the horse's centre of gravity and too near the loins.

Sitting in this way makes you both difficult and uncomfortable for the horse to carry. Have you ever carried a heavy pack on your back which seems to be hanging down too near to your waist? It feels uncomfortable and difficult to carry so you hitch it up higher, closer to your shoulders, nearer to your centre of gravity and it immediately becomes both more comfortable and easier to carry. You are the 'heavy pack' on your horse's back. Make sure that you are in the easiest and most comfortable place for your horse to carry you.

When the horse's hollow back is the *cause* of the problem and its head in the air the *result*, you must encourage the horse to raise the part of its back behind the saddle and step under more with its hind legs. You will need to sit well forward in the saddle and, to obtain the best and quickest results, to keep your seat right out of the saddle. It is easier to do this if you shorten your stirrups to jumping length so that you can adopt jumping position and stay in it. Keeping your weight forward, out of the saddle, walk your horse on a 20-m circle on a very light rein contact. Working in circles encourages the horse to step forward and under with its inside hind leg and to carry itself. Let it feel that you have 'allowing hands', which will encourage it to step forward and lower its neck and head.

When this is working well in walk on both reins and the horse feels relaxed and is beginning to take a longer stride, try the same thing in trot, still keeping your weight well forward and your seat out of the saddle. You will be holding yourself in balance over the horse's centre of gravity without rising to the trot.

Most horses will go hollow-backed in downwards transitions. To help to avoid this, keep your weight forward and out of the saddle as before and, as you ask for a downwards transition from trot to walk or walk to halt, bring the horse smoothly on to a smaller circle. It will then step under more with its inside hind leg, making it easier for it to keep the roundness in its back. Use this turning in to get the horse to slow down of its own accord. Do *not* use the reins to slow down or the horse will go hollow.

Let the horse feel how much easier and more comfortable it is to go in this rounder way.

The rider getting even a fraction behind the movement has a very obvious effect on most horses. Have you ever trotted across a school to change direction and, as you changed diagonal, got behind the movement (perhaps coming down with a bit of a bump on the horse's back) and felt it go hollow-backed immediately, come above the bit with its head in the air and possibly quicken its stride?

The position of the rider in relation to the horse's centre of gravity is the key to good riding. The rider's ability to sit quietly in balance and adjust that balance smoothly and accurately as the horse changes gait and/or direction is absolutely essential. Without this ability, you are unlikely to improve a horse with any of these problems.

The horse must be going calmly and rounded correctly on the flat in all three gaits of walk, trot and canter before you think of jumping. Do not use sitting trot because at this stage the horse is likely to stiffen its back and go hollow again.

Trotting poles, especially on a circle using a 'fan' of poles (see page 282) can encourage a horse to round its back and lower its head. They usually work well with a horse whose problem starts with a hollow back and they can be introduced earlier.

A fussy, excitable horse whose problem starts with its head in the air, however, may be made worse by working over trotting poles too soon because of its natural tendency to rush.

Head in air, hollow back

These problems go together so often that they can be considered as 'cause and effect' in whichever order they are creating a problem.

If it is head in the air that is leading to hollow back, one of the following causes is probable.

- sharp teeth or wolf teeth (see page 108);
- sore corners of lips (see page 79);
- a too-severe or uncomfortable bit;
- the rider's hard, rough or unsteady hands;
- poor conformation, such as a ewe neck, in which the topline of the neck is concave and there is often a large bulge of muscle on the underside of the neck. A thin, weak neck, with the head set on so that its natural carriage is high, often occurs with a ewe neck. When looking at horses loose in the field, take note of any which, in play, fling their heads up and back towards where a rider would be sitting. This natural action often denotes a future problem when ridden. It may be possible to overcome this tendency but it could be a very long-term project. If possible, avoid buying a young horse showing this behaviour.

An older horse with a ewe neck, with no muscle on top of its neck and a thick bulge under its neck, is a sure indication that it has been allowed to go in an incorrect outline for some time. It may be strong and keen and have learnt to put its head up and lean against a running martingale or even more so against a standing martingale. It may be a thick, bullocky type of horse which uses its strength and muscle to get its own way.

The same conformation and incorrect outline of concave topline of neck and bulge of muscle underneath can be seen on hot, fussy Thoroughbred types which skit about all over the place and are very difficult to guide accurately.

In all of these cases the high head carriage is causing the hollow back.

There will be tension in all of these horses. Get expert help to find out the main cause of the problem.

- If the teeth are sharp ask a vet or equine dentist to rasp them or deal with any problems.
- See page 111 if the corners of the lips are sore.
- See page 76 for advice on bits and their fitting.
- If the rider's hands are a problem, get expert help. Try holding the reins so that they come from the bit into your hand between your index fingers and thumbs and leave them by your little fingers. This way of holding the reins will allow you to be far more supple and sympathetic in all your arm joints, particularly your shoulders. Stiffness in the shoulders often prevents a rider's hands from following the natural movement of a horse's head, resulting in a jerky, loose–tight contact on the horse's mouth. The reaction

of a sensitive horse is to put its head up in the air so that the jerks come on its lips instead of on the more sensitive bars of the mouth.

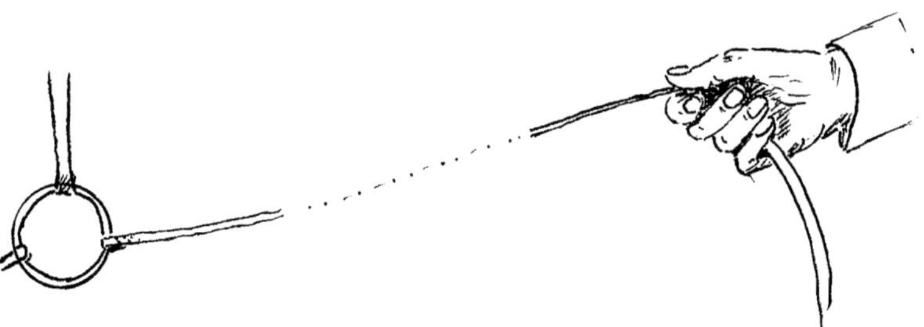

If you feel you are a bit heavy handed or are stiff in wrists, elbows or shoulders, try holding your reins like this. You will be amazed by the difference it will make to you and to your horse.

A horse with its head up in this position in order to evade the bit is far more difficult to stop or guide. The head-high position is often accompanied by swinging the hindquarters to one side or by swinging them from one side to the other to evade control by the rider's legs.

When the more obvious possible problems of teeth, lips, bits and hands have been identified and improved as far as possible, a long-term plan for correction is necessary. To get rid of the tension and encourage the horse to lower its head and lengthen the top of its neck, it can be lunged in an enclosed area or the corner of small paddock in just a cavesson.

Some horses may not be controllable in a field in only a cavesson. Such horses will need a small fenced-in area in which to be safely lunged or, if you have a small, safe, enclosed area, they can be loose-schooled (see page 162). With no contact at all on their heads, they may relax more quickly.

As soon as possible the horse can be ridden in the same schooling area that was used for lungeing or loose-schooling, where it has already learnt to relax. Ride at a walk on as light a rein contact as possible and sit quietly in balance with your horse. See if weight forward and seat out of the saddle give a better result.

Gradually ask the horse to halt or change direction to your voice, weight and leg aids, all used very gently and tactfully with little or no rein contact. When the horse will circle, halt and change direction without tensing up or raising its head, introduce a little rising trot (sitting trot at this stage may produce tension in both rider and horse and can be tried later). If the horse tenses or raises its head too much, revert to walk and try again later.

Head in the air and hollow back are almost always accompanied by short jerky steps in all gaits. The hoofbeats are hard and loud. When the strides become longer, as the horse begins to lower its head, and the hoofbeats

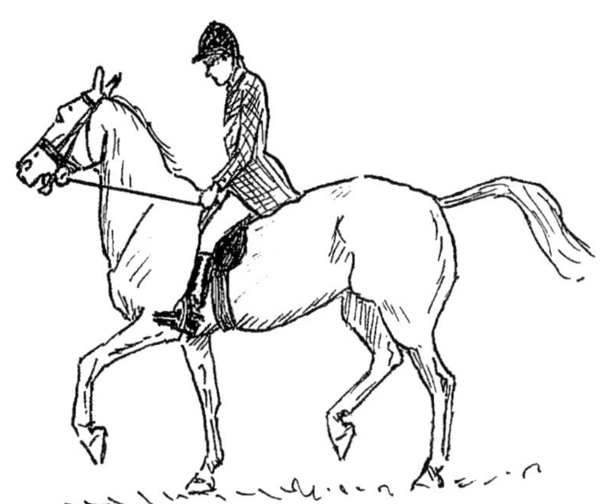

Head in air – hollow back. The rider is stiffening his shoulders, elbows, wrists and hands and pushing downwards. He is bracing himself against his stirrups and so is sitting towards the back of the saddle.

sound quieter, you know you are starting to make some progress in improving the horse's way of going.

Some horses relax and learn more quickly with no bit in their mouths and the reins attached instead to the rings of a correctly fitted drop noseband (fitted high enough so that it rests on the bone of the nose, not restricting the passage of air through the nostrils). If in doubt about safely controlling the horse like this, have a bit in its mouth and use two sets of reins, one pair attached to the bit and one to the noseband and only use the bit reins in an emergency.

A Market Harborough (see page 266), fitted by an expert and, at first, used only under their supervision is, in my opinion, the best aid to improving this problem once the horse has relaxed and is not fighting the rider. It is not something that you should suddenly put on a very excitable, scatty, head in air horse, however, as some horses of this type may panic, run backwards and lose their balance when incorrectly introduced to this item of equipment.

As soon as possible, hack the horse out gently, concentrating on keeping it relaxed and trying not to allow it to go with its head in the air by riding it forward and having little or no rein contact at first. Alternate hacking and schooling and gradually introduce the gaits of trot and canter.

WANDERING

Young and unschooled horses find it difficult to go in a straight line. If possible, at first use a natural path, furrow or wheel mark and, with hands and legs, ride the horse straight along this. Try to use your legs more than your reins to keep the horse in a straight line. Ride it forward so that it is held between your legs and your hands. Start in walk then progress to trot and canter if the horse will remain calmly in a rhythm. Still use your natural 'guide lines'. Next use markers and ride straight from one marker directly to the next. Markers help you to have an exact aim and to know that you are riding accurately.

If you are riding in company, do not allow your horse to follow directly behind another horse. Make it take its own straight line slightly to one side of the other horse. At first, using the natural guide of something like wheel marks will help.

A well-schooled horse will go in a straight line on a loose rein, controlled only by your legs.

SIGNS OF TIREDNESS

Reaching when tired

In walk or trot a tired horse may stretch its head forward and down, reaching at the reins every few strides. This is a much slower and gentler movement than the reaching and diving (see page 225) which nearly pulls the rider out of the saddle. It looks more like the stretching of aching muscles. Dismount and lead the horse.

Stumbling when tired

A very tired horse begins to lose the natural rhythmic sequence of foot movements and so will stumble and may nearly fall because it will be slow to bring another foot forward quickly to save itself in the normal way. The horse may feel that it is almost fumbling along.

In both of these cases, dismount and lead the horse, loosening its girth a few holes before you do so. Horses which show these signs of tiredness are getting too much work for their stage of fitness, too much work for the food they are receiving, too much work for their age, their rider is too heavy for them or they are not well. Worms or anaemia can both cause abnormal weakness and tiredness in horses.

Brushing when tired

A horse which does not normally brush may do so when tired. It may become less active in its movement and slightly unbalanced. This will alter its normal foot flight so that one foot will knock the opposite leg.

Horses which stand with their toes out in front (see page 00) are more likely to brush. Horses which stand cow hocked (hocks turned in) are more likely to brush behind. The lower, inside part of the fetlock joint is the place most commonly hit by the shoe on the opposite foot of a tired horse.

Buffing

Another form of 'interfering' seen on tired horses is the white line on the inside of the coronet caused by buffing. This can be seen in front and behind but is commonest behind. The mark is made by the shoe of the opposite foot and may sometimes wear so deep a groove that it draws blood. Buffing is often seen on horses which have been doing a lot of school work and circling, especially if they are not used to it. It is often seen, for instance, on ponies towards the end of several days of Pony Club camp.

A horse which does not normally brush or buff probably just needs a few days of rest. If the problem is more frequent, see Brushing on page 139.

Clicking and forging

These names are given to the noise made when the toe of the hind shoe as it comes down catches on the toe of the front shoe as it is being picked up.

A horse may click or forge when tired because a tired horse often starts to go on its forehand. The forelegs are therefore a little slower to pick up and so the hind legs catch up with them.

It can be a sign that the horse's feet have grown too long and it needs shoeing. Sloppy riding can also allow a horse to go in this way.

Resting two legs at once

A tired, leg-weary horse may be seen in a field or stable resting two legs at the same time. One foreleg is stuck out in front with the foot flat on the ground and the diagonally opposite hind leg is also resting, hock bent and toe only on the ground.

NB: this action of resting a foreleg is quite different to the stance of an unsound horse 'pointing' a foreleg. When a horse is 'pointing' to take the weight off a painful foot, it will rest only the toe of the front foot on the ground. It will be standing square behind with both hind legs sharing its weight equally.

Lying down

If a horse is seen lying down a lot during the day in field or stable, when it does not normally do so, this can be a sign of tiredness. If your horse has had hard or long work in the past few days, this is likely to be the cause. If this is not the case, the horse may be feeling unwell, so keep a careful eye on it. It can also be a sign of laminitis (see page 144).

EVADING THE BIT

Horses evade the bit for many reasons.
 1 The rider's hands are too hard and strong.
 2 The rider's hands are unsteady and therefore the contact of the bit with the horse's mouth is often loose, tight, loose, jerky.
 3 The horse's mouth is sore at the corner (See Split Lip, page 111.)
 4 The horse has sharp teeth. (See page 108.)
 5 The bit does not fit the horse (See Bitting, page 76.)
 6 The bit is hanging too low or too high in the horse's mouth. (See page 77).
 7 The bit is too narrow, sharp and severe on the bars of the horse's mouth.
 8 The bit is too thick to be comfortable in the horse's mouth because this horse has a very thick tongue.
 9 The horse is frightened of being ridden in a curb bit.
10 The horse has protruding glands on each side of the throat, just behind the long, curving cheekbone. When it lowers its head to come on the bit these glands are pinched between the curve of the cheek bone and neck muscle.

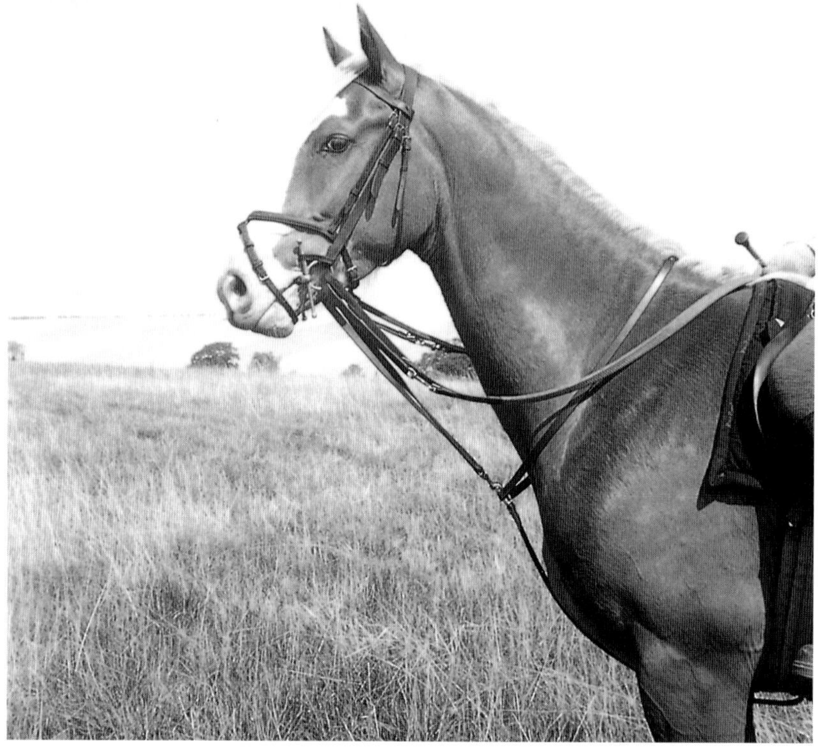

There is a weak topline to the neck and a bulge of muscle under the neck. The horse is being worked in a Market Harborough to correct this.

11 The horse has a ewe neck and has developed a large bulge of hard muscle under its neck which prevents it from lowering its head and lengthening and arching the top of its neck. This incorrect muscle development can be the result of 1, 2, 3, 4, 5, 7, 9 or 10 above.

What you need is expert help from a rider whose horses you have seen going calmly and happily and who seems to ride them effectively without any visible aids. It is not easy for an inexperienced person to pinpoint the problem you are having. It may be you, it may be the horse or it may be a combination of several of the things I have suggested.

1 and 2 Your hands are too strong or are giving an unsteady or uneven jerky contact on the bit. (This may be particularly true in sitting trot if you find this difficult.) Try holding the reins so that as they come from the horse's mouth they enter your hands via your index finger and thumb and leave your hand by your little finger. Hold your hands so that your palms and fingernails are facing upwards. You will find that, in this position, your wrists, elbows and shoulder joints are all much freer and more supple so it is easier for you to follow the movement of the horse's head. The horse moves its head most in walk. It is easiest to sit quietly and balanced in the

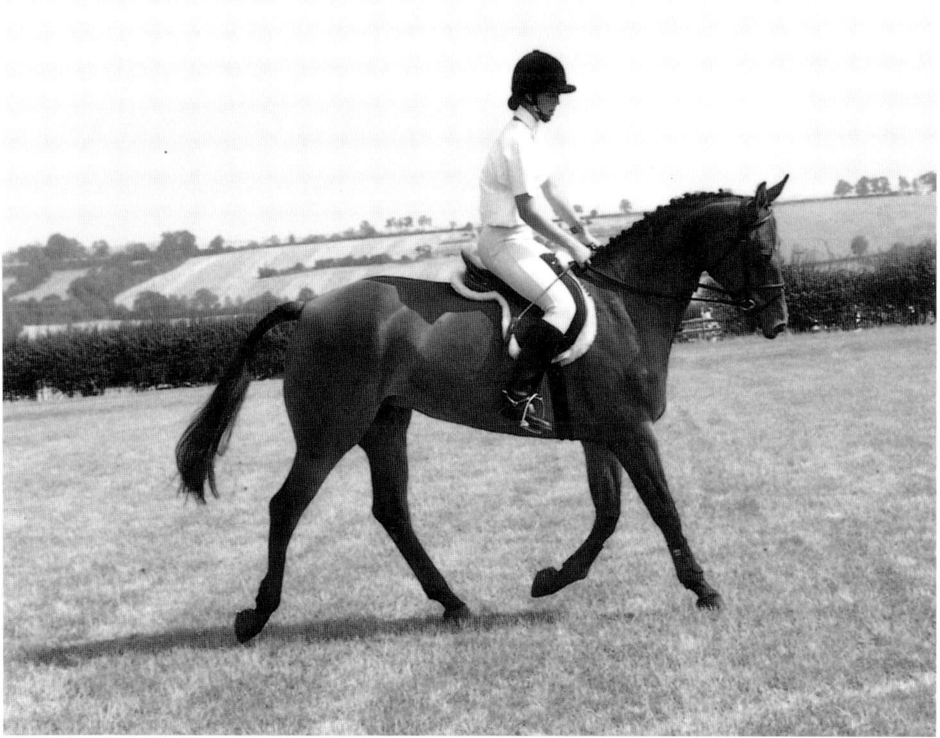

The rider is stiffening her hand and wrist in trying to 'ask' the horse's head down.

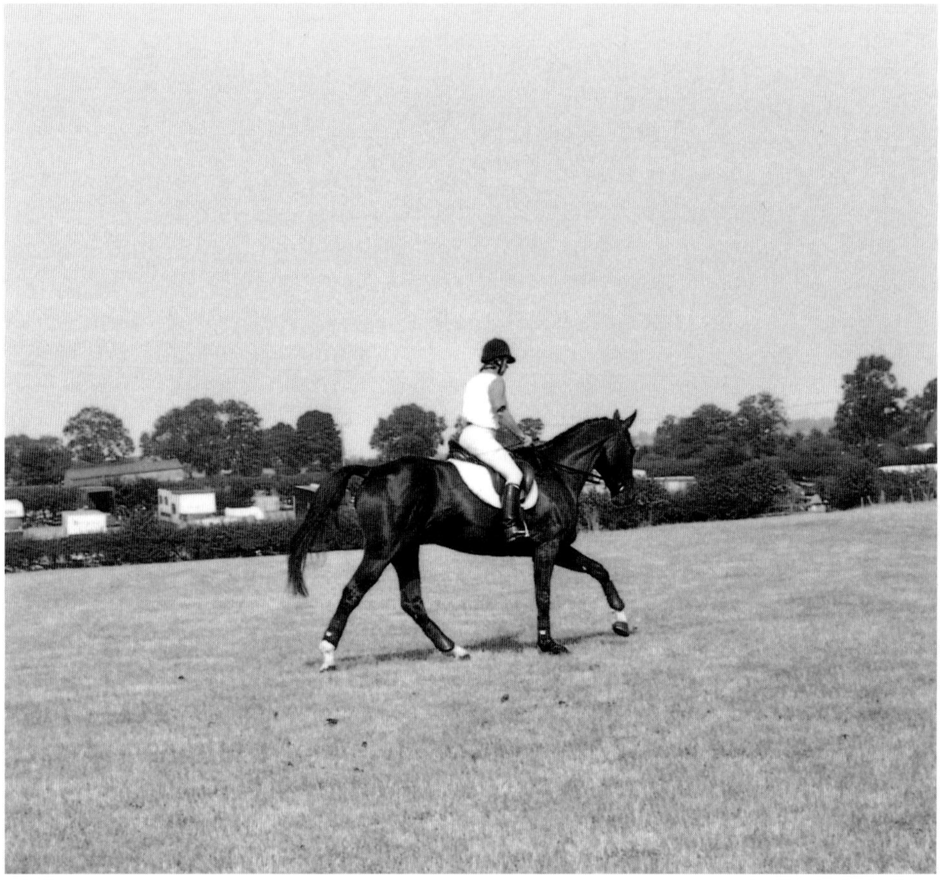

The horse is stepping under with the inside hind leg and is accepting the bit happily.

saddle at walk so practise in this gait. Remember that your hands belong to your horse's mouth and must follow it at all times.

3 Examine the corners of the lips and right inside where the lip has a double fold back which may be split.

4 Get a vet or horse dentist to inspect the teeth.

5, 6, 7 and 8 Get an expert to check your bit and its fitting.

9 Try riding the horse in a snaffle bit. If you are worried that it is too strong for you in a snaffle, ride it in a small, enclosed area. It may take several days or a week before the horse will relax and lower its head in a snaffle or you may find an almost immediate difference.

10 Protruding glands are usually an on-going problem.

11 This can have started with naturally bad conformation or be the result of many of the items in my list. (See Hollow Back Head in Air page 240; Head in Air, Hollow Back page 243; Ewe Neck, page 6; and Market Harborough, page 266.)

TONGUE OVER THE BIT

A horse learns to get its tongue over the bit to avoid pressure on its tongue. A horse which gets its tongue over the bit is more difficult to control.

The habit very often starts if the bit is fitted too low in a young horse's mouth. Once learnt, it is very difficult to cure.

A jointed bit which is too wide for a horse can cause this problem because the V of the joint hangs so low in the mouth that it is very easy to get the tongue over. Many big Thoroughbred horses have very narrow mouths and need only a pony-size bit yet, because they are 16 h.h. or more, they are put in a full-size bit. This is especially true with racehorses where, as they are turned, you can often see three inches of bit hanging out of their mouths on one side.

A straight-bar or half-moon bit gives more direct pressure on the centre of the tongue than a jointed bit. Even though these bits hang higher in the mouth than the centre of a normal jointed bit, some horses still object to them and get their tongues over.

A French snaffle with cheeks hangs high in the horse's mouth, held up by small leather loops attached to the cheekpieces of the bridle.

The soft, figure-of-eight-shaped, double joint in the mouthpiece allows room for the tongue and does not have the 'nutcracker' action of a single-jointed bit. I have found this bit, with cheeks set a hole higher than normal, to be the most successful cure for the tongue-over problem.

(The Dr Bristol, also double jointed but with a flat, sharp-edged centre plate is *not* suitable.)

Special bits can be bought whose purpose is to prevent a horse getting its tongue over. Some have a grid which lies on the horse's tongue above the bit. There is also a rubber Juba tongue port which fits on to a straight-bar or half-moon bit and lies along the tongue above the bit. It is not successful on a jointed bit.

A thin metal extra mouthpiece, roughly in the shape of a W and attached by its own leather headpiece, can be used in conjunction with any bit. The centre part hangs higher in the mouth.

A horse must open its mouth slightly to manoeuvre its tongue up and over the bit so sometimes a fairly tight drop noseband in conjunction with a French snaffle with cheeks does the trick. If given the chance, however, most horses will revert to this habit.

LEANING ON THE BIT

Horses lean on the bit for one or more of the following reasons.
- The horse wants to go faster and the rider holds it back with an even, dead pull which it learns to lean on.

- The horse's conformation makes it heavy in front so that its centre of gravity is naturally too far forward. It may have big, thick shoulders and weak hindquarters. It may be built higher in the hindquarters than at the withers. It may have a thick, heavy neck or a very big head. Any of these conformation problems will make the horse heavy on its forehand and looking for something to lean on for balance – often the bit.
- The horse may have been ridden at too fast a pace. It may have learnt that if it keeps trotting fast it can keep its balance if it leans on the bit and so feels very heavy on the rider's hands and shoulders.

The main problem in each case is the horse's centre of gravity being too far forward. The horse is literally tipping forward on to the bit to keep its balance and is allowing the rider to take its weight and hold it up.

If a horse is leaning on the bit and therefore on your hands, you cannot stop it doing so by holding it back more nor by trying to lift its head up higher. Its hind legs are left behind and it is trundling along on its head!

You must get it to move its centre of gravity further back, step under its body more with its hind legs and carry itself without leaning on you. A horse which is on its forehand will often click and forge (see page 151), names given to the noise made when the toe of the hind shoe, as it is going down, catches on the

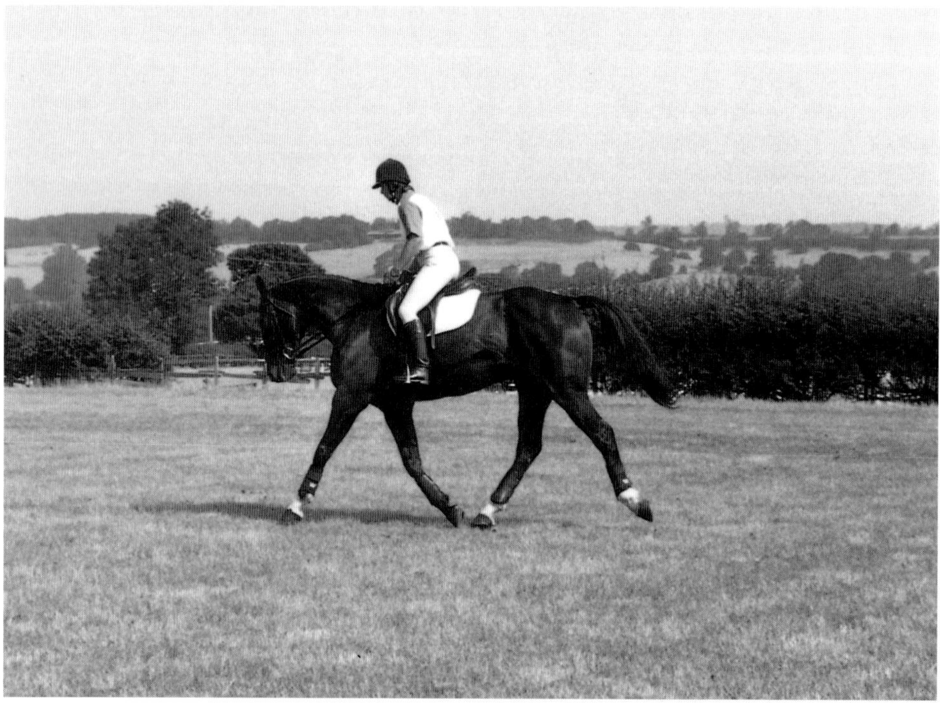

The horse is trotting too fast for its stage of schooling, pushing itself on to its forehand and leaning on the bit.

toe of the front shoe as it is coming up. As your horse improves and begins to carry itself, instead of leaning on you, it should cease to make this noise.

Most horses lean more on a straight-bar or half-moon, unjointed bit so use a jointed bit. If the horse is used to a normal jointed snaffle with rings and no cheeks, change to a jointed snaffle with cheeks. The cheeks are kept in place close to the cheekpieces of the bridle by little leather keepers on each side of the bridle. A cheek snaffle with keepers will sit higher in the mouth than an ordinary jointed snaffle (see diagram, page 76). It will feel different so the horse will not be as likely to lean on it. By the same token, if the horse is used to a cheek snaffle, change to an ordinary snaffle because it will also feel different and make the horse think.

Ride the horse on a 20-m circle in walk, slightly raising your inside hand as you do so. This will allow the horse to step under its body and forward with its inside hind leg. This is the first step towards moving its centre of gravity further back. Stepping forward and under with its inside hind leg is essential to improving the horse so be very careful not to lower your inside hand as you ask the horse to turn on a circle or you will completely block that inside hind leg and actually prevent it from stepping forward and under.

The fault of lowering the inside hand on turns and circles is one of the commonest faults in riding and can be seen in all gaits.

Decrease and increase the size of your circles on both reins and ride the horse forward with your legs into a steady but active walk. Repeat the circle work in trot, again being careful not to lower your inside hand. If the horse tries to hurry do not hold it back but make the circle smaller. See which works best for you and your horse, rising trot or sitting trot. Horses which are trying to hurry and go faster are usually better ridden in rising trot and slower horses in sitting trot. If, as you change direction from one circle to another, the horse tries to rush as soon as its head and body are in a straight line between the two circles, only change direction in walk. Ride your downwards transitions by turning in on to a smaller circle and use your voice to ask the horse for a slower gait. Use as little rein as possible. You should very soon begin to feel that the horse is not leaning on your hands so much. This is partly because you are not giving it the opportunity to do so and partly because it should, by now, be finding it easier to carry itself because it is stepping forward and under more with its hind legs.

Reining back (see page 272) for a few paces then immediately going forward into trot on a circle can give you and the horse the feeling of balance and self-carriage which you are aiming for. When the horse reins back, its hind legs are right up under it and its centre of gravity is automatically moved further back as long as it does not rein back with its head between its knees. If it does do this you cannot use rein back as a method of improving its balance.

Keep the pace of trot steady but active. If the horse keeps trundling along at a fast trot, it will not improve so quickly. At a slow but active trot, it has to carry itself.

Once the horse is light on trot circles, start to ride straight lines but revert to the circle and make it smaller as soon as the horse gets heavy again in front. If you have been using rein back successfully, turn in on to the circle then ask for a few steps of rein back. Ride a straight line on the long sides of a marked-out school of 20 x 40 m and ride circles on the short sides. Ride straight across the diagonal using a circle before and after.

Canter is the most difficult gait in which to keep a horse light in front. The horse must now lower its hindquarters and lighten its forehand, something that a problem horse will find very difficult. To canter, the horse has to lift and round its back just behind the saddle. It will find this far easier to do if your weight is forward out of the saddle. Put your stirrups up two holes, which will make it easier for you to sit forward and in balance. Ride a 20-m circle in rising trot and, as you ask for canter on the same circle, bring your weight forward and a little more into your inside stirrup iron. Only have just enough rein contact to guide your horse on the circle. If it tries to hurry, make the circle smaller. As long as it is not hurrying or leaning on you, canter two or three circles one after the other, then walk and give the horse a rest. Keep your seat out of the saddle before you ask for canter, during canter and when you ask for trot.

When you feel that the horse is carrying itself and finding canter easier, you can gradually and gently sit down into the saddle after the first few strides of a good canter. Hopefully, you will soon be able to sit normally throughout all gaits but horses which have been allowed to become heavy on their forehands and have leant on their bits for years can take a very long time to improve.

PULLING, RESCHOOLING AND CONTROL

If your horse is always pulling at you and trying to go faster and faster, you will find it difficult to ride in balance. In canter, you may find the horse difficult to control.

The problem is usually tension which can have several causes: worry, fear, excitement, discomfort.

- **Worry** A rider who does not sit in balance with the horse, in such a way that their two centres of gravity coincide, can have an adverse effect on the horse. An uncoordinated, tense or nervous rider can upset a sensitive horse.
- **Fear** A rider who is rough with hands, legs, spurs or whip can thoroughly upset any horse.
- **Excitement** A horse which has been raced about, allowed to trot flat out and canter on every bit of grass it is hacked over may pull out of excitement.
- **Discomfort and pain** A horse may try to run away from the pain of a badly fitting saddle, a back problem or a painful bit.

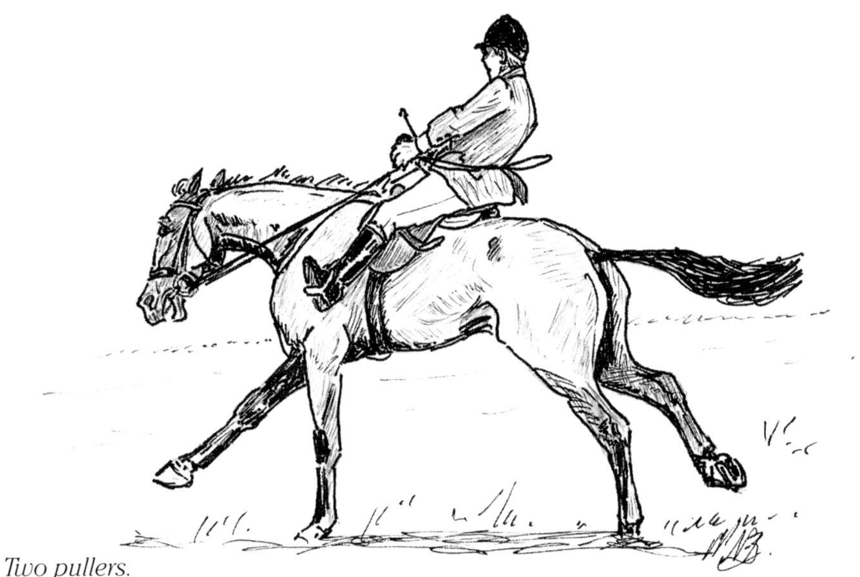

Two pullers.

All of these horses will be tense but their way of pulling will vary. Some will try to lean on the rider's hands, set their necks against the rider's hands and go faster and faster. Some will reach and dive their heads downwards and try to pull the rider out of the saddle and so get a longer rein which will enable them to go faster. Others will canter on the spot, head up or up and sideways, throw their heads up violently or shoot sideways, one way and then the other. Neither a more severe bit nor giving them a good gallop until they are tired is the answer. Unfortunately for the horses concerned, both of these suggestions are often made.

First check that the horse's mouth and lips are not sore or being pinched and that its teeth are not sharp and cutting the inside of its cheeks. Check the fitting of the saddle, check for any discomfort on or beside the spine or for inward pressure just below the withers. Check for girth galls.

You are more likely to be able to teach a horse to relax if it lives out or is at least turned out for part of each day. Shutting a horse in a stable for 23 hours a day creates tension.

Lunge the horse quietly. Many horses relax on the lunge and only tense up when ridden; others will tear round frantically on the lunge as well. If lunged quietly every day in an enclosed ring, most horses will begin to settle into a rhythmic trot and will eventually walk of their own accord. For many days, or even weeks, a very tense horse will still set off at a flat-out trot on the lunge. Your aim must be to have a calm, relaxed horse which will move off at walk. You need to lunge a strong, excitable horse in an enclosed area because it is very difficult to control a horse which can only think of going faster and faster. In an open field, it is likely that you will let go of it, so only lunge this type of horse in an enclosure.

Riding a tense, pulling horse

Ride in an enclosed area because the horse will soon realise that there is nowhere to go. Sit forward with your weight out of the saddle. Ride in circles at walk. If your horse keeps breaking into a trot, keep your weight forward, gently steady the horse to walk on a smaller circle, use your voice, say 'W–A–L–K' and give it a looser rein immediately it walks. Do this by pushing your hands forward, not by constantly lengthening and shortening the reins. The action of shortening the reins is a 'go, go' signal to any badly schooled horse, so avoid this.

When the horse will walk in circles in both directions with a low, relaxed neck and head carriage and no tension in its back, gently sit down in the saddle. Make sure you sit well forward in the saddle and do not slide to the back of it, legs forward, and get behind the movement as this will upset a sensitive horse.

Try a few steps of trot, again with your weight forward out of the saddle. Work on a circle and turn the horse inwards on to a smaller circle to slow it down. A few steps of trot then walk will have a calming effect if you keep on doing this. The horse will not get excited because it knows that it is soon going to be asked to walk again. Circle in both directions, first 20 m, then down to 15 m, and, at first, walk as you change the rein between your trotting circles. The action of changing your aids and weight as you change direction will make some horses shoot forward. Use rising trot as sitting trot tends to cause tension in this type of horse, especially if the rider is inclined to stiffen and bounce. If you want to try sitting trot, sit for only a few paces then rise for several. Try the rhythm of rising, sit, sit, sit, rise. This is good for the rider's feel for rhythm and also good for giving them a feeling of being in balance with the horse.

A tense, excitable horse will only improve if ridden by a calm rider capable of sitting in balance with the horse and of smoothly co-ordinating their aids.

Transitions

Teach your horse to slow down to your voice aid and to you sitting down gently in the saddle and slowly moving your shoulders and weight back. Practise walk to halt first. Use no rein or as little as possible at first and then progress so that the horse answers to just your voice and weight.

Riding out

Find out if your horse is calmer and more relaxed alone or in company. If in company, only go out with one other calm and steady animal which will go in an even rhythm. Its rider must understand how you want to improve your horse. Some horses go more calmly when in the lead; others feel safer and relax more when following another. Find out which is best for your horse. At first, practise calm walking and short trots, then transitions from trot to walk to halt. If there is a suitable place and your horse remains calm, you can trot in a circle in one direction while your companion goes in another but, at first, stay within sight of the other horse.

If your horse is calmer alone, practise all the things you did in the enclosed schooling area when riding out.

- **Canter** When your horse will stay in an even rhythm in trot with a light contact on the reins, you can try canter. Alternate riding out and schooling sessions so that the horse will continue to improve in calmness, rhythm and balance in both situations. Towards the end of one of your schooling sessions in the enclosed area, try a few steps of canter. Make as little fuss as possible about this. Keep your body forward, stay in rising trot and, as you approach a corner, move your weight a little more into the inside stirrup iron and forward and use a high, quick voice to say, 'Can–ter'. If the horse just trots faster, quietly bring it on to a circle and ask again in the same way but this time steady your horse slightly with your reins as you ask for canter. Alternatively, ride a 15-m circle in rising trot and, as you ride towards the side/fence on your circle, ask for canter in the same way. Going towards the side/fence makes the horse 'back off' slightly and encourages it to canter without trotting faster.

  Most horses go more quietly if you keep your seat out of the saddle in canter. If you have any problems and the horse tenses and tries to rush, leave it and try again in a few days. You cannot slow a tense horse down by holding it back. If all is well, canter only two or three steps then turn in on a circle and slow your horse down to trot with your weight and voice, sit gently in the saddle, move your weight back a little more and use your voice for walk. Keep on doing this as long as the horse remains calm. Knowing that it is always going to trot or walk again after just a few steps of canter will help to stop it rushing. Try cantering on the short side of the school and trotting on the long side using a 15-m circle in trot before and after each canter to steady and rebalance the horse. Still keep your seat out of the saddle in canter.

Use circles and serpentines in rising trot, being careful to change diagonal very gently and making sure that you stay in balance with the horse when changing diagonal. If the horse shoots forward as you change diagonal, it shows that your co-ordination and sense of balance are not good enough. In this case it is better not to keep changing the diagonal. Your seat should go down gently, just to touch the saddle, as the horse's outside diagonal pair of feet go to the ground in trot. (To change diagonal, sit gently for two beats then start rising again.)

Think and feel what is happening under you. Know what your horse is thinking and feeling. Be patient. Your horse will tell you whether you are riding well or badly! If it shoots forward with head up as you change direction in rising trot, you have probably got behind the movement (at one step of trot your bottom will have bumped the saddle instead of just touching it lightly). You may have changed direction and changed your aids too suddenly. Ride the horse straight for several strides after a turn or circle and before the change of direction to give both you, and then the horse, time to change your bodyweight smoothly.

If, as you trot across the school or up the centre line and approach the wall or fence, the horse changes its bodyweight from left to right, moves its head from left to right or cocks an ear back towards you, it is saying, 'Help, which way do you want me to go?' You have not warned and prepared it soon enough for the change of direction. This is particularly obvious when you watch someone riding serpentines. In this exercise you must change your weight and your aids smoothly as you cross the centre line so that the horse has time to understand what you want and prepare its body for the change of direction. If you ride a serpentine correctly, the horse will go smoothly and confidently forward, often keeping its ears pricked throughout the changes of direction. This shows that it is happily thinking forward, understanding what you want it to do next.

Ride in balance with the horse so that your centre of gravity is directly above its centre of gravity. Imagine that the horse is going to be 'whipped out' from under you. You should land in balance on your feet. This applies whether you are riding with longer stirrup leathers when schooling or with shorter leathers for jumping. It applies at all gaits, going up- and downhill and over a jump. You must change your weight and centre of gravity smoothly and gradually to indicate an increase of pace (a little forward), decrease of pace (a little back), change of direction (a little towards the direction in which you want the horse to go). The horse moves under your centre of gravity as it carries out your wishes and, once more, your two centres of gravity coincide. This is the ideal and if you really think and feel what you are doing and see how the horse responds to your slightest weight movement, you will be surprised to find it is not difficult.

Serpentines, turns and circles

Your weight should be a little more into your inside seat bone. Don't lean, think 'inside heel down'. As you straighten the horse your weight must be central, equal in both seat bones, and as you prepare to change direction you must put more weight smoothly into the new inside seat bone. Only your *weight* is transferred so do not lean your body over to one side – sit upright.

When your horse turns or circles, its inside hind leg must step forward and under. If you drop your inside hand (one of the commonest riding faults), you will stop the horse stepping forward and under. Think of lifting your inside hand to encourage and allow the horse to step forward and under with its inside hind leg.

When the horse is going calmly and in a rhythm, think about getting it to bend in the direction in which it is going by asking a little with the inside rein and allowing a little with the outside rein. You must do this because when you ask the horse to bend, and therefore slightly shorten the inside of its neck, it also has to lengthen the outside of it. Keep a contact on the outside rein and never allow your outside hand to cross over the central line of the horse's neck.

Cantering out on a hack

Keeping the horse calm and controlling it
Always trot first and do not canter until the horse is going calmly in an even rhythm. At first canter uphill, with your seat out of the saddle, at a slow, steady pace. The uphill slope will slow the horse down naturally. Walk after cantering. On the flat, canter for only a few yards so that the horse does not have time to get excited. Keep your seat out of the saddle. Never canter towards home and never canter up level with another horse. If you are riding out with others, ask them not to overtake you at canter. Do not ride out with people who cannot prevent their horses from 'tanking off'.

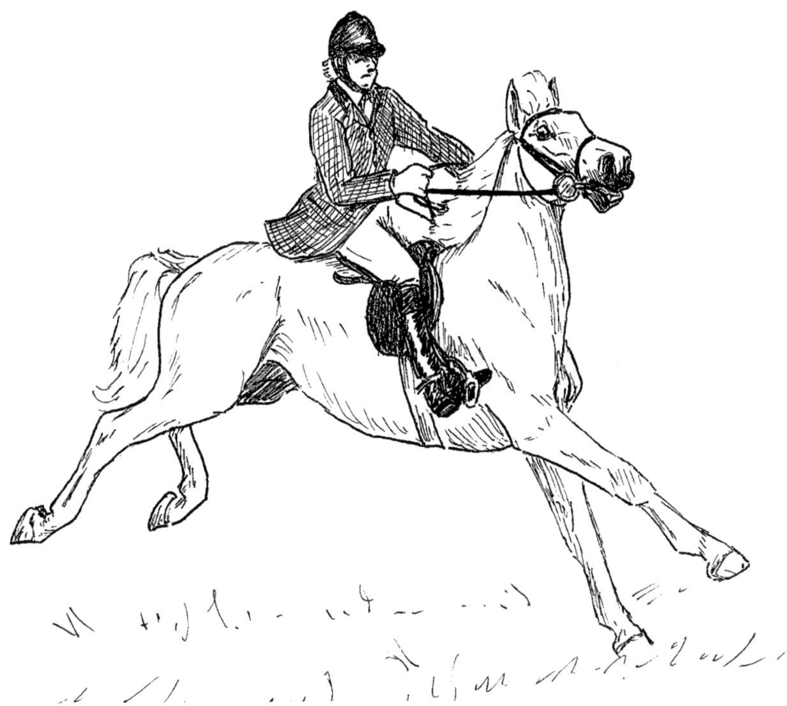

This rider is being carted. The horse's head is up beyond the angle of control and its mouth is open. The rider is leaning back, bracing herself against the stirrups and tugging at the reins.

Learn to check your horse in a perfect rhythm at every stride of canter. Your hands must be used in rhythm with the canter stride – steady, steady, steady. You must check the horse as it is finishing one canter stride and before it starts the next. This rhythmic steadying is to ensure that each canter stride stays the same length as the previous one. Horses do not normally get out of control very suddenly. They gradually get into a longer and longer canter stride until the rider cannot control them. This is caused by an out-of-rhythm pull-and-let-go action on the rein, often with the rider standing up and bracing against the stirrups or by a frantic tugging or a dead pull on the reins. Your reins must be short enough before you start cantering because if you move your hands to alter your reins at canter, the horse will take the chance to lengthen its stride very quickly.

You cannot improve a pulling, excitable horse by riding it once or twice a week. It needs to be ridden every day and two shorter sessions will improve the horse more quickly than one longer one.

How long will it take to feel an improvement? It depends on the horse and on the knowledge, feel and experience of the rider. There should be a difference within two weeks but a lasting, real change in mental attitude and behaviour could take a year of consistent work.

Control

When riding a very strong horse that you know will be difficult to control, ride with your stirrups one or two holes shorter than usual. This will give you a firmer seat and you will be less likely to be pulled forward out of the saddle. Shorten your reins before you trot or canter or, as you move your hands to do this, the horse may take the chance to get into a longer stride and quickly become out of control.

To steady a very strong horse, with a short rein, brace your weaker hand against the top of the horse's neck just in front of the withers so that the horse cannot pull you forward. With your stronger hand take, take, on the rein in rhythm with the stride. Try to prevent the horse getting into a longer and longer stride. Try to keep each stride as short as the one before. If you miss steadying for even one stride or if you attempt to move your hands to alter your rein length, the horse will go on, out of control. This method of control requires knack, feel and timing more than strength.

Many horses try to hurry in the first few steps of a new gait. Check the horse with your voice and with a feel on the reins, using them in the rhythm of the horse's stride. As the horse begins to slow down, lighten your hands and maintain a gentle contact on the horse's mouth. Teach your horse to trot and canter at an even pace by gently checking it when it tries to hurry and easing the contact when it responds. It will learn to carry itself in balance without leaning on your hands or trying to hurry. It will learn to stay in rhythm at any gait you choose. Once you can feel balance and rhythm in yourself, and then

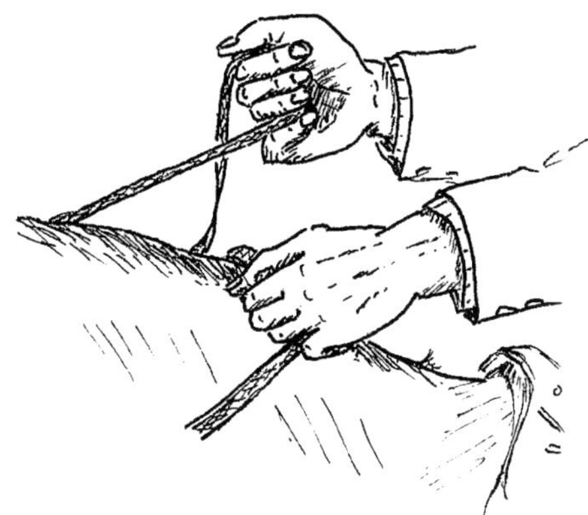

The left hand is braced against the horse's crest. The right hand steadies the horse in the rhythm of its stride.

in your horse, you will make rapid progress.

Some horses will, without warning, suddenly try to take off flat out from walk. A sound in the hedge, a puff of wind, any excuse will do when a horse is feeling very fresh. You may have been walking, quite relaxed on a long rein, and be taken by surprise. Quickly bring your horse round in a short, tight circle, with its head on your knee. This will slow it down and give you a few seconds to organise your reins and regain control. If you try to steady it in a straight line with the reins too long, it will have got going quite fast by the time you have shortened your reins and it will then be much more difficult to steady it and once more be in control.

IMPROVING A HORSE'S OUTLINE

A poor outline could be the result of poor conformation, bad training or temperament? The commonest problems are head in the air, ewe neck, hollow back or all three. So, where do you start?

I would start with temperament. If the horse is tense and worried and hurries along with a short, jerky stride, you are not going to improve anything until you can get the horse to relax. No correct outline or good paces will come from schooling in its present tense state. Hack out in a mild bit on as loose a rein as possible. Get your weight out of the saddle and sit forward off its back as much as possible. Encourage it to lower its head as much as it can. Walk up and down hill over all sorts of ground. Encourage it to use its head, neck and back by walking up and down hills and over rolling ground.

You will feel the tension going out of its body. You will feel its stride lengthening. You will feel it beginning to step under with its hind legs. Only then can you do all these things in rising trot. Guide and control your horse as much as possible by small changes of your weight, moving towards the direction in which you want to go, and also by your voice. Reins are likely to create tension so, where possible, avoid using them. Canter uphill, always trotting first and not cantering until the horse is trotting calmly in rhythm. When your horse will hack about in a calm and relaxed way with a low head carriage and will allow you to take a little contact on the reins without tensing up, you have a choice as to your next step.

This choice is also available to the owners of the horse with the poor conformation of ewe neck or hollow back and those which have developed in this way through incorrect training. If the horse has no tension problems, it can start one of the following forms of retraining immediately.

1 School the horse to go in a long, low outline by riding it forward into a light contact when out on hacks. Then, when it will lower its head and stride out, begin to ride it on large circles and serpentines. Ride it forward into a contact so that it eventually begins to go forward and down on to the bit. It will take a very long time to get a result because the horse has probably developed a bulge of muscle underneath its neck and nothing on top. Until the muscle underneath the neck has softened and begun to disappear, the horse will find it very difficult, and even uncomfortable, to carry out your wishes. It will constantly try to evade your hands by coming up and back towards you with its head. When doing this, it will still be using the muscle under its neck and the more it does it the longer it will take to reduce this muscle.

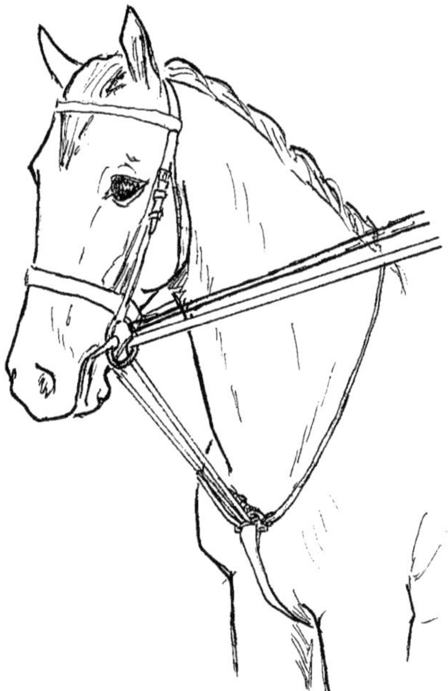

Running reins should, for safety, be attached to a strap between the forelegs and used with a neckstrap. Always use with a normal rein.

2 Accept that a 'gadget' may produce the correct result more quickly. I have, however, seen far too many horses hacking out with inexperienced riders holding their heads down (often almost between their knees) with running reins held far too short and tight. The horse is forced into an unnatural, cramped position and held there continually, forced to shorten its stride and 'mince' along. It is a sad sight indeed. I would not recommend a running rein for anyone other than a very experienced trainer of horses who has extremely good hands. An inexperienced rider can have the running reins far too tight, they can have one rein far tighter than the other, they can shorten the horse's stride and, by holding the horse in a cramped position, cause it actual pain. They can also be quite unaware of the harm they are doing.

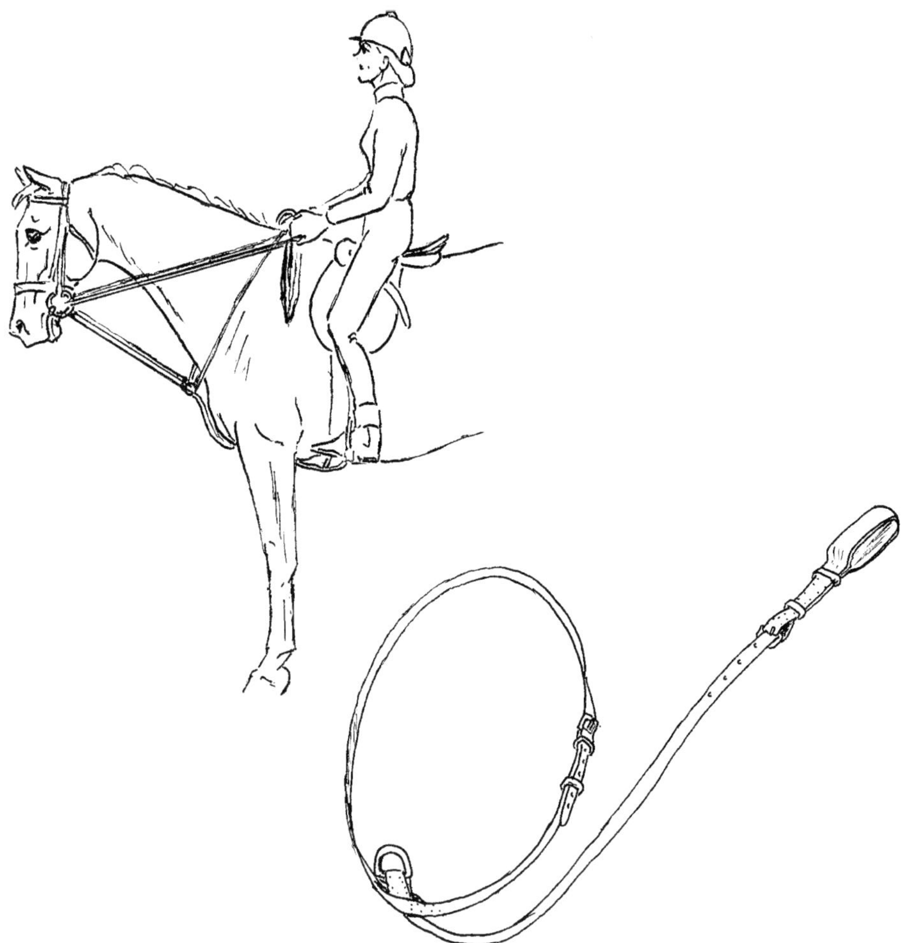

A running rein attached to a centre D in the neck strap is safe because it cannot then hang down low between the forelegs. This method also allows the horse to go forward freely.

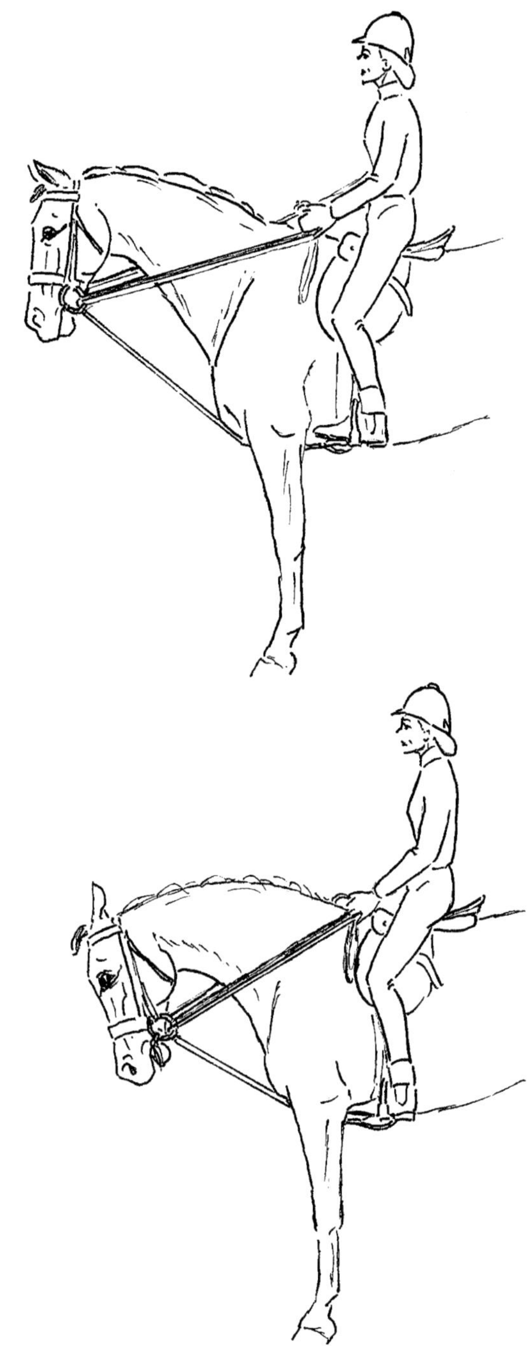

correctly used

incorrect
the horse's head is
being pulled down

Running reins correctly used, above, and incorrectly used, below, where the horse's head is being pulled down. When correctly used, running reins allow the horse to go forward more freely. If they are held too tightly, the horse may develop a 'broken' neck where the highest point is on the crest instead of the poll.

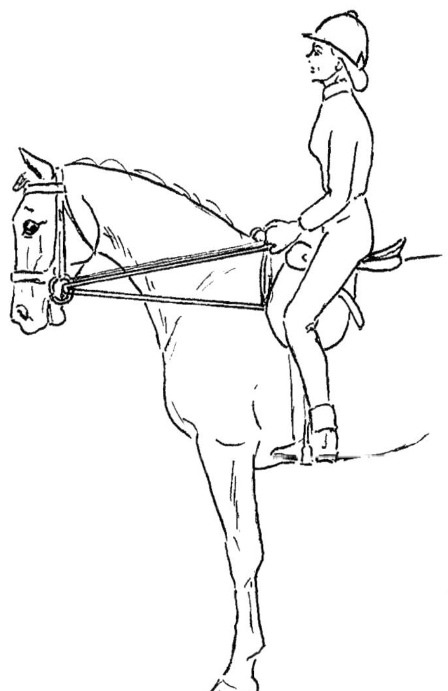

This method can shorten the stride and restrict the shoulder.

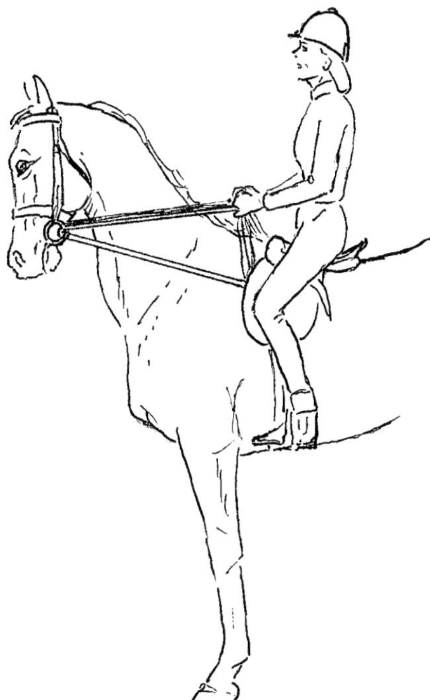

If used incorrectly it can also shorten the neck and bring the head up and back towards the rider.

Market Harborough

One gadget which, once fitted correctly, cannot be accidentally or deliberately made more severe by the rider is a Market Harborough. This form of martingale is rather like a running martingale but instead of the two divided straps ending in rings, the straps are longer and end in clips. The straps pass through the rings of the snaffle bit, from inside to outside, then clip on to an ordinary pair of reins which have three or four metal Ds sewn on to each rein.

To introduce a horse to a Market Harborough, have someone experienced in their use present to adjust it really loosely and watch the horse's reaction. The rider holds and uses the reins in the normal way. The Market Harborough only comes into action when the horse throws its head up. This causes pressure on the mouth to ask the horse to lower its head and lengthen the topline of its neck. A very few horses do object to a Market Harborough and may throw their heads up and then rear or run backwards. The rider must be warned of this unlikely reaction and told immediately to push their hands forward (to prevent any further action of the Market Harborough on the mouth) and to ride the horse forward strongly with their legs.

Once the horse is accustomed to the feel of the Market Harborough, it should be adjusted so that the normal rein comes into action just before

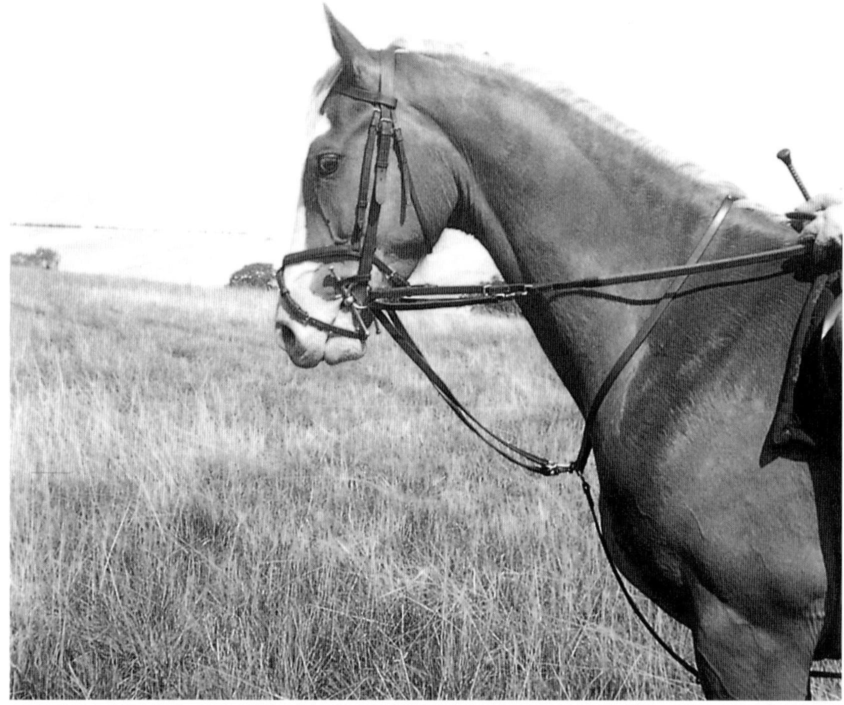

This Market Harborough is too loose to have any effect.

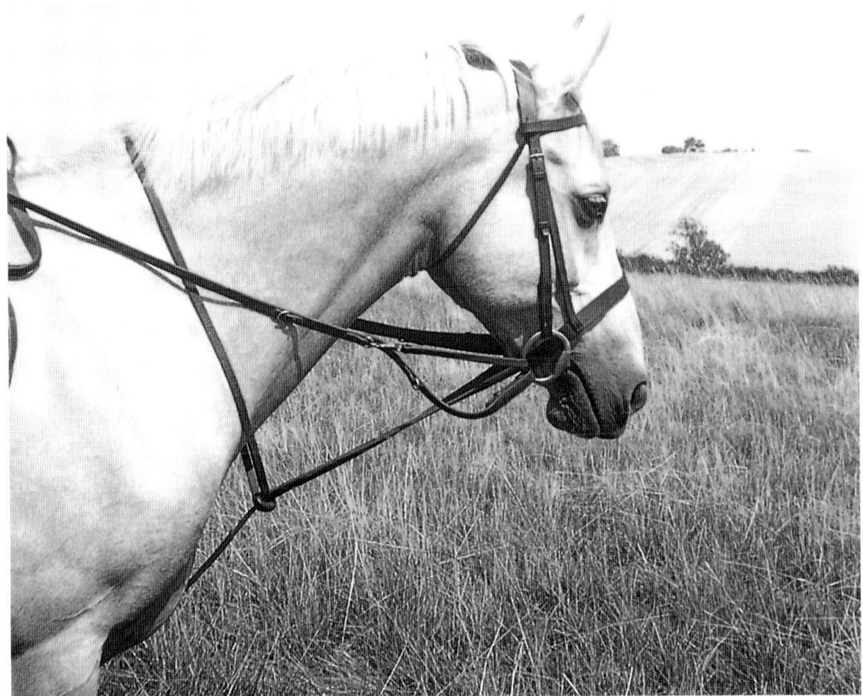

This Market Harborough is too tight, coming into effect before the bridle rein.

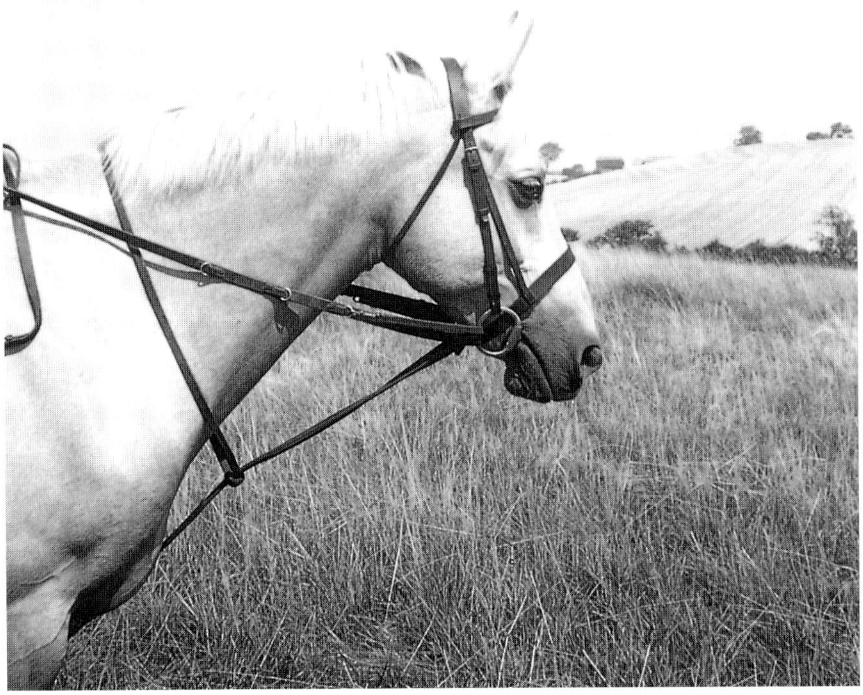

A Market Harborough correctly adjusted.

the Market Harborough and so that the Market Harborough only comes into action when the horse tries to put its head up to evade the bit. A Market Harborough corrects the horse directly from the bit. (See also Martingales.)

Martingales

A standing martingale, which is attached to the girth and the noseband, is a solid fixture which the horse learns to lean against. This creates a large bulge of muscle under the neck. Horses which have learnt to misuse standing or running martingales can easily be recognised by the bulge of muscle under their necks, which is obvious even when they are turned out in a field. A standing martingale does not correct a horse, therefore I would not recommend its use.

A running martingale can correct a horse and give a rider more control by helping to keep the horse's head down in a normal position, but it will not correct a horse with a large bulge of muscle under its neck, a horse which has learnt to come up and back towards the rider with its head.

A Market Harborough will correct this problem. The bulge of muscle under the neck will go and there will be a gradual build up of muscle on the topline of the neck. Once this is established, the horse will find it more difficult to bring its head up and back towards the rider.

How long will it take? This depends on the horse and the rider. A horse which quickly accepts the action of the Market Harborough and soon ceases to try to bring its head up and back towards the rider will show a softening of the bulge of muscle under its neck within two weeks of daily use. The build up of muscle on the top of the neck should begin to show within a month.

The ability of the rider comes into play because they must be able to ride the horse forward into a steady, even contact from their hands through the reins to the horse's mouth.

An unstable rider, out of balance with the horse and whose reins go loose, tight, loose, tight, is not going to succeed. A child or adult who is not very experienced but who rides gently and carefully will get a result and can do no harm with a correctly adjusted Market Harborough to which the horse has been introduced by an experienced rider.

At first hack out in it, then proceed to schooling, using big circles and serpentines. As the horse's outline improves, the Market Harborough may be shortened one D as, with the improvement in the horse's outline, the normal rein will be found still to come into action just before the Market Harborough.

The Market Harborough allows the horse to stretch its head and neck forward and down as much as it likes. It only prevents the horse from putting its head up high. For this reason, it is also suitable for schooling a horse when jumping and for giving a bit of extra control to a child or adult on an excitable animal, for instance out hunting.

USING HALF-HALTS

Halt-halt is the name given to the steadying and rebalancing of a horse before, during and after changes of pace, gait, direction, gradient or when approaching a jump. The rider rides the horse forward into a slighty holding hand, thinking 'whoa' without actually stopping. It is so slight that, while the horse should be aware of the aid and respond to it, it should be invisible to the eye of anyone watching. The hands must be light and have, if anything, an upward feel; definitely not a downward one as this will make most horses come above the bit (see pages 243-5) and go hollow.

By using a half-halt the rider is encouraging the horse to step under a little more with its hind legs, so putting its centre of gravity further back and thus lightening its forehand, making it ready to carry out your next instructions.

TRANSITIONS

Downwards transitions

Downwards transitions are full of problems. If a horse drops raggedly into a downwards transition, you may need to ride it forward more with your legs. If you are going from canter to trot, think 'trot *on*'. If you are going from trot to walk, think 'walk *on*'.

You may be lowering your hands as you use your reins to slow down. This action blocks the horse's forward movement and causes it to change gait suddenly. Think of lifting your hands slightly as you ask the horse to change gait.

You may be moving your weight too suddenly in the saddle so that the horse responds jerkily.

You may not be using half-halts (see above) to warn and prepare the horse for the change of gait so that it is taken by surprise and does not respond smoothly.

Horses often come off the bit in downward transitions. This can be because the rider has not used enough leg to ride forward into the downward transition and so keep the horse on the bit. It can also be because the rider has stiffened and lowered their hands, uncomfortably increasing the pressure of the bit, which the horse avoids by bringing its head up. This is a very common rider problem.

Improve the quality of your downwards transitions by asking for them on a decreasing circle. Think of riding forward and on, and of lifting your hands slightly to counteract the tendency to lower them. The act of riding on to a decreasing circle encourages the horse to step under with its inside hind leg, so putting its own centre of gravity further back (necessary in smooth downward transitions) and enabling it to carry itself smoothly into a slower gait.

Upwards transitions

The commonest fault here is going too fast in one gait before changing up into the next.

Half-halts are essential (see page 269) to steady the pace so that the rhythm and length of stride stay the same right up to the change of gait. Trot to canter is the biggest problem. Here, horses, and particularly ponies, can be seen trotting faster and faster until they finally fall into canter.

This is most often a rider problem. The rider's reins are in loops and they are using their legs frantically. They are actually asking the pony to trot faster and the pony does just that. Ride the animal in a circle in trot, preferably sitting, and keep the contact on the reins so that your hands are saying, 'Don't trot fast' while your legs are saying, 'break into canter'. If you suddenly release the feel on the reins as you ask for canter, the horse or pony may continue to trot fast or may go into two or three strides of long trot before it canters.

Keep the contact on the reins as you ask for canter and ease it only very slightly to allow the horse to continue in canter. To keep canter on a slightly lazy animal, think of every stride of canter as being the first stride and ask and ask and ask for canter.

With a horse which tries to go a little faster, it will be necessary to use half-halts in rhythm with the beginning of every canter stride.

It will be best to work on a circle.

GETTING THE CORRECT LEAD IN CANTER

Most horses have a favourite leg to lead on – usually the near fore. With some horses it is a real problem to get them to lead on their off fore.

Canter is a three-time gait. If you want your horse to canter with the off fore leading, it must take the first step of canter with its near hind. The off hind and near fore come next, moving together, and the third beat is made by the off fore leading leg (so called because it appears to step out in advance of the other foreleg in canter).

Normal canter aids with the off fore leading

Steady your horse in sitting trot with your left rein. Ask for a slight bend to the right with your right rein. Put a little more weight into your right seat bone to make it easier for the horse to take the first step of canter with its near (left) hind leg. Keep your right leg on the girth and use your left behind the girth to ask the horse to step into canter with its near (left) hind leg. Ask for canter as you go towards a corner or as you turn towards home.

If you sit heavily to the back and left of the saddle, you will make it difficult for the horse to take the first step of canter with its off (right) hind leg.

If you feel on your left rein, you will make it difficult for the horse to bring its off hind forward to take the first step of canter because its head will be bent to the outside.

Make sure you are not causing the problem by doing either of these things.

Ways of teaching your horse to lead on its off fore in canter

- Ride a circle to the right in trot near a hedge or fence and ask for canter on the part of the circle where you are just approaching the fence. Make sure your horse is bent to the right and that you are allowing with your left rein. Sit forward with more weight in your right stirrup. Use your right leg on the girth to keep the horse going forward and ride in rising trot. (Trot is a two-time gait, the legs moving in diagonal pairs.) Keep your weight forward and put more weight into your right stirrup. Feel on your right rein and ask for a slight bend to the right and, as the left diagonal (near fore and off hind) begin to come to the ground, use your left leg behind the girth. This will encourage the horse's near hind (which at that moment is free to make a change of gait) to take the first step of canter.

- Sometimes you can get canter with the off fore leading by asking as described above but using your right leg to ask for canter. See what works best for your horse. You will see both methods used by show jumpers.

- Ride across a grassy, sloping (not slippery) field in trot with your horse's off (right) side uphill. Use the same aids as in the first method above to ask for canter. The downward slope by its near hind makes it easier for the horse to use that leg to start canter. The uphill slope near its off fore makes it think about keeping its balance by cantering with the off fore leading.

- Use a sloping pole in a corner of the school or field. The outside of the pole should be on the ground at the foot of a wing or cone. The inside end should be raised by 45–91 cm (1½–2 ft) on a jump stand. Trot round on the right rein and, exactly as you come to the pole, ask for canter with the off fore leading, using the preparation and aids as in the first method described above. If the horse lands on the correct lead, keep cantering. The reason for using this sloping pole is that you want the horse to strike off into canter with its near hind leg. The horse, however, wants to strike off into canter with its off hind leg but the higher part of the pole nearest to its off hind leg will make it believe that it will bang that leg if it uses it. The very low part of the pole near to its near hind leg looks safer and will encourage it to use the correct leg to begin canter.

  The rider must be experienced enough to time the exact moment to ask for canter accurately and to co-ordinate the preparation and aids for canter.

- A lazy or laid-back horse can be encouraged to start canter with its near hind by using all the preparations as in the first method described above, plus putting both reins in the right hand and hitting the horse once, behind the saddle, with a whip held in the left hand. Again correct timing is essential as the horse must be hit in trot exactly as the left diagonal (near fore and off hind) are just coming to the ground. At this moment the near hind is free to take the first step of canter.

- Try to get canter directly from walk with no trot steps.

If your problem is getting your horse to canter with the near fore leading, try all of these methods but the opposite way round.

REIN BACK

Teach a horse to rein back in hand first. Turn it away from the door of the stable or, if you are outside, away from the direction in which it would like to go so that it is thinking a little bit back behind it. Stand in front of it but slightly to one side, put one hand on the bone of its nose just above the nostrils and the other in a fist on the point of the shoulder of whichever foreleg is standing slightly forward (that, naturally, being the first one it will move). Push back with both hands at the same time saying, 'Back' in a slow, deep, distinctive voice. Use your toe to press on the coronet of the foreleg which will take the first step back. Be patient, go slowly and take one step at a time, changing the shoulder and coronet that your fist and toe will press on as the horse takes each step. Two or three steps are enough at first. Stop, lead the horse forward, reward it with a rub or a stroke and a quiet word. (Do *not* give titbits as they are the cause of many problems, see page 159.) Repeat this exercise two or three times, always in different places.

When the horse is responding well and happily, put a bridle on it and gradually cease to use your toe or fist and begin to put very slight pressure on the reins so that the bit works as it would if you were riding. Still use the command, 'Back'. Be prepared to go back a stage if you have problems.

Now ride your horse in a place where you have often practised backing in hand and ask it to go back with you on board. (Obviously, you must teach your horse to halt and stand still before you try to teach it to back.)

It is very important that your legs are absolutely still, just holding the horse's sides. If you use your legs, the horse will think you want it to go forward and will do so, but you will be feeling on the reins at the same time, asking it to go backwards. This action of 'go forward' from your legs and 'stop' from your hands will puzzle and worry the horse which may well think, 'The rider's legs say go forward, but the rider's hands and the bit in my mouth say don't go forward; there is only one way left to go so I will rear and go up'. This is a very common situation for some unfortunate horses and ponies. The rider must *not* kick. The legs must close quietly on the horse's sides to keep it straight and to control how fast and by how many paces it goes back.

Ride forward into a normal halt, using one side of the school or a fence to help to keep the horse straight. When the horse halts, keep the contact on its mouth and keep your legs quiet on its sides. Bring your weight forward very slightly so that it is easier for the horse to lift its back just behind the saddle in order to take backward steps. Say 'Back' in your usual voice and gently feel on the reins as you have done from the ground. No force should ever be used. If you have trained your horse properly and taken sufficient time for it to learn this lesson, it should back quietly, step by step, at a touch. After two or three steps, close your legs a little more and ask your horse to go forward into a normal halt.

Always do some normal halts after rein back so that the horse will not anticipate rein back when you have, in fact, only asked for halt, and thus learn to run back out of hand.

If the horse's hindquarters begin to swing sideways, correct them with a little more pressure behind the girth from the leg on that side. Do not correct the position of the hindquarters with your reins. If the horse constantly swings its hindquarters in one direction, you may be using too much leg or too much rein on the opposite side. If your horse does not understand your aids for rein back when ridden, an assistant can help you by pushing on the horse's nose and point of shoulder and tapping its coronet as you did when on the ground.

Sometimes, in a dressage test for instance, you may be asked for an exact number of rein back steps. If you have been asked for four steps back, close your legs and ride forward as the horse just begins to start the fourth step back. It should then take that fourth step and stop or go forward again according to your instructions and aids.

STIFFNESS

Suppling exercises will help to improve a horse that cuts corners or falls in on circles (see page 278).

Making the circle bigger by leg yielding

To teach a horse to keep the correct bend when following the arc of a circle, and to become more supple by stepping forward and under with its hind leg, you can start by riding it on a 10-m circle at walk. Keeping the bend throughout its body, neck and head, perform a half-halt, maintaining the bend with your inside rein and using your outside rein for the half-halt. Then, keeping your outside leg on the girth, use your inside leg slightly behind the girth to ask your horse to move forward and sideways.

A horse can only respond to your inside leg's request to move its inside hind leg forward and sideways if you ask as that leg is about to come off the ground. If you ask when the horse's weight is on that leg, it cannot respond.

To move sideways successfully, it is necessary to know exactly what is happening under you, particularly when each hind leg is about to come off the ground. You will feel a fractional lifting under one seat bone as the horse lifts its hindquarters on that side in preparation to taking a step. It is at this moment that you must use your leg on that same side.

Most horses are more supple to the left (perhaps because we tend to start them off as youngsters by leading them from that side), so start this exercise on the left rein. You do not need to kick or pull. If you train your horse gradually and co-ordinate and time your aids correctly, it should happen quite easily.

Keep the correct bend with your inside hand and leg. Your outside hand steadies the horse and your outside leg controls the horse's hindquarters.

Your hands must allow the forward movement, but the outside hand checks it fractionally for a second or two, in rhythm with the horse stepping forward and under, when you use your inside leg at the correct moment. Your weight should be slightly into your outside seat bone, the one that the horse is moving towards. You are not *stopping* the forward movement, you are merely changing it to forward *and* sideways.

As you use your outside hand, fractionally before your inside leg, think 'check and over', 'check and over' in a steady rhythm. At first, ask for only a few steps forward and sideways, then continue on the slightly larger circle that you will now be on. Next, ask for a few more steps forward and over until the horse will go smoothly and in rhythm from a 10-m circle to a 20-m circle. Repeat on the other rein.

This sideways action, looking away from the direction of movement, comes naturally to a horse. You see a horse doing this when it shies at something or when another horse threatens to kick it when they are loose in a field.

When the horse is going really well in walk, the same thing can be done in trot, sitting or rising. See which works best for you and your horse.

The horse will not find it nearly so easy to make the circle smaller still keeping the inward bend and following the arc of the circle while looking in the direction in which it is going.

Leg yielding down a school

Again, you are not stopping the movement but are changing it to forward *and* sideways. The horse's neck and head will be bent slightly away from the direction in which it is going, so it is a movement that comes naturally to the horse, except that its body is kept straight and parallel to the sides of the school or a marked-out arena. It is much easier to ride this movement towards a solid wall or fence than away from it.

If you are riding in a marked-out area of 20 x 40 m, just after you have passed A or C, turn on to the three-quarter line, parallel to the long sides of the school, keeping the bend in the horse's head and neck that you asked for on the turn. Give the horse a few strides to straighten its body by using your outside leg. Ride a half-halt, check the horse fractionally with your outside hand while keeping the bend with your inside hand and use your inside leg to ask the horse to step forward and over as it begins to pick up its inside hind leg. Use your outside leg to control its hindquarters. Your weight should be a little more into your outside seat bone, the one that the horse is moving towards.

Again, think 'check and over', 'check and over' as you use your aids in a co-ordinated rhythm. You are not stopping the forward movement; you are changing it to forward and sideways in the same rhythm as before.

The horse should move on two tracks – the forelegs on one and the hind legs on the other.

Again, at first ask only a few steps, then go straight, then ask for a few more. There should be no need to pull or kick. If you have trained your horse carefully and patiently, it should happen easily. When the horse is going well in walk, leg yielding can be done in trot, sitting or rising. See which works best for you and your horse.

Shoulder in

Here, exactly the same principle of co-ordinated, rhythmic aids applies. Most horses, however, do not find this exercise quite as easy as the ones described above.

Ride the horse on to a 10-m circle at walk in one of the corners of the school. Keep the bend and arc of the circle throughout the horse's body, neck and head as you come out of the circle with the horse's outside hind leg on the outside track of the school and its body at an angle of 30 degrees to the side of the school. Your inside hand keeps the bend, your outside hand checks the horse to prevent it from going forward towards the centre of the school, your inside leg asks the horse to step sideways and under, your outside leg controls the hindquarters and how fast the horse goes sideways. Your weight is slightly more into your outside seatbone, the one that the horse is moving towards.

The biggest problem is that nearly all horses want to go forward and away from the track. If you find that you are having to use too much rein to prevent this from happening, that the horse is getting in any way tense or upset or that you are getting overanxious or frustrated, leave it as you will do more harm than good. Work on the other exercises a little longer.

If all is going quite well, however, continue for a few steps and then either allow the horse to go straight and forward on to a larger circle or bring its forehand back on to the track so that the horse is proceeding straight along the outside track in the normal way. In both methods, use the next corner for a 10-m circle from which to start the exercise once more if you wish to do so.

I have found it easier to teach horses by the second method because if they know that they are going to come out of this rather difficult movement by coming back on to the track, they will not perpetually be trying to go forward towards the centre. Horses that are brought out of the movement either by going straight and forward *away* from the track or forward on to a bigger circle do seem to be waiting to be allowed to go forward or will even anticipate this and not settle to the movement in the same way.

This movement is on three tracks. The outside hind leg is on one, the inside hind leg and outside foreleg are on the second and the inside foreleg is on the third track.

No pulling or kicking should be necessary. If you need to use strong aids, you are doing more harm than good.

Serpentines and serpentine circles

Serpentines are S-shaped exercises in which you ride the horse in walk or trot straight across the centre of the school and then ride a half-circle as you come towards the side. They help to supple the horse because each half-circle is in a different direction. There must be time to straighten the horse, which is necessary before asking it to change its bend for the next half-circle.

Forming a full circle within each of the loops of the serpentine and riding what I call 'egg-timer' serpentines, where you go diagonally across the school each time, enabling you to fit in many more almost three-quarter circles, will also help to supple your horse.

These variations help to keep the horse listening to you and thinking about what you are going to ask it to do next so the horse is less likely to become bored with its schoolwork.

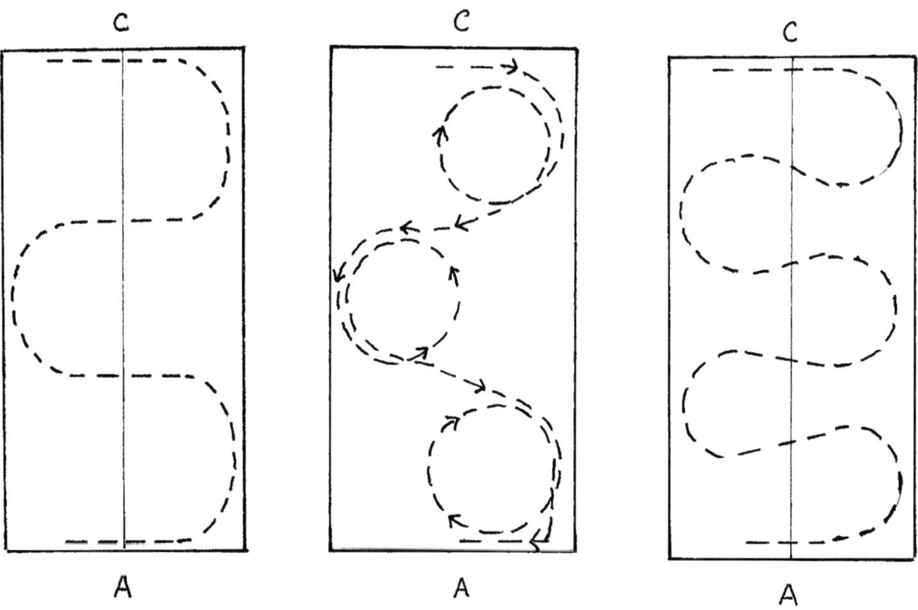

A serpentine.   *A serpentine incorporating circles.*   *An 'egg timer' serpentine.*

TURNS AND CIRCLES

Remember that *before* you start your turn, you must ask the horse to move its inside shoulder a little away from the direction in which you want it to go and begin to bend its head and neck towards the direction in which you want it to go. If you do not do this, your horse will soon learn to lead with its inside shoulder, looking away from the direction in which it is going as it turns. You are then very likely to have the same problem with the inside shoulder falling in on circles. This habit makes it very difficult to keep a horse out on the true track of, say, a 20-m circle.

Wrong bend

If you have difficulty in getting your horse to bend its head and neck correctly towards the way it is going in turns and circles, read Cutting Corners or Falling In on Circles (page 278) Hanging (page 221) and Running Sideways (page 222). The same method of riding and the same ways of correcting the problem apply.

Changing the bend

Your horse cannot instantly change from one bend to the other, it must go straight for a few strides first and then be asked for the new bend. Half-halts (see page 269) are needed *before* you straighten the horse, *as* you straighten it, *when* it is straight just before you ask for the new bend and *when* you have got the correct new bend. Half-halts are tiny, invisible, rebalancing aids that are used all the time in riding, which only you and your horse are aware of, but they will make the riding and performing of this quite complicated movement much easier for both of you. The horse has to change its balance and its whole head, neck and body position, so this needs careful, thoughtful, well-prepared riding.

When you are riding on a circle to the left, or turning left, you must sit with fractionally more weight on your inside seat bone. This does not mean that you are leaning to the left or moving your seat in the saddle; you are simply conscious that your left seat bone is carrying a little more of your weight. It sometimes helps if you think of putting your left heel down a little further (but without pressing more on your left stirrup). As you straighten your horse, your weight comes central again, equally on both seat bones, and as you ask for the new bend to the right, you sit with a little more weight on your right seat bone. This changing of your weight must be very, very gradual and must synchronise with the horse's changing of its own bodyweight under you.

If you are riding serpentines in a marked area (see page 276), you will ride the horse straight as you cross the centre of the school and your weight will be central as you cross the AC line at X. As soon as you have crossed the centre line, change your weight and aids for the new bend and direction and watch your horse's ears. If you have changed your weight and aids soon enough and given a clear indication of what you want, a horse with pricked ears keeps them pricked. If you have not, the horse will cock an ear back at you as if to say, 'Hey, which way do you want me to go now?' If, after crossing the centre line, you approach the wall or fence on the opposite side without having changed your weight and aids soon enough, the horse may cock both ears back and alter its weight and head position quickly from left to right saying, 'Help, which way *do* you want me to go?'

Note and feel if your horse carries out your instructions calmly, happily and in a rhythm because you have warned it soon enough, prepared it well and given your aids clearly. If it goes out of rhythm, ears cocking backwards and forwards, weight changing from one side to the other, these are sure signs that your riding of these movements is ill-coordinated, unbalanced and ill-prepared.

Cutting corners or falling in on circles

This is a very common problem. The horse falls into the circle through its inside shoulder and often looks to the outside as it does so.

Start in the stable with the horse in a headcollar or bridle. Stand on the near (left) side of the horse with the left rein or halter rope in your left hand and ask the horse to bend its head and neck slightly to the left. Make a fist with your right hand and nudge, nudge, nudge the horse just behind the girth area on the near side to ask it to move its hindquarters away from you. (If you simply press your fist on the horse's side it will tend to lean back on you.) If this does not work, nudge with your right hand in a fist just in front of the girth area and just behind the elbow. (This is one of the most sensitive areas on the horse.) Repeat from both sides until the horse will move away from your fist as soon as you apply it.

Next, with both hands positioned as before, walk the horse forward then apply your hand 'aids' and ask the horse to move forward and sideways away from you. Repeat from both sides until the horse responds smoothly and willingly.

Many horses will cut corners or fall in on a circle when being schooled as they begin to turn towards home or towards other horses.

They must be taught not to do this at the slowest possible gait, which is walk. Carry your whip in your inside hand with the whip vertical so that the tip of it is touching the horse's shoulder. Get the horse evenly bent to the inside throughout its head, neck and body and, before it approaches the area where it begins to cut in and lose its correct inside bend, tap, tap, tap with the whip on the horse's shoulder while using your whip hand to ask, ask, ask the horse politely to continue to bend to the inside.

It may be necessary to carry your whip hand out a little way from the horse's

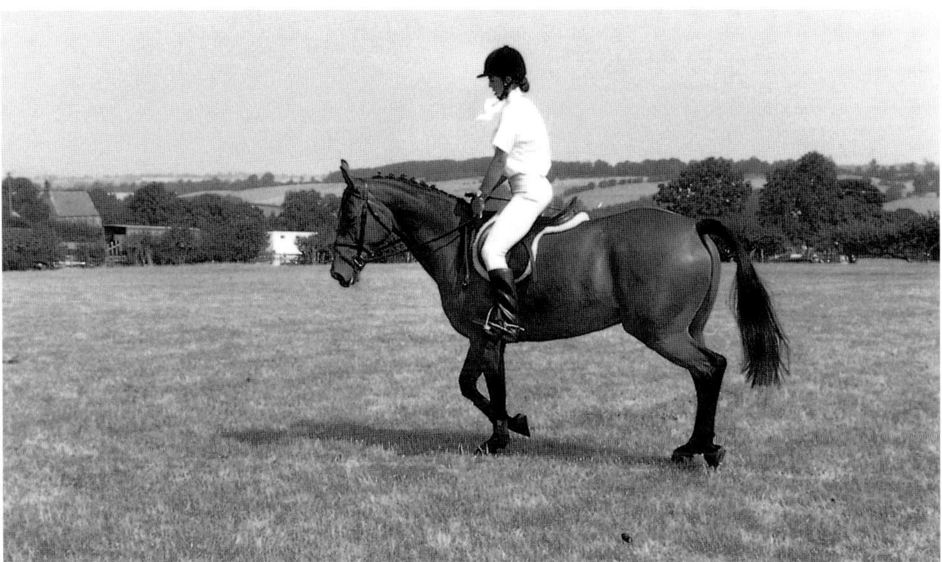

The horse is falling in on the circle. Its weight is on its forehand. The rider has stiffened her shoulders, elbows and wrists.

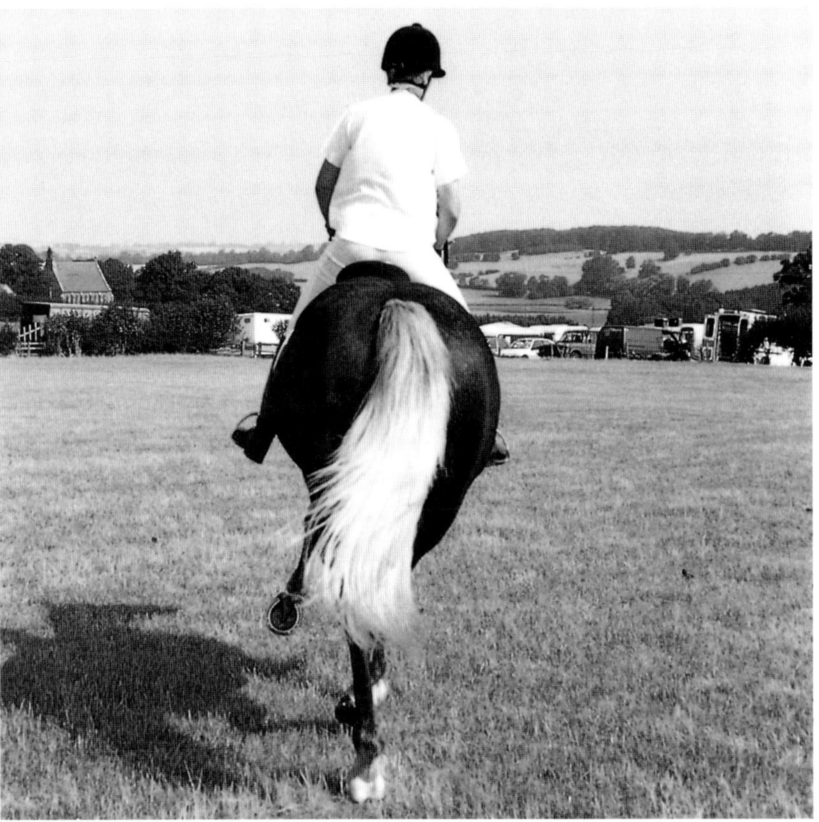

The rider and the saddle have slipped to the outside on the circle.

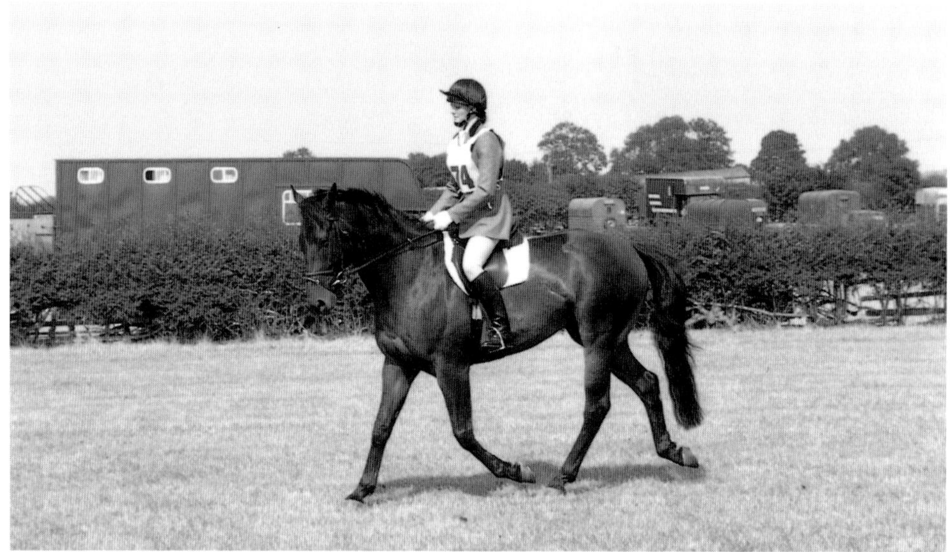

This horse is going nicely. The rider is sitting in balance with her horse. She has sympathetic hands, with a straight line through elbow to wrist to the horse's mouth.

neck so that your wrist movements can make the tip of the whip tap the horse's shoulder. The same hand has to ask for the inside bend so the tapping must be done by movement of the wrist (the little finger tilting in towards the horse as the thumb tilts away from it). If you jerk the horse's mouth it will be confused and cease to go forward so your aids must be very co-ordinated. Your outside hand controls the amount of bend in the beck. Your inside leg on the girth is used to keep the horse going forward and to help to prevent its tummy bulging to the inside. Your outside leg prevents the hindquarters swinging out.

Do not work in trot until you can control the horse accurately at walk. Each time that you school the horse, start in walk and remind it of the correct way of going before you progress to trot. Perfect it in trot before you attempt canter. Always start the work in walk because it is then easier to control the horse. If you start each session correctly, the horse will learn quicker.

Repeat this exercise on both reins. When the horse is responding well in walk, try the same exercise in trot.

Next progress to leg yielding (see page 273).

Note: some horses become frightened and upset by a whip tapping near their elbow so start very gently. If the horse becomes worried and upset, do not continue with this method.

If the horse is unworried by the long whip, you can carry a whip in each hand and thus avoid having to change one whip over.

10 JUMPING

TROTTING POLES

Horses can be thoroughly upset by being asked to *walk* over poles set at *trotting* distance. They cannot help knocking a pole or putting a foot down on one because the distance is impossible for the four-time walk stride.

The normal setting for trotting poles is 1.5 m (4½ ft) apart for the average 15 h.h. horse. A larger animal or a long-striding animal may want them further apart; very small ponies will need a shorter distance.

When your horse is going forward well in a steady, rhythmic trot, its hoofprints should be seen in the centre of the gap between each two poles if they are the correct distance apart for your horse.

If the first hoofprint is correct but the next hoofprint is seen before the centre of the gap, the distance is too long. If the first hoofprint is correct but the second one is seen after the centre of the gap, the distance is too short for your horse.

If your horse tries to rush and seems panicky and worried, work over one pole and, keeping the same rhythm of rising trot, turn in very short to the pole. The horse will then not have so long to look at it and think about rushing.

Next work over two poles at 2.7 m (9 ft) apart. The larger gap between the two poles will make the horse feel less restricted. When it is going confidently and steadily, put in a third, middle pole and add a fourth at the end if you want to.

If horses with different lengths of stride are working at the same time or if you want to progress to teaching your horse to shorten or lengthen its stride, use three poles in a fan shape, setting the inside ends at 30 cm (1 ft) apart and the outside ends at 1.8 m (6 ft) apart. Use striped poles of white and one other colour if possible because you can then follow the colours as you ride what should be part of a perfect circle. Pass over each pole at a point that is exactly the same distance from the end so that the strides are the same length. This does require very accurate riding but it is a useful exercise for improving both rider and horse. Small ponies can go over the narrower distances on the inside. Large horses can go over the wider distances towards the outside.

281

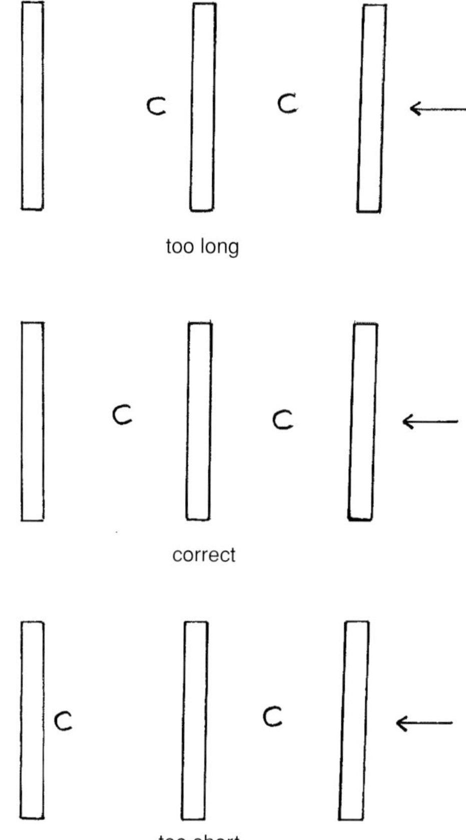

Trotting poles.

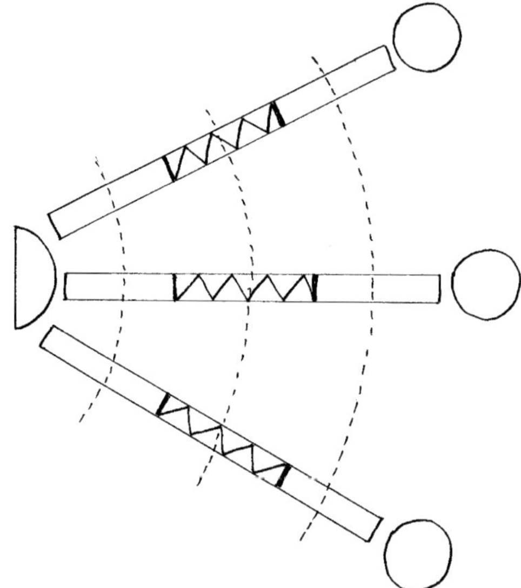

Fan trotting poles.

It will help to keep the horse straight if you have a marker at each end of trotting poles.   The poles should be round, not square, as a sharp edge could bruise the underside of a horse's fetlock joint.

Setting the poles at the correct distance is very important to build a horse's confidence. If a pole is knocked slightly out of line, it must be readjusted.

If a horse constantly knocks poles from sheer laziness, raising them 15 cm (6 in) on blocks can gain the horse's attention.

You want your horse to round, raising its back and lowering its head and neck, over the poles. This is easier for the horse if you ride in rising trot.

Trotting poles are an excellent preparation for jumping. They can be used to teach a rushing horse to become more steady by turning it in very short to them. They can also be used to make a clumsy horse think where it is putting its feet.

REASONS FOR REFUSING AND RUNNING OUT

Your horse will not learn to jump properly until it is going calmly in a rhythm at all gaits on the flat. It must be supple enough to change the bend in its neck and body when it changes direction. It must increase and decrease pace calmly and with obedience. It is the way the horse is going on the flat when approaching a fence that produces a good or bad jump, a refusal or a run out. If you want a safe, confident, willing jumper, spend time on its flat work first.

There can be several reasons for a horse refusing to jump:
- spookiness, fear of the appearance of the jump;
- fear of being jabbed in mouth by the rider if it does jump;
- fear of the too-severe bit in its mouth;
- fear of being unable to stretch out its head and neck in order to jump because the rider is holding the reins short and tight all the time;
- fear of pain in feet, legs or back on landing from the jump;
- being asked to jump too high or too wide for its age, experience, the hard state of the ground or the ability of its rider;
- a nervous rider clutching the reins and hoping the horse won't jump or even actively using the rein to stop it jumping;
- a horse may have been overjumped, day after day, backwards and forwards over and over again until it gets absolutely fed up and says 'no', possibly refusing even to approach the jump.

In making the following suggestions I am presupposing that you have got your horse going calmly and obediently on the flat and over trotting poles (see page 281); that is has the mildest possible bit in its mouth and that you are a confident, capable rider who enjoys jumping.

Spookiness

Many horses have been allowed to get into the habit of refusing first time, looking at and sniffing a jump then, having decided it is safe, going over it at a second attempt.

This very common habit can be cured by keeping the jumps really low – so low that if the horse does stop it can be made to climb over from a standstill. The horse must learn that it has got to get to the other side somehow the first time it is put at a jump. The rider must sit forward with the horse because it may do an enormous leap over the jump from a standstill or it may just climb over. If you sit as if you are expecting a large jump, you are safe whichever method the horse chooses to negotiate the obstacle.

Your legs must ride the horse forward and help to keep it straight. Your hands on the reins must have just sufficient contact to prevent the horse from trying to turn away from the jump but be ready to push forward towards its mouth to allow it complete freedom of its head and neck and no pressure on its mouth when it does jump or climb over the fence.

First ride the horse through the gap between two uprights at walk and then trot. Only when it is going completely confidently without attempting to slow down or hurry at any point should you put your cross poles in the gap.

Start with a small cross pole which encourages the horse to go straight for the lowest part, the centre. When you introduce any kind of filler, make sure that it is very small and in two separate halves so that you can set these up with a gap of at least 1.2 m (4 ft) in the centre between them. Leave this gap completely without poles – empty.

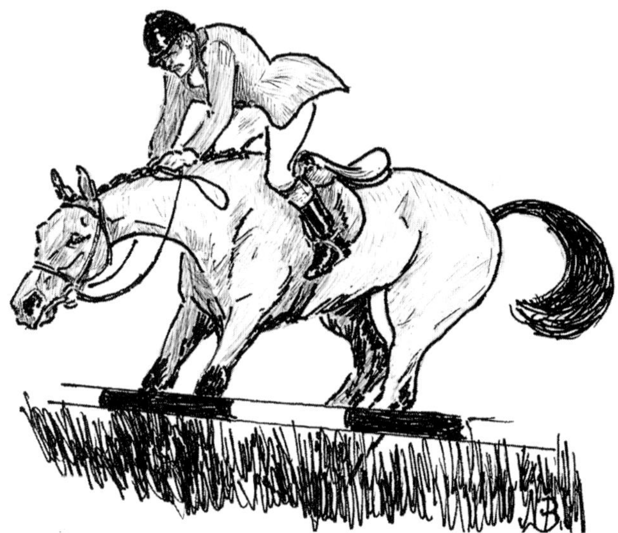

If the rider is in front of the movement in the approach, they will be in trouble if the horse does not jump.

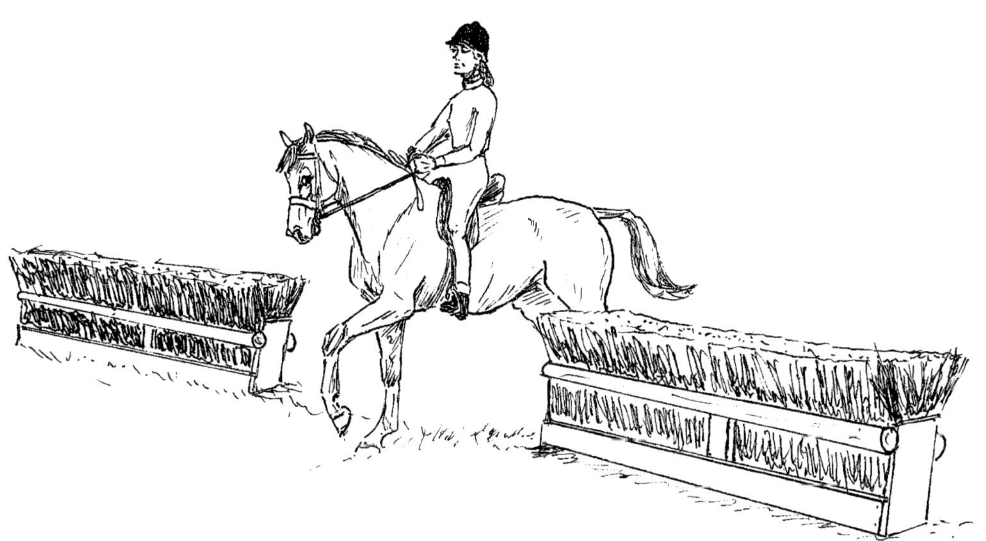

To give a horse confidence, open up a gap between the two halves of a brush fence or wall and ride through the gap several times before closing the gap and fence. Start with a fence that is lower than this one.

The rider's stirrups are really too long for jumping. She would feel more secure and find it easier to sit in balance with her horse if she put her stirrups up by two or three holes. She looks rather stiff, tense and nervous. Perhaps she is not looking forward to jumping?

Very gradually, bring the fillers closer together until they are touching. If, at any point, the horse hurries or slows down, showing that it is worried, don't close the gap any further.

This method can be successfully used with branches, birch bundles, stuffed sacks, tyres, bush fences, wooden walls or wooden fillers. Aim to jump the greatest possible variety of tiny fences, always going over them at the first attempt. If you have a refusal it is your fault; you have asked too much too soon or you have not warned and prepared the horse for the jump. Only when the horse will jump any small obstacle first time and with complete confidence should you go higher or wider.

Fear of being jabbed in the mouth or restricted by a rider holding the reins short and tight

At small shows it is, unfortunately, a common sight to see animals being charged at the practice jump flat out only to stop at the last second. They really want to jump but they daren't because they know that they will get a painful jab in the mouth if they do so.

There should be a lot of movement in a horse's head and neck when it jumps. Before it takes off it slightly lowers its head and neck then it raises its head and neck and puts its centre of gravity further back towards its hindquarters. These go lower as it bends its hocks and raises its forehand ready for the upward thrust from the hind legs at take off. As the horse goes up in the air, it stretches its head and neck out and continues to do so over the top of the fence. As it lands it brings its head up slightly to help it to rebalance just before the hind legs land. The rider must be able to sit in balance over the horse's changing centre of gravity during the jump. They must have supple shoulders and elbows to allow their hands to follow the horse's mouth and not interfere, even the tiniest bit, with its freedom to use its head and neck when approaching and during the jump.

Fear of a too-severe bit or being restricted by the rider's hands

A horse which is frightened of a too-severe bit will often rush at a jump flat out and either stop dead at the last second or hurl itself into the air with a hollow back, flinging its head up and back towards the rider in a vain attempt to avoid the agonising jab in the mouth which it has learnt to expect. If the rider is either nervous or insecure in the saddle, they are not going to be capable of regaining the confidence of this horse. It must have a rider who can sit in balance with the horse, independent of the reins, and who is not in the least

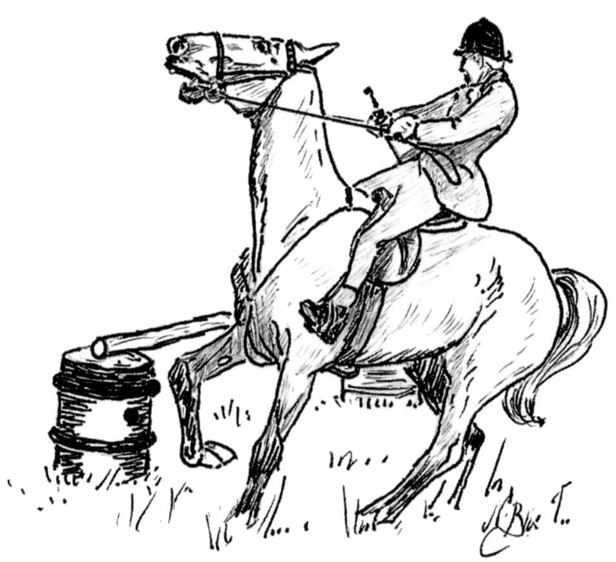

This rider has heavy hands and is out of balance, leaning back against the stirrups and hanging on to the horse's head so that it could not possibly jump.

nervous. The horse will need riding on the flat in as kind a bit as possible and schooling over trotting poles (see page 281) and small fences at trot only, by a rider who will never, ever, under any circumstances pull its mouth or restrict the use of its head and neck. If it continues to try to rush at its fences with the thought, 'I hate this, it's going to hurt so let's get it over quickly', refer to the section on rushing fences (page 296).

Napping or rearing to avoid jumping

This reaction is invariably caused by frightening or painful experiences which the horse connects with jumping. (If the horse also rears or naps on the flat, see Napping, page 199, and Rearing, page 229.) If the horse only naps or rears when asked to jump you must take time and give the matter thought to regain its confidence. Perhaps it only connects a rider with this horror of jumping, in which case dismount and lead it on a long rein over the poles on the ground, first in walk, then trotting, stopping frequently to stroke and praise it. Progress to lungeing over poles, then very small jumps. (See page 167.)

Make sure that the horse is always relaxed and calm and seeming to want to go forward. Some horses may accept this different approach to jumping immediately, others may take a long time of leading before they will jump happily on the lunge.

Just before you ride your horse over a pole, repeat leading it over it as a reminder, then ride it over the same pole in walk and trot and gradually include the fences you have lunged it over. If all is well, very tactfully introduce different small fences. If you have the slightest setback, be prepared to go back several steps and be quite exceptionally careful never to touch the horse's mouth when jumping and not to ask too much too soon.

One of the greatest pleasures is to ride a horse which used to nap, rear or refuse to jump and which now pricks its ears and goes forward willingly and with confidence saying, 'Oh yes, I want to jump'.

Being allowed to run out

Some horses start running out for the reasons previously mentioned – mainly pain, fear or perhaps boredom. Some learn to run out because the rider has their reins in loops and is not guiding the horse on an accurate track, holding it between legs and hands to bring it exactly to the centre of the fence. If continually ridden on loops of rein, the best of animals will soon learn to take the easiest route – round the side of the jump.

If a horse has learnt to run out it may nearly always run out to the same side, say, to the left. To correct this, when the horse does run out to the left, turn it to the right and bring it in on a right-hand circle. If it is always more inclined to run out to the left, try to approach your fences with a fraction more contact in your right rein and use your left leg more strongly. Carry your whip in your left hand and tap the horse on the left side of its neck or hold the whip out in your left hand so that you can be sure that the horse knows the whip is being carried on the side it was running out towards.

Fear of pain on landing

In the summer the ground often becomes hard and can be painful for horses with foot problems. If you notice that your horse shortens its stride on a hard tarmac road and lengthens it and goes more freely on the grass verge or actually *tries* to go on the grass verge in preference to the hard road, this shows that the jar of the hard surface is uncomfortable or even painful. This condition may be more noticeable when the ground everywhere hardens up in a hot, dry summer. The horse may shorten its stride to the little steps of a quick, stilted trot. The difference will really be noticed if it is then ridden on a soft surface such as an indoor school or outdoor sand area.

A horse which shortens up on hard going to this extent is likely to find landing from a jump really painful and may refuse or run out in anticipation of this pain. Many older horses compete with enthusiasm until the ground is hard, then don't want to jump. It is not fair to try to beat a good horse round a course of jumps under these circumstances. It can go on to have a useful home with a rider who hunts in the winter and only show jumps indoors, or with someone who only wants to hack quietly in the summer.

Rubber pads between the shoe and the foot can help a little but, in my experience, the horse always thinks that jumping is going to hurt and it often feels so different to its usual bold, free-going jump when on soft ground that it is no pleasure to ride on the hard anyway.

Much the same reaction will be felt if the horse has any problem in its forelegs which causes pain on landing. NB: always check a horse's forelegs for heat or swelling *before* you ride it and, even if it is sound, do not jump a horse which has had heat or swelling in a leg in the past week.

If there is the possibility that your horse, which has previously been jumping willingly and confidently, could be refusing because its back hurts, see Back Problems, page 118.

Being asked to jump too high or too often

It is rarely necessary to school your horse over the height or width it will have to jump in a competition. It is unfair on a willing animal to jump it higher and higher or wider and wider until it does eventually refuse. Your aim should be a well-rounded jump from a horse using its head and neck with freedom and confidence, approaching and leaving the fence in an active, yet calm, even rhythm.

A nervous rider

A rider who is nervous and secretly hopes that the horse will refuse, or who actively pulls the reins to stop it jumping, is a total disaster for any animal. Do not ride a horse towards a jump unless you *do* really want to get to the other side.

Riders who do not want to jump and who actually make their horses refuse are often seen in the hunting field. At shows, frightened children, overhorsed by overambitious parents, can be seen riding at the first fence hoping that their pony will refuse, either because to the rider the fence seems enormous or because the rider knows that they cannot control the pony as it races round the course far faster than they want to go.

Boredom from overjumping

Horses suffer to a certain extent from overjumping. This can be done by practising day after day, perhaps over the same fence, higher and higher or wider and wider until a previously willing horse has had enough and says 'no'.

Ponies are often really badly treated by unthinking, unsupervised children. The parents may not be very knowledgeable. They buy a pony for their child who treats it like a machine. It was probably a willing pony which enjoyed jumping when it was first purchased but it has been soured and disillusioned by a thoughtless, unsupervised child who has jumped it for hours at a time day after day, higher, wider, faster. It has been whipped round and suddenly put a fence, turned in at every angle, some impossible, ridden by friends, perhaps indifferent riders, all squabbling about whose turn it is to jump the pony next. Is it any wonder that a previously willing little pony, which used to enjoy jumping, now not only refuses but probably tries to tip its rider off as well? Unfortunately, this situation is all too common.

Do not believe your child when it says it must practise jumping its pony every day. Twice, at most three, times a week is quite enough and then for a short time only with a maximum of jumping 20 times on each occasion. For the pony's sake and the child's safety, an adult should be present when a child jumps. Put yourself in your horse's or pony's place. Would you enjoy jumping under the same circumstances? Would you be happy and confident? Wouldn't you like a rider who sat in balance, wanted you to jump and allowed you the freedom of rein to stretch out your head and neck and never jabbed your mouth and then allowed you to stop when you had done your best and jumped well several times?

RUNNING OUT

Horses can run out for any of the reasons given on page 283 but they can also run out because they have been allowed to do so and have learnt that it is an easier option than jumping.

If there is nothing in the section on refusing which seems to fit your horse or you, its rider, we shall assume that it has learnt that running out is the easier option.

As you approach a jump, your horse does not look at the jump because it has no intention of going over it. It simply looks for the best way to avoid and go round the jump. It is your job to beat the horse at its own game.

Make it easier for the horse to go over the jump than go round it. Build the jump with high, very long wings or build it against an existing high, solid fence (not barbed wire or any form of wire) where you will only need to make one wing. Use poles, barrels, branches, big fillers, anything to make the wing appear a formidable obstacle to try to run out round.

At first have nothing on the ground between your jump stands, then a small cross pole. You should feel that the horse is now beginning to look at the gap where the jump will go and not look for a way round it.

Gradually begin to use a few, different, small fences, all with big wings. Make sure the jump always looks more inviting and seems the 'easier option' than going round it. Give your horse lots of verbal praise, strokes and rests on a long rein at walk as a reward. Do not ask too much or go on too long. As you progress, learn to keep your legs on your horse's sides and a contact on your reins in the approach to a jump. Your horse then feels that you are controlling it and keeping it on the track which you want it to follow by holding it there between your legs and hands. It will therefore be less likely to try to take command and run out.

Running out at doubles

Most horses learn to run out at doubles because the rider does not think ahead and plan a track correctly. If you keep looking at the two parts of the double as you turn towards them and make sure that, when you ride at the jump, the centre of the first part is exactly in line with the centre of the second part, your horse is much more likely to jump both.

If, when on the left rein, you turn in too soon, the horse will see the first jump but then, straight in front of its eyes, will be the gap to the right of the second jump so it will naturally go for that inviting gap and run out to the right of the second part.

If you turn in too late and overshoot the centre line to both jumps, your horse will see the first jump but then, straight in front of its eyes, will be the gap to the left of the second jump, so it will naturally head for that inviting gap and run out to the left of the second part.

Some horses are worried by the fences being close together so, instead of setting the fences at one non-jumping stride apart (5.5–7 m or 18–23 ft according to the length of stride of your pony or horse), set them at two-non-

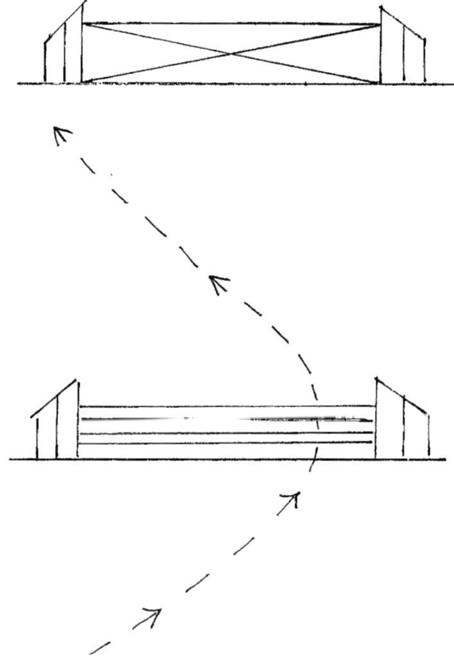

An incorrect approach to a double. The horse will see the gap to the left of the second fence and aim for that.

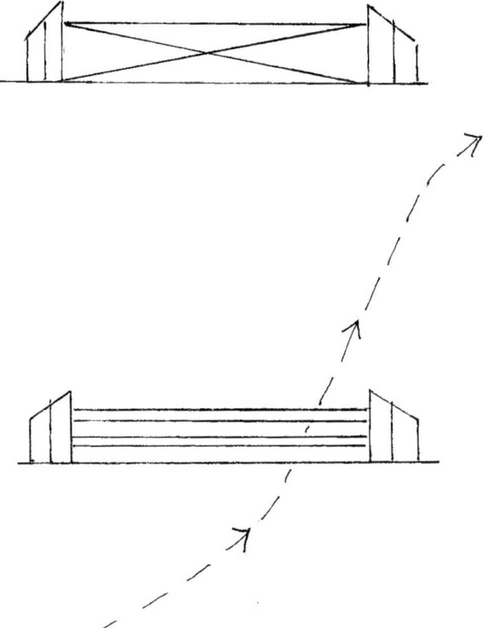

Here the horse will see the gap to the right and aim for that.

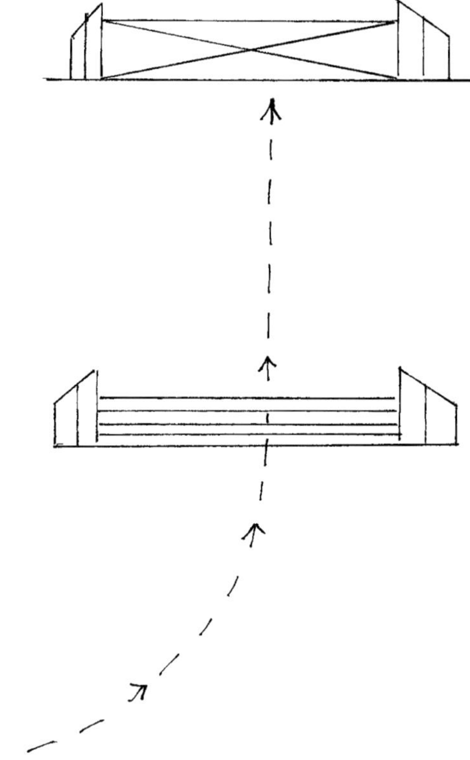

A correct line for a double. The horse will be looking at the centre of the second fence.

jumping strides apart (8.2–10 m or 27–33 ft according to the length of stride of your animal).

If your horse has been consistently stopping or running out at the second half of a double, build up its confidence by making the double very low. Come in on a circle so that you jump the second half alone two or three times. If you then jump both parts in the usual way the horse will almost always go happily over them both.

JUMPING FLAT – HOLLOW BACKED

Horses which rush, are held on too tight a rein or which are frightened of their mouths being hurt often jump flat or hollow-backed. Read the previous pages to see if anything relates to your horse's problem and use the corrections suggested there if relevant.

Your horse needs to learn to round its back and use its head and neck correctly, lowering the neck and stretching it out instead of adopting its present style of flat or hollow back and head and neck held stiffly in the air as it jumps flat and long.

The first thing to do is to get the horse going correctly on the flat (see Hollow Back, Head in Air, page 240 and Head in Air, Hollow Back, page 243).

When your horse is going correctly on the flat, work over trotting poles (see page 281) then small fences approached at first in trot from a 20-m circle. Going away on the same circle on landing will help to keep your horse round. A placing pole on the ground 2–2.7 m (7–9 ft) before the fence, according to the size of your horse/pony, and approached in trot will encourage the animal to meet the fence correctly and round its back over it. Always approaching fences from a circle and leaving them on the same circle encourages roundness. Working from trot means that the horse has to make a greater effort and so is more likely to round its back and use its head and neck. Your hands must always allow and encourage the horse to stretch and use its head and neck so there must be no backward restriction. If it tries to go too fast, approach the fence from a small circle so that the circle, not the reins, will slow the horse down.

Building up to three 'bounce' fences 2.4–3.6 m (8–12 ft) apart, according to the length of stride of your pony/horse, is a good way of encouraging a horse to use its back, head and neck and really 'round' as it jumps.

Build a jump 30–60 cm (1–2 ft) high to suit your pony/horse. Put a placing pole on the ground 2.4–3.6 in (8–12 ft) before it. Having negotiated this successfully, put a second fence where the placing pole was and the same size as the first fence and put a placing pole before this fence. The horse will find it

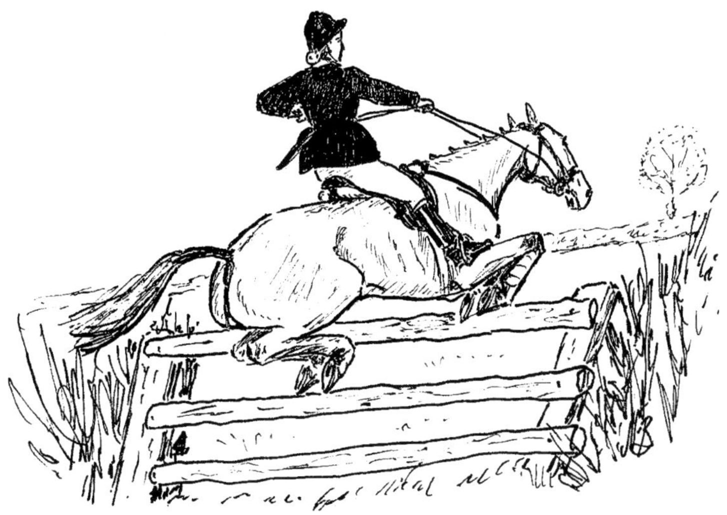

This horse is jumping flat. The rider has been left behind but has slipped the reins so that the horse's mouth is not jerked.

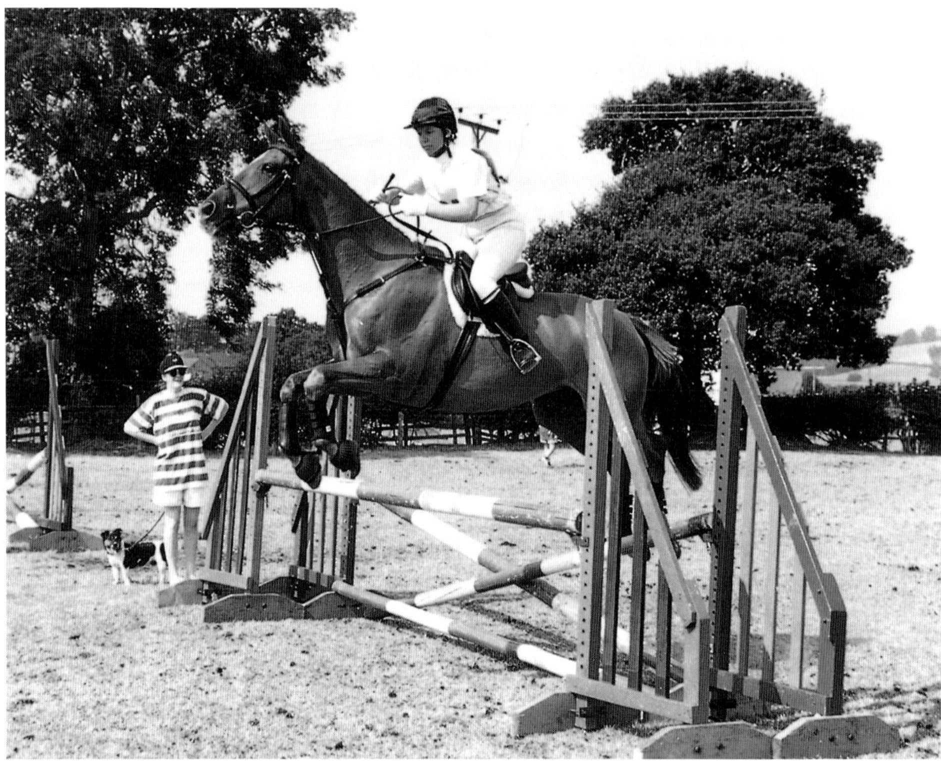

This horse is jumping with a hollow back and its head in the air.

easier if you now approach in canter because canter is the same action and rhythm as jumping. Having negotiated these successfully (two or three times if the horse seems puzzled or has any difficulty whatsoever), put a third fence where your last placing pole was. The horse lands and takes off again without any non-jumping strides in between so it really has to use its back, head and neck to maintain the continual jumping movement for three fences. You will find that you, the rider, will also have to be supple and well balanced to follow the movement of three jumps in rapid succession.

If the horse was uncertain to start with, go back to one jump and placing pole when you change the rein.

CURING A HORSE WHICH DOES NOT WANT TO JUMP

Obviously, this depends on the cause of the problem, how long the problem has existed, the temperament of the horse and the ability of the rider or instructor.

The quickest reaction that I ever got was at a show where I saw a pony refusing even to go forward in the direction of the practice jump. The child's mother was watching her efforts so I offered to help. For once, my offer was accepted. (However tactfully and politely I have offered to help, I have often been told to clear off and mind my own business!)

I saw that the pony was being ridden in a Pelham bit with a very tight curb chain and the only rein was attached to the small, bottom, curb ring of the bit. (The cheek of a curb bit acts as a lever; the longer the cheek, the greater the leverage.) This combination of curb rein only and tight curb chain was very severe and the pony was too frightened of what was in its mouth to go forward. I removed the curb chain completely and attached the single rein to the large top ring of the bit so that the bit would now act as an unjointed snaffle. I explained what I was doing and why I thought the pony was behaving as it did. The mother then told me that the pony was entered in the Working Hunter class which started in fifteen minutes' time! I told the child to ride on a long rein and use her legs to encourage the pony to follow me. I led it forward a few steps then let it go and it followed willingly. I ran a few steps and it trotted with me. We then walked over the pole on the ground. She trotted the pony round in circles by herself and it began to go freely as it gained the confidence to lower its head on finding there was no pain.

It trotted over the pole then over a small cross pole. By now it was already pricking its ears and wanting to jump. It had to jump 76 cm (2 ft 6 in) in the ring so I put the practice jump up to 60 cm (2 ft) and it sailed over. I then looked for something else for it to jump and saw a suitable log which it jumped with confidence and enthusiasm. To everyone's delight it then went into the ring, jumped a clear round and came second in its class.

I have seen the same pony on several occasions since, competing success-fully and jumping with confidence.

An amazing difference can be made to most animals in an hour if you follow my suggestions about going back to the beginning of jumping, having won the horse's confidence on the flat first.

Depending on the temperament of the horse, the cause of the problem, how long the problem has existed and your patience and ability to ride with feel and sympathy, you should achieve excellent and lasting results in from a few days to a couple of weeks with all except the most difficult of horses.

JUMPS AND STANDS

You need not buy expensive show jumps to school a horse over. Junk yards and rubbish tips often contain very suitable materials. Make sure, however, that there are no nails or sharp edges to damage the horse. Leftover paint can be mixed together to make more of the same colour. Jumps must look solid, not knock down too easily, have solid-looking wings or uprights which are higher than the fence, must be wide enough and must look inviting to jump.

Narrow jumps, flimsy poles with no fillers or the whole jump at the same height with no uprights will all tend to make the horse careless or teach it to run out.

Start low – it is better to jump 60 cm (2 ft) the first time than 1 m (3 ft 6 in) at the third attempt!

Rushing fences

Why does a horse rush at a jump?

- It loves jumping and can't get enough of it.
- It has been badly frightened while jumping and wants to get it over with quickly.

In both cases it must learn to go calmly and in a rhythm on the flat by riding it in and out and round jumps but never over one. The rider must be capable of sitting in balance with the horse and having sympathetic hands. Do not hold the horse back or steady it with the reins as this only makes things worse when keen or worried horses tense up and try to go faster. Use the turns and circles round and among the jumps to slow it down and continue to work in rising trot until it becomes calm or tired and wants to walk. Ride the horse out on exercise as usual but include work among the jumps every time it is ridden. Depending on the temperament of the horse and the ability of the rider, sooner or later the horse will start to go quietly and calmly.

When this happens you can begin to ride the horse between the wings or uprights without even a pole on the ground. Some horses will immediately start to rush again and must go back to stage one, going round the jumps for a few minutes before you try again. Others will remain calm and can progress to cross poles. Always work in rising trot because horses are less likely to tense up in rising trot than sitting and so is the rider. Have a metronome in your head and try to keep an even rhythm in the approach and on landing, reverting to circles without jumps if the horse hurries. Do not hold the horse back; use circles to slow it down when necessary. Progress until the horse will jump a course of fences calmly in trot, circling on landing and between fences immediately the horse starts to hurry.

Canter over one fence at a time, approaching and leaving it on the same circle. Use circles between fences. Having cantered over one, trot over the next. Think of rhythm and calmness always. Take the horse to strange places and work steadily through the same system, going as far back in the work as is necessary to start each occasion calmly. At a show, try to work through the system over the practice jump or take your own jump for that very purpose.

You should be able to obtain a calm, rhythmic, first round but the horse may get excited if you have to go in for a second round. Obviously, it will be a long time before you can take the horse 'against the clock' without undoing all the good you have done so far.

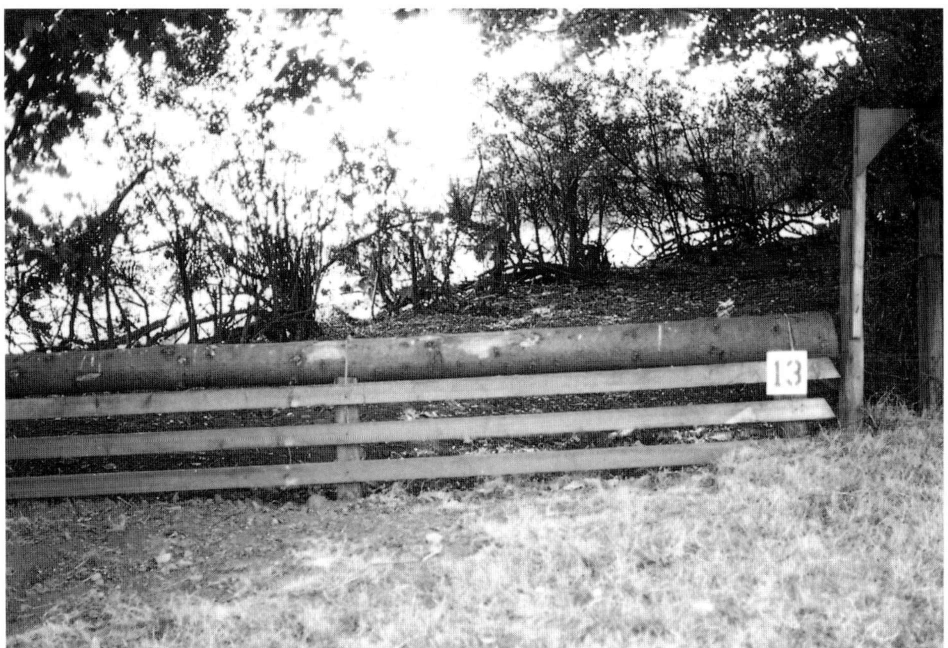

A well-built fence but it is uninviting because it leads into a wood and the horse will be asked to jump into the darkness.

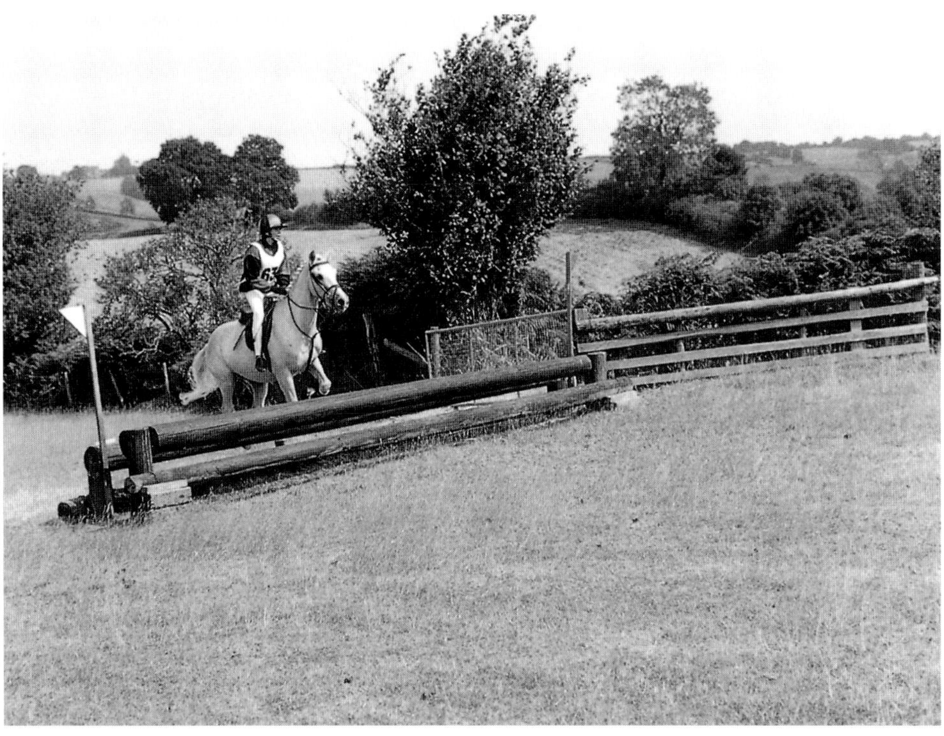

A well-built cross country fence to encourage both horse and rider.

Experienced, balanced, sympathetic riding is absolutely essential to improve any horse suffering from any of these problems.

BUCKING ON LANDING AFTER A JUMP

This habit can have several causes.
- The animal has learnt that riders can be easily dislodged at this moment (this is particularly true of some ponies).
- The saddle does not fit and is pressing down hard and painfully on the horse's backbone with the jar of landing from the jump.
- The rider is unbalanced, behind the horse's centre of gravity and jolts down hard on the horse's back as it lands. (See Sitting in Balance, page 241.)
- The rider is unbalanced, too far forward in front of the horse's centre of gravity and flops on to the horse's neck as it lands. (See pages 306-7.)

The horse that is deliberately trying to dislodge its rider must have a strong, competent rider to correct it. They must ride the horse forward strongly as it lands, keep their heels well down and get the horse's head up as they ride it forward. Turning the horse on to a circle as it lands, but still riding it strongly forward, can help.

Children need more assistance with a quick, naughty pony. Some will buck the child off or buck then drop a shoulder to remove the child. Others will stop dead as they land, hump their backs and put their heads almost between their legs to ensure that the child goes straight on into the ground. It is often difficult to find a small enough but capable rider who is also brave enough to have a go at curing this habit.

Side reins or strong cord can be attached to each side of the bit, taken up through the loops on each side of the brow band, then knotted on the pony's crest halfway between its ears and its withers. The ends can be attached to the Ds on each side of the front of the saddle or to the stirrup bars. (If you use these, make sure that the cord does not also go round the stirrup leathers. These *must* be free to slide off with the stirrups if the child should get a foot caught up.) Adjust the side reins so that the pony can use its head and neck just enough to jump but cannot get its head down.

Lunge it over small jumps in the side reins without a rider. It may still try to buck on landing and find it difficult to do so or it may not even bother to try when there is no rider.

NB: with the pony which stops dead, humps its back and puts its head down when landing, you may find that the side reins pull the saddle quite far forward in front of the pony's withers, especially if it has not got much shoulder.

It is not fair to try to make a child jump a pony which you know can and will try to buck them off on landing. Would you like to jump a horse which did this constantly?

In case the saddle is the cause, check it for comfort by putting three fingers under the front arch when there is no numnah under it. Keeping your fingers there, stand up in the stirrups and lean forward. Your fingers should not be pinched between the saddle and the horse's withers. If they are, take the saddle for restuffing. If possible, get the saddler to look at the saddle on the animal. He or she can then see if it will be necessary to stuff it at the back also so that it still sits correctly on the horse and enables the rider to sit in balance. Putting in a lot of stuffing only in the front can cock the saddle up in front and make the rider slide to the back of it.

RESCHOOLING A HORSE THAT REFUSES TO JUMP

I have had animals which would not even go near a pole on the ground. Some got excited and worried just at the sight of it; others became wooden and 'muley' according to their temperaments. They had either been jabbed in the mouth in the past when they did jump or beaten up when they refused out of fear, discomfort or confusion.

Hopefully, you will not have got your horse into this state but you may have bought one or been asked to ride one which behaves in this way.

The first thing to do is to win the horse's confidence on the ground in stable and field. Lead it about; ride it about. Make life calm, happy, peaceful, interesting and enjoyable by going for relaxed, quiet hacks in company. Have sympathetic hands and sit in balance with your horse (see page 241).

Put two long poles on good, level ground, end to end with a 30–61 cm (12–24 in) gap between them. Lead your horse round the field and then through the gap. Walk in front of the horse with a long, slack rein so that it just follows calmly. Gradually close the gap until the two poles are touching.

Repeat the exercise in exactly the same way when riding the horse, starting with a 1.8 m (6 ft) gap between the poles. Now use single poles with a cone or stand at each end to discourage the horse from running out. Your hands must be sympathetic and 'allowing', encouraging the horse to go forward. Repeat the exercise in rising trot. Include small logs, a flat plank on the ground, anything the horse can safely walk or trot over. You are doing the right thing if you feel that your horse now *wants* to go forward over the poles etc. In rising trot, gradually introduce small cross poles (which encourage the horse to go straight for the centre). Introduce tiny brush fences, walls or fillers on their own by at first setting them well apart with a 1.8 m (6 ft) gap between the two halves. The horse can see a clear way forward through this gap and does not feel trapped. Gradually close the gap, putting uprights at each end of the fence to discourage the horse from running out.

Sit in balance with the horse and never, under any circumstances, pull its mouth when it jumps.

Work it in a steady, forward-going rhythm of rising trot. If it tries to rush, come in from a circle and, on landing, go away on the same circle. Do not hold the horse back or it will become apprehensive once more. (See Rushing Fences, page 296.)

Do not ask too much too soon. Do not keep changing riders. The most experienced, balanced rider with sympathetic hands should ride the horse throughout its reschooling period.

Your aim is to have the horse going calmly and confidently forward, enjoying jumping many different, *very small* fences.

THE RIDER

BALANCE

This section really is the most important part of this book!

Some horses are born naturally well balanced. You can spot them as youngsters in the field, galloping about, twisting, turning, stopping suddenly, always graceful and light on their feet.

Others lumber along on their forehands, unable to stop or turn quickly, carried on by their own momentum because their centre of gravity is naturally too far forward.

The rider can be as one with a naturally well-balanced horse or they can destroy that horse's good balance by not sitting and riding above the horse's centre of gravity.

The horse that is naturally unbalanced and on its forehand can be improved by a knowledgeable, thinking rider or made much worse by a rider who sits out of balance with it.

When a person carries a heavy pack on their back, they arrange it most carefully so that it will be central over their spine and directly above their centre of gravity when they walk on the flat. If they go up a steep hill, they will lean forward a little and hitch the pack a little higher up their back so that it is still above their new centre of gravity which has moved forward because the backpacker has leant forward to go uphill.

If the pack bounces about or continually slips to one side, the person carrying it will try to fix it so that the weight remains stable in the same place because this will make it far easier and less tiring to carry and the backpacker will be more sure footed. A pack sitting lop sided or suddenly slipping down or sideways really unbalances the person carrying it. It is annoying, uncomfortable and sometime painful because being constantly crooked strains the muscles of the back.

You, the rider, are the 'pack' on your horse's back. Are you easy to carry, sitting quietly and central over the horse's centre of gravity, ready to adjust your body position smoothly by going with the horse as it turns and circles, goes uphill and down or over jumps? Or are you crooked, sitting heavy behind the movement (behind the horse's centre of gravity) so that it has to cope with your shifting weight as well as the extra strain you are putting

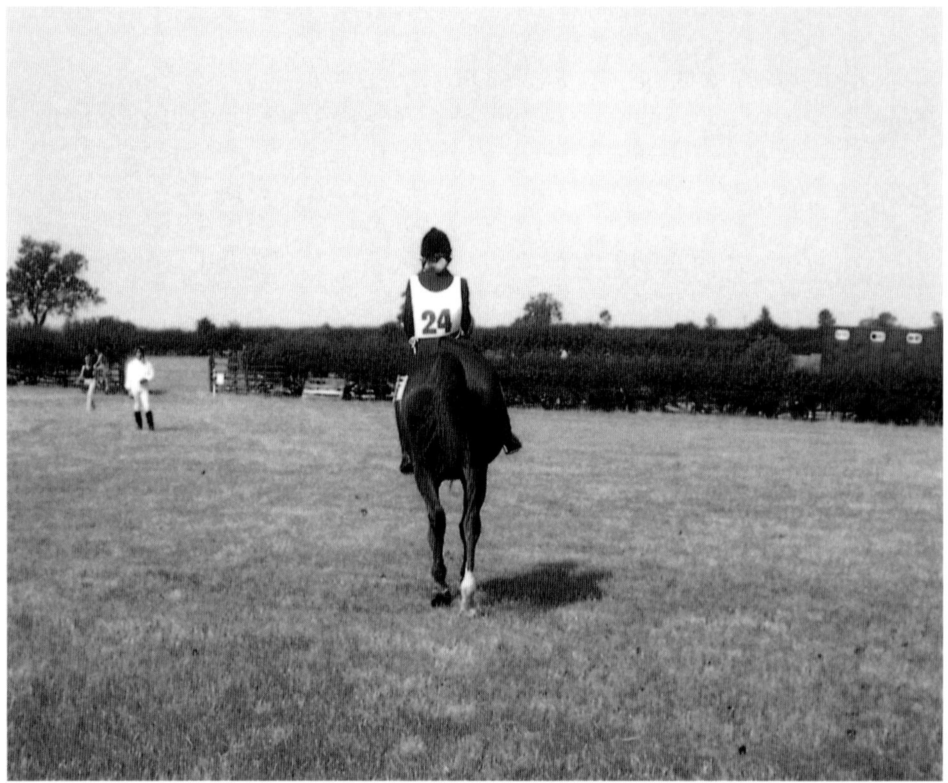

This rider is sitting very crookedly. Note the level of her feet.

on the area of its back behind the saddle? Are you slow to adjust to the horse's movements or are you so unaware of its ever-changing balance that you make no attempt to do so, just letting it carry you as best it can while you become an uncomfortable burden for it, often sitting in quite the wrong place?

I cannot overemphasise the importance of sitting in balance with your horse. If you do not learn to feel this 'oneness' with a horse, when you are both in balance together, you miss out on so much of the pleasure of riding.

An unbalanced, uncoordinated rider can cause 90 per cent of the problems some horses demonstrate when ridden. A sensible, well-schooled horse sold to such a rider can change in only a few days and become a mental and physical wreck in a month. This is no exaggeration – I have seen it happen many times. The probably expensive horse or pony goes reasonably well initially but with a puzzled look in its eye and uncertain movements at the first show it is taken to. A week later, at the next show, it is refusing, running out, being hit and shooting about with its head in the air. It is in a mental turmoil through no fault of its own but the new owners say the horse is no good and that the previous owner has sold them a 'wrong un'. They sell it and buy another and, sadly, the same thing happens again. I have seen this happen and it really saddens me.

Sometimes knowledgeable local people will buy the unfortunate animal and in a month or so it will reappear looking relaxed and happy and once more going with calm confidence on the flat and over jumps because this new rider is sitting quietly in balance with the horse using co-ordinated aids. The rider is thinking ahead, warning and preparing the horse and, with tactful leg and hand aids and smooth body movements, telling it what they want it to do next.

A sensitive horse will try to remain under your centre of gravity so that if you lean slightly left, the horse goes lefts. If you put your weight back slightly, the horse slows down. If you put your weight forward slightly, the horse goes forward.

Think about this section of my book next time you ride. Do nothing with your reins or legs, just slowly change your weight and centre of gravity at walk and notice the effect it has on your horse. Its ears may go back towards you as it wonders what you are doing. The length of its steps may alter, it may move sideways, turn, stop or go forward according to your body movements. The very slightest change of your weight affects a sensitive horse and it will learn to respond to it so that your leg and rein aids are of less importance and the horse appears to the onlooker to respond simply to your thoughts. This can be almost true because as you think of what you want the horse to do you will often subconsciously move a muscle or change your weight a fraction and the horse responds to this.

These remarks do not apply only to dressage and high-powered competition riders. They apply to, and can be felt and learnt by, any child of seven on a woolly pony or an adult beginner. When you sit on a horse, learning to feel what is happening under you, and why, is the most important lesson of all.

The rider's weight

The rider's weight affects everything the horse does and, if used thoughtlessly or incorrectly, can cause problems for the horse. Many riders are totally unaware that their body movements have the slightest effect on the horse and don't realise that they are the cause when a horse responds to the rider's movement by doing something quite unexpected.

Used correctly, smoothly and thoughtfully, your body weight is an essential aid to any horse's performance. The slightest movement of your body, backwards, forwards and sideways, affects the horse enormously. The horse can feel, and learn to respond to, the slightest alteration of the rider's weight. A horse so schooled can be totally thrown, both mentally and physically, by a rider who has no knowledge of, or feel for, the skill of using their weight as a carefully controlled, minute aid. The new partnership can be disastrous and the horse will be blamed.

SADDLES

A saddle which helps you to sit in balance with your horse is essential.

Riding on the flat

The deepest point of the seat should be within 15 cm (6 in) of the stirrup bars. If the saddle tilts so that your seat slides to the back of it, you will be sitting behind the horse's movement, behind its centre of gravity, with your lower leg forward. You will probably be sitting with a collapsed back.

To be comfortable for the horse to carry, you should sit centrally with your centre of gravity directly above the horse's centre of gravity. If you look at a rider sitting correctly on a horse, they should be in such a position that if, in imagination, you whipped the horse out from underneath the rider, they would land in balance on their feet.

A bad saddle will give you backache because your muscles will be constantly tense as you try to hold yourself in a correct position in spite of the saddle.

Most people can afford only one saddle so this has to be a general purpose saddle which is forward cut enough to give your knee support when you pull your stirrups up a couple of holes for jumping. If you try to jump at your normal length, you will become wobbly and unstable when you lean forward.

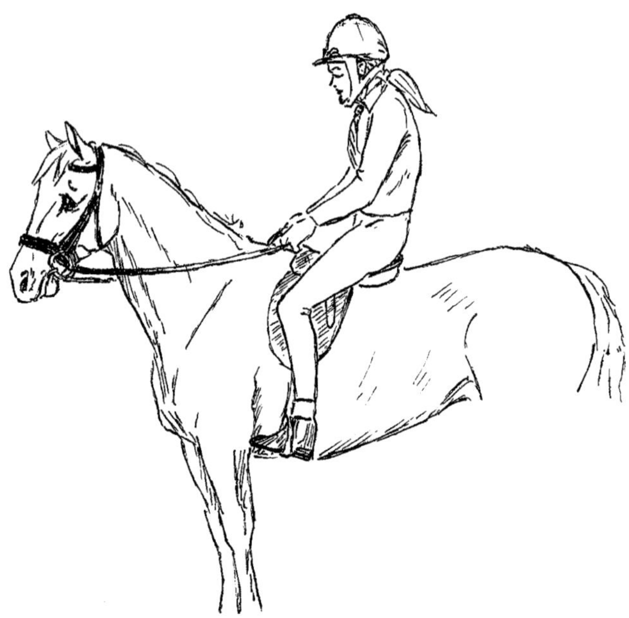

This rider is sitting with a collapsed back. Her seat has slipped to the lowest point – the back of the saddle.

To stay in balance when your shoulders and upper body come a little forward, your seat must move back a little. When jumping, your shoulders and upper body must come forward a lot so your seat must therefore move back quite a lot for you to stay in balance. You can stay balanced for a greater range of movement if your stirrups are shorter. You are then able to close the angle between your body and the top of your thighs and that at the back of your knee, between the bottom of your thighs and your lower legs, and still remain stable and balanced. (See page 318.) The lowest point of a GP saddle will be a little further back than a dressage saddle that is intended purely for flat work.

Watch other people riding, at a local show for instance, where there are people of all ages and standards. Notice which riders are in balance; which are behind the horse's movement, sitting on the back of the saddle, probably with a collapsed back and lower leg forward; which are tipping their upper bodies forward, with lower leg too far back and probably also having too short a rein. Imagine whipping their horses out from underneath them and think how they would land on the ground. The balanced riders would land on their feet and remain there, the one sitting at the back of the saddle, with legs forward, would be sitting on the ground, with legs forward; the rider who is tipping forward would be lying on their face, with legs back.

The saddle may be the culprit as it is extremely difficult to learn to ride properly in a badly fitting saddle.

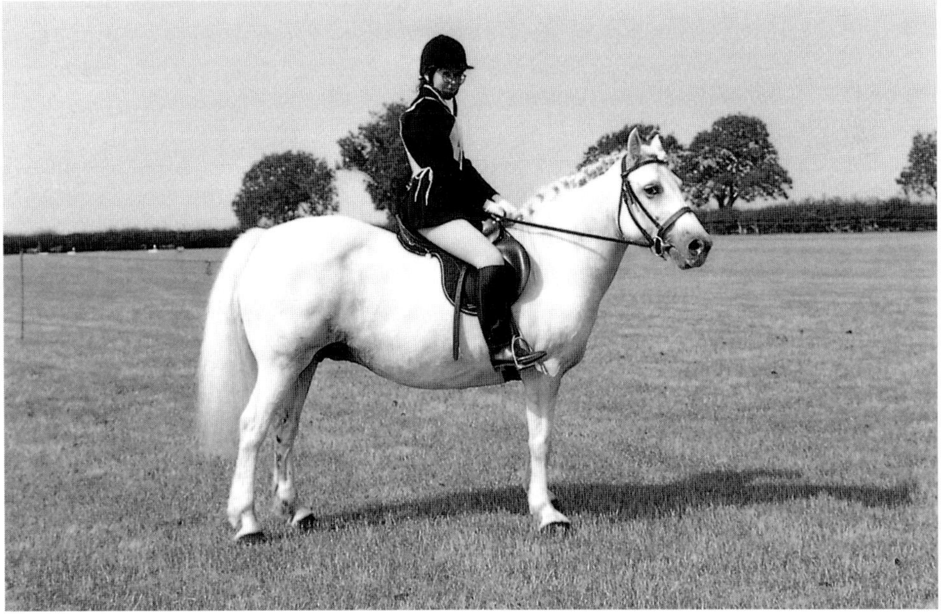

The rider is sitting on the back of the saddle with her lower leg forward. If you whipped the pony out from under her, she would be sitting on her bottom on the ground.

There are, of course, other possibilities.

- A nervous rider may lean back and brace their feet against the stirrups, so forcing their lower leg forward and pushing their seat back in the saddle. They will also be behind the movement and out of balance with the horse but the saddle is probably not to blame.
- The rider's reins are too long but, instead of shortening them when trying to control and guide the horse, they bring their hands back towards their body to enable them to have a contact on the horse's mouth. They then lean their upper body back to get it out of the way of their hands. This rider will also be behind the movement of the horse and out of balance but for a different reason. This problem can often be corrected very easily by putting elastic bands on the reins at the shorter length at which you want the rider to hold them. The hands will thus be kept much further forward and this will also bring the upper body further forward.
- A rider tipping forward may be the result of sitting in a saddle which is too high at the back and which tips them forward on to their fork but this is not a common cause.
- A horse which is higher in the hindquarters than at the withers can tip a rider forward.
- A nervous rider can hold the reins too short, making the rider reach forward and bring the upper body forward in order to do so. This is one of the commonest causes of tipping forward out of balance and in front of the horse's movement.

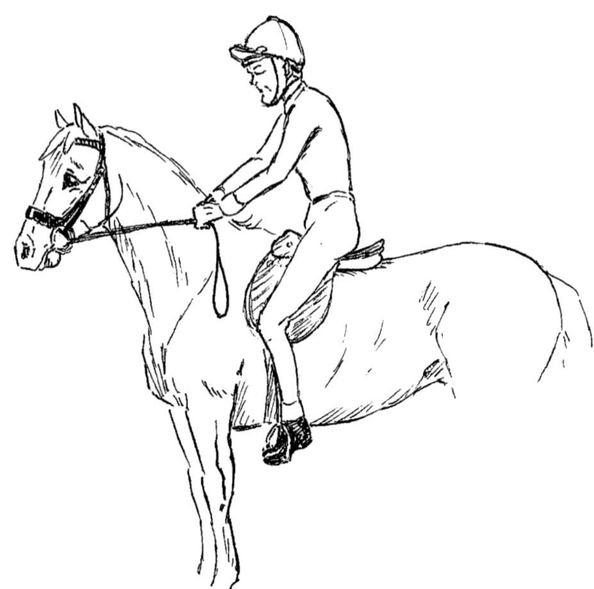

The reins are too short; the stirrups are too long; the rider is tipping forward on to her fork.

● Another very common cause is having the stirrup leathers one or two holes too long so that the rider has to reach for the stirrups with their toes. They find that if they tip forward on to their fork, they can reach the stirrups more easily, so this is what they do. They are then out of balance and in front of the horse's movement.

The unbalanced rider leaning back is not only out of balance themself but because their centre of gravity is now too far back, they are also out of balance with the horse and are therefore totally upsetting its centre of gravity which will also be too far back. This rider will be very hard work for the horse to carry uphill because the rider's weight will be towards the horse's loins (behind the saddle). When our backbacker is walking uphill, where do they

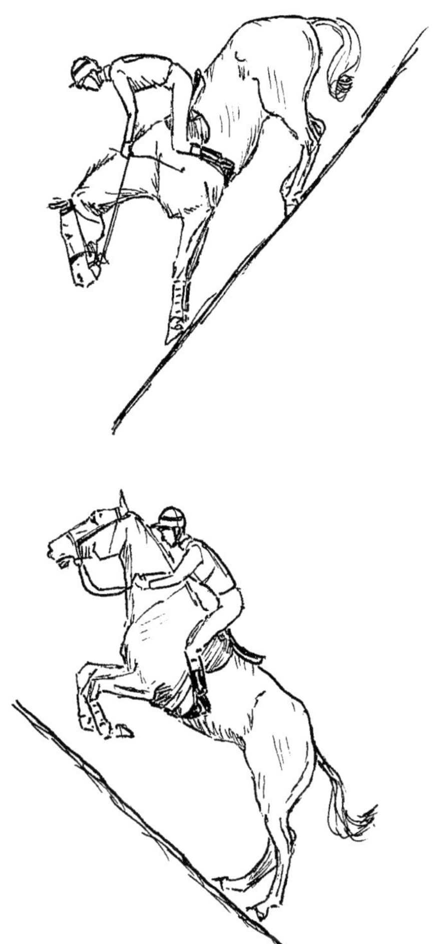

Go with your horse and allow it to have freedom of its head and neck.

hitch the pack on their back? They hitch it forward, towards their shoulders, so that when they lean forward to go uphill, the weight of the pack will still be over their centre of gravity. When a horse goes uphill it lowers its head, stretches its neck out and down and puts more weight into its shoulders, thus moving its own centre of gravity further forward to make going uphill easy. You, the rider, must sit forward above the horse's new centre of gravity if it is to carry you with the least possible effort.

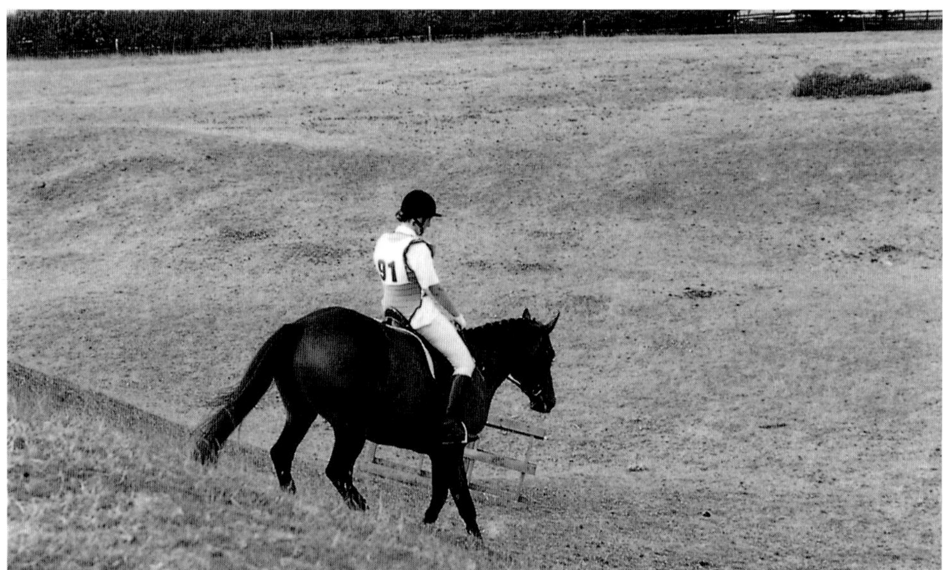

This rider is leaning back and putting her weight over her horse's loins.

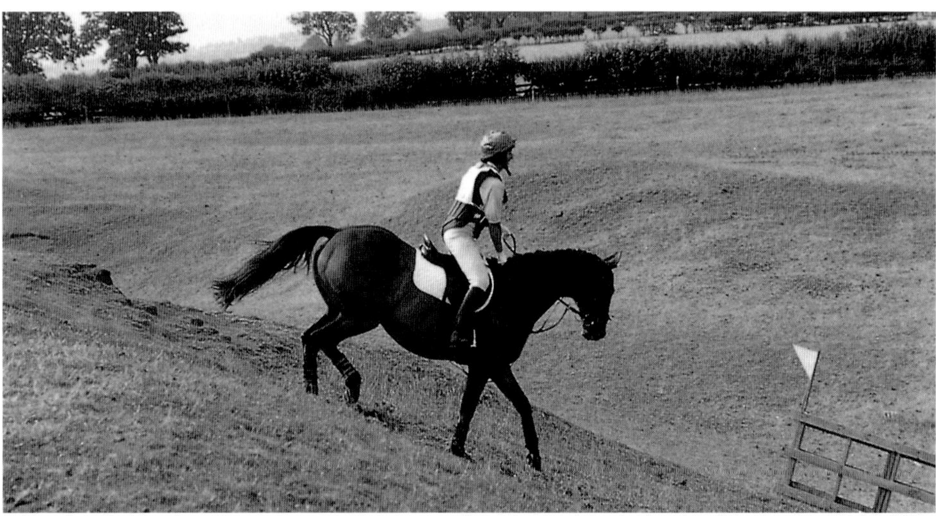

When going downhill sit forward and allow the horse to use its head and neck to balance.

A long day's ride, a long cross country course or a long day's hunting can be much less tiring and much less likely to cause stress and possible lameness through strain on muscles, joints and ligaments if the rider is sitting in balance all the time that they are on the horse's back.

THE RIDER'S HANDS

The rider's hands can cause many of the problems horses have when ridden. Unbalanced riders often save themselves by holding on with the reins. A sudden jerk on a horse's mouth, carrying almost the full weight of the rider, can very nearly pull the horse over.

A rider clutching the reins tightly and kicking with their legs is saying 'stop' and 'go' at the same time. This is what many riders do when the horse starts to shy at something. They clutch and tense up. The horse senses the rider's nervousness and is therefore more frightened because fear is infectious. Under these circumstances, the horse is unlikely to go forward so, with the rider pulling and kicking both at the same time, it may well go backwards whereupon the rider tightens the reins even more. The horse is by now probably beginning to panic and may go backwards into a ditch or into a passing traffic. It has learnt that if something in front frightens its rider, its rider is likely to hold it tightly and frighten and confuse it, so it may begin to shy more in anticipation of what is to come and start to run back as soon as it sees something it does not like the look of. It is the rider who has created this all too common situation.

If your horse raises its head slightly and pricks its ears at something spooky ahead of it, talk to it calmly, use your legs and seat to drive it strongly forward and have only a very light contact on its mouth. The horse *must* feel that your hands are allowing it to go forward and that your legs and seat are also asking it to do so. Do not try to force it to go close to the frightening object. Your aim is simply to get the horse past this without the horse going backwards or trying to whip round. Use your hands to keep it facing in the right direction if it tries to turn but the second you have corrected its direction, push your hands forward and allow it to go on in the direction you want it to go.

Overstrong hands teach horses to nap, rear, whip round and go backwards. A rider with sympathetic hands, who sits in balance on a horse, will soon cure these problems. In most cases they are not the horse's fault.

Some unfortunate horses are sold by one ignorant, rough rider to another. The poor horse is labelled as a 'rogue who needs some sense knocking into it'.

Quiet, patient, yet firm riding by a rider sitting in balance with the horse and riding with hands which the horse feels are allowing it to go forward can sometimes win the horse's confidence in only a few minutes.

If horses have been ridden by strong-handed, clutching riders for months or even years, the mental problem has probably become deep-rooted and will

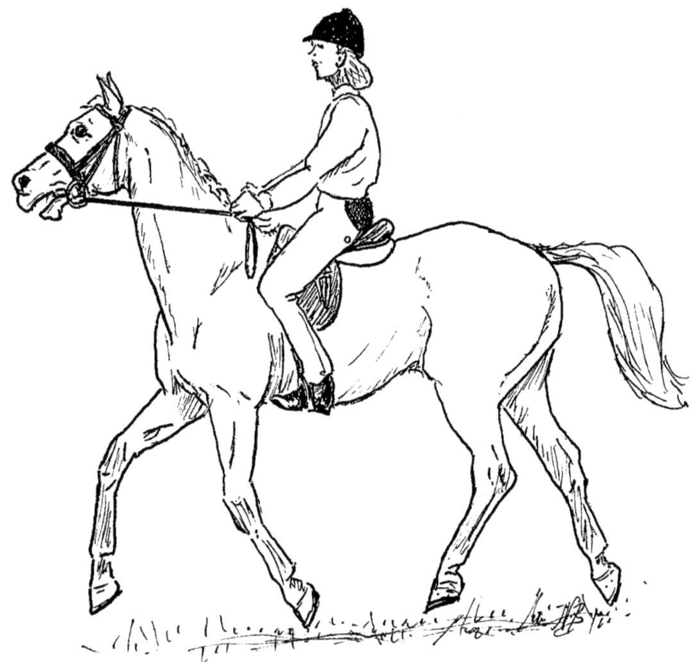

The rider is trying to pull the horse down on to the bit.

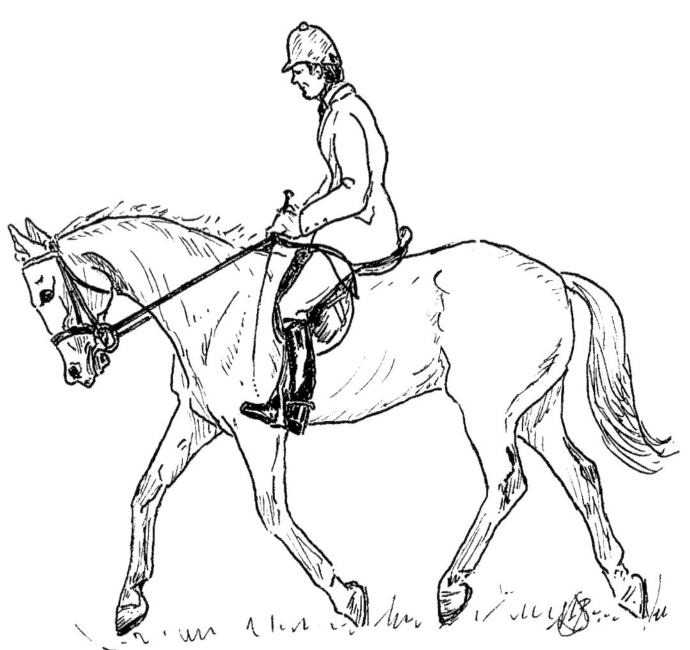

The rider has fixed hands, elbows and shoulders. She is bracing her feet against the stirrups. The horse is overbent and is leaning on the rider's hands.

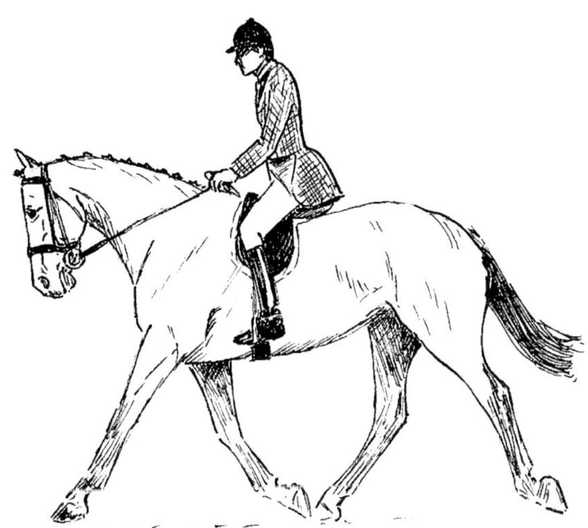

The horse is going forward happily. The rider has sympathetic hands. Note the straight line through elbow, hand, bit. However, the horse's head is slightly behind the vertical and the rider's heel is coming up.

take longer to eradicate. The horse may also revert to its previous behaviour as soon as it is ridden again by a nervous or strong-handed rider using unco-ordinated aids.

The horse gets blamed but most of the problems have been caused by a rider.

THE RIDER'S LEGS

The rider's legs should rest gently against the horse's sides. Because a horse's rib cage is rounded, your lower leg will come away from the horse's side if you tighten your thigh and grip with your knee. Relax and allow your legs to follow the contour of the horse's body. Your legs indicate your wishes by squeezing or nudging the horse's sides. It should rarely be necessary to kick.

A well-schooled horse should move away sideways from your leg when asked by a squeeze given more strongly by one leg only.

If you shorten your reins and take a strong feel on the horse's mouth, it is likely to go backwards unless your legs are urging it forwards more strongly than your hands are steadying it.

Your legs should be much more influential in guiding your horse than your hands. A horse which has been schooled to answer to the leg is a pleasure to ride and can be ridden smoothly and accurately. A rider who uses their legs to control the horse probably has light, sympathetic hands which do only ten per cent of the guiding and controlling.

Many riders use their hands and reins for 90 per cent of the controlling and guiding of their mount. They 'steer' the horse with their hands and only use their legs to ask it to go faster. A horse which has been ridden in this way is difficult to keep in a straight line and also difficult to control as it swings its hindquarters all over the place because it is unused to a rider's legs controlling them.

RHYTHM

Think about and feel the rhythm of your horse's strides at different gaits. Be aware of the four-time beat of walk, with each foot moving independently.

In the two-time beat of trot, the legs move in diagonal pairs and even out hacking you should frequently change diagonal by sitting for two beats. If the horse has nearly always been ridden on one diagonal, it will at first probably feel slightly different when you change on to the diagonal that it is not used to carrying you on. If you persevere and ride even more often on that diagonal, you will eventually feel it become more comfortable for both of you. (If your horse feels *extremely* uncomfortable on one diagonal, see Back Problems, page 118.)

The three-time rhythm of canter is started off by a hind leg, then a diagonal pair, then the so-called leading leg. In reality, this comes last in the sequence but is called the 'leading' leg because it appears to come out further in front and 'lead' the canter.

Use your hand, leg and body aids in rhythm with the horse's stride. The knack of steadying a horse and controlling it accurately comes through the experience of riding in rhythm with the horse, not through strength.

Many horses which are used to being ridden by a knowledgeable rider who understands the rhythm and action of each of the horse's legs at any given time and rides accordingly, are thoroughly upset by an uncoordinated rider. Major behavioural problems can occur and then the horse is blamed – not the rider.

WEAK ANKLES

Some riders have weak ankles which collapse painfully outwards and put more of the rider's weight under the little toe than where it should be, under the big toe. This is not something which can be corrected simply by telling the rider to put more weight into their big toe. It is a very painful problem. The tilt of the head of the stirrup iron makes an enormous difference so using built-up treads, which are higher on the outside, near the little toe, can help.

If the stirrup leather is narrower than the slit in the stirrup iron through which it passes, the stirrup iron invariably slips to the inside of this slit as you

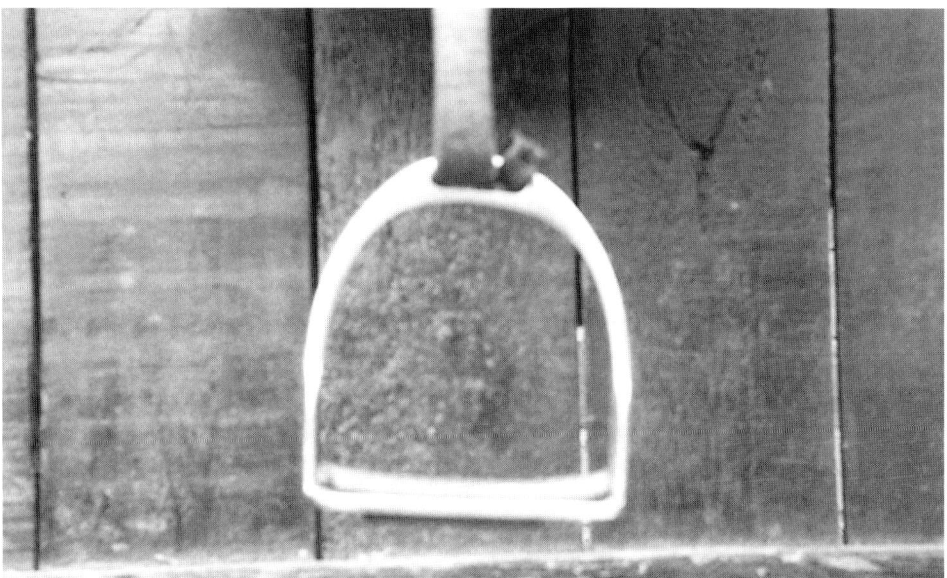

A piece of leather has been threaded through the inside of the stirrup slit to make the stirrup iron hang at the correct angle to avoid strain on the ankle joint.

ride. This causes the head of the iron to tilt so that its lowest point is on the outside, throwing your weight on to your little toe and tilting your ankle outwards. A small piece of thick leather can be threaded through the slit in the stirrup iron in the area nearest your big toe and the ends sewn together. The stirrup leather will now stay in the slit in such a position that the outside of your iron, nearest your little toe, supports your foot and ankle and does not tilt downwards. This small adjustment has a truly amazing effect on this problem. It is something that is seldom thought about yet it makes all riders feel more secure. If your own stirrup leathers are narrow enough to move about in the slit in the stirrup iron, try this out. However, people riding serious dressage or wanting a very supple knee may not like the feel.

This weakness of one or both ankles can be found in riders of any age and until you have suffered from it you have no idea how painful it can be. Lace-up boots can help to support an ankle.

An elastic bandage, put on in a figure of eight round the instep and the ankle, can be cut to a length that will support the ankle yet still fit inside a boot. The boots might need to be made of rubber or a size too big.

THE RIDER WHEN JUMPING

The following is a list of useful points to bear in mind.
● Check your girth.

- Shorten your stirrups by one to three holes because you will then find it easier to remain in balance with your horse and will feel more secure.
- Check that the loop of the end of your reins cannot catch round your toe now that you have shortened your stirrups. If it can, put a knot in the end of the reins. (See photograph, page 84.)
- Only jump if you really *do* want to get to the other side first time. Many jumping problems that show up in the horse are caused by the rider being nervous, not *really* wanting to jump and conveying this message to the horse through their body, legs and *hands* on the reins.
- Start low enough so that you and the horse are happy.
- Do not jump until you can ride your horse calmly and accurately in turns, circles and straight lines in walk, trot and canter on the flat.

The approach

- The slower you go, the more control you will have. The faster you go, the more control the horse has. For example, it can run out more easily.
- If you approach a fence and jump it from trot you will feel the sudden acceleration and thrust as the horse takes off. You must be ready for this and go forward more to go with the horse. NB: this is particularly true when jumping ditches. Think of them as a large, high jump and sit accordingly and you are more likely to go with the horse and stay on.
- A jump from canter is usually smoother because the jump is just a larger canter stride. Because the horse is going faster there is not such sudden acceleration.
- Look ahead to the next fence as soon you have landed. Look at the track you intend to ride to it.
- In the approach do not swing out beyond the centre line of the fence. Do not cut in short.
- Steady and rebalance the horse between fences but keep riding forward to maintain impulsion.

The rider's weight

- When you are riding in a straight line your weight should be central.
- If you want to turn left, put a little more weight into your left stirrup when beginning to prepare for the turn. A horse learns to recognise this change of weight as an indication of which way you want it to go next.
- If you are approaching a fence on the left rein, near fore leading, but your next fence is away to the right, you can influence the horse to change legs in the air and land with the off fore leading ready for the right turn.

  To do this, change your weight very smoothly as the horse takes off, look right, think right, ride right.
- If your horse lands from a fence with the near fore leading and the track to

the next fence is on a right turn, check the horse to the fewest possible steps of trot and ask for canter with the off fore leading immediately.

- If your horse constantly changes leg in the air and always lands with the same leg leading there are two possible causes:
    1. You always sit crooked with weight over to one side and the horse is responding to this.
    2. The horse feels discomfort when landing on the other leg.

Get someone to check your position from both in front and behind. Many people always look down the same side of their horse's neck when jumping and this must make their weight unevenly distributed.

If you are not the problem, have the horse checked.

Balance

- To be in balance with the horse you must be sitting directly over its centre of gravity. The two of you must be as one.
- If you are behind the movement:
    1. it is more difficult for the horse to jump;
    2. you are very likely to get left behind and catch the horse in the mouth;
    3. you will feel unsafe and will therefore stiffen and tense up more next time you approach the fence.
- If you are in front of the movement you will not interfere with the horse so much. Some horses, however, will refuse and duck out at the last moment if they feel a rider in this position.
- If you approach the fence with a contact on the horse's mouth and are riding it forward into the fence then, suddenly, at the last or second last stride, drop the contact on the reins, perhaps to hold the mane or a neckstrap, and cease to use your legs so that you can cling on with them, your horse may refuse.

From feeling a contact with your hand and feeling your legs encouraging it forward so that it is looking and thinking forward to the fence, the horse is suddenly left with nothing. Its mind goes *back* from the fence to you. It thinks *back* to you: 'What has happened? Where are you? What shall I do?' By the time it arrives at the take-off point it is still thinking *back* to you so it refuses.

Think *forward*, ride *forward* and keep your horse thinking *forward*.

Using a whip

- If a horse refuses, never hit it when it is facing *away* from the fence.
- Only hit it if you are certain that the refusal was the horse's fault.
- To reapproach the fence, circle and, as you come towards the fence on the circle, hit the horse once, hard, then ride forward using your legs.
- To use a whip effectively you must put both reins in one hand and use the whip behind the saddle to urge the horse to go forward.

- If you use the whip when only two or three strides from the fence, the horse may suddenly think *back* to you and the whip, instead of forward to the fence and so stop because its mind was not on the fence.
- Hitting a horse at take off needs expert training. I have often seen people hitting the horse when it is already in the air.

  Hitting the horse at take off tends to make it jump flat and can make it panicky and with a tendency to rush its fences. 'Why do you hit me when I jump? I'll try to go faster.'
- You cannot make a horse jump by hitting it. Patience, thought and thorough schooling must be used to gain the horse's confidence so that it *wants* to jump.

Being jumped off

This is a very common problem with riders who are learning to jump or who have become nervous about jumping. They are frightened and worried so, as they approach the jump, they lean back and brace their feet against their stirrups with their lower leg forward as if to delay the moment of take off.

The thrust of the horse's hindquarters at take off makes the saddle seat hit the rider on the bottom and, at least, throw them up in the air, at worst, throw them right off. It is a vicious circle because on the next approach they are even more frightened and so lean back even more so that things get worse.

To teach someone to jump or to regain their confidence you must have an animal which will approach a jump calmly but willingly and will always go over the jump first time.

Put the rider's stirrups up one or two holes according to the length at which they normally ride. Get them to ride about at walk with their weight forward on to their knees, thighs and stirrups. Tell them to cock their bottoms up in the air, well clear of the saddle, and bring their shoulders down closer to the horse's neck. Tell them to imagine that there is a low tunnel and they must duck down to avoid the roof but must still look ahead. Do the same thing in trot on the flat over a single pole. Use very low jumps, preferably cross poles which encourage the horse to go straight over the lowest part in the centre. Have good wings or sloping poles to help to guide the horse into the jump.

The rider must stay in balance over their own feet, leaning forward and holding the mane in the approach, over the jump, on landing and for a few strides after landing. *It is a very long, low tunnel!*

People often feel more secure holding the mane, which is more stable than a neck strap, which wobbles about. Keep the jumps very, very low until the rider feels safe, goes forward and stays forward and wants to try something more difficult. They can stop holding the mane as soon as they feel safe and balanced enough for there to be no risk of them jabbing the horse in the mouth when it jumps.

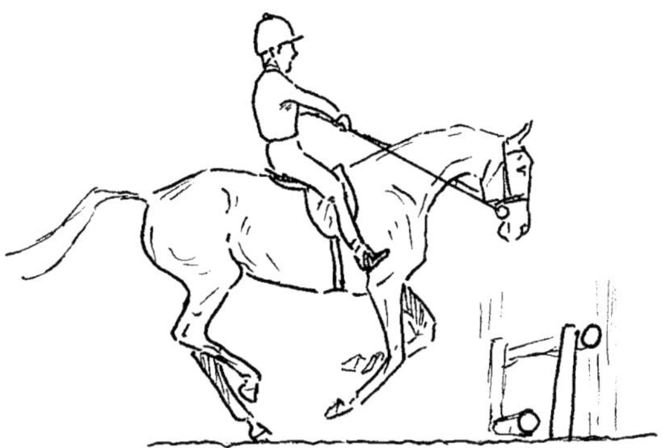

A nervous rider sitting back behind the movement coming into a fence.

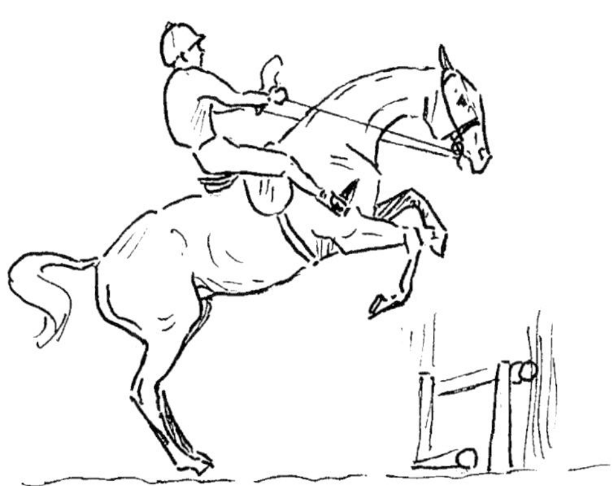

As the horse takes off the rider is thrown further back and is completely left behind hanging on by the reins.

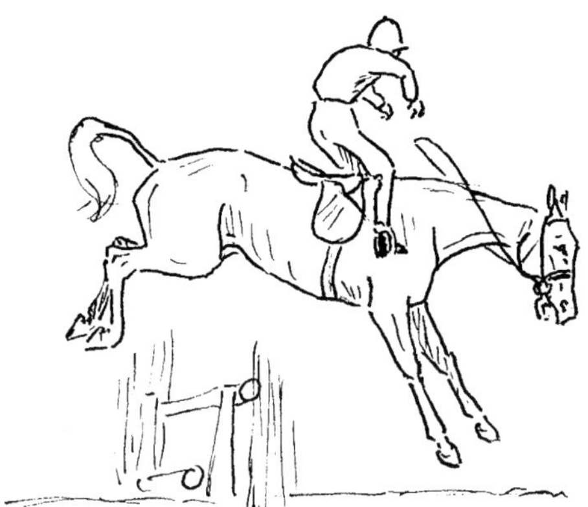

As the horse lifts its hindquarters to jump, the saddle hits the rider's seat. The rider is thrown up into the air and off the horse. It has been an unhappy experience for both of them.

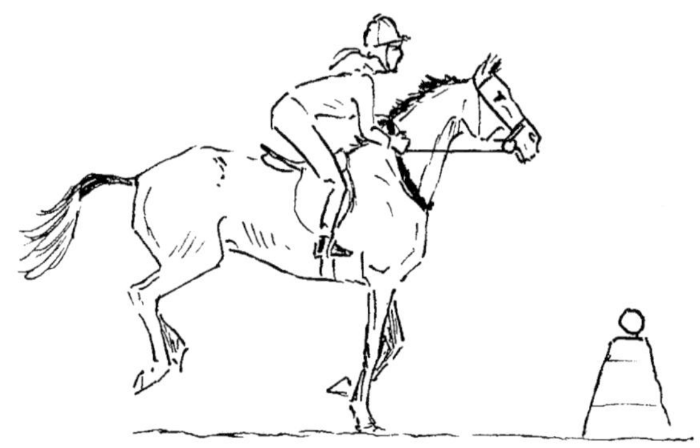

When learning to jump, sit forward in balance with the horse. Hold the mane or a neck strap.

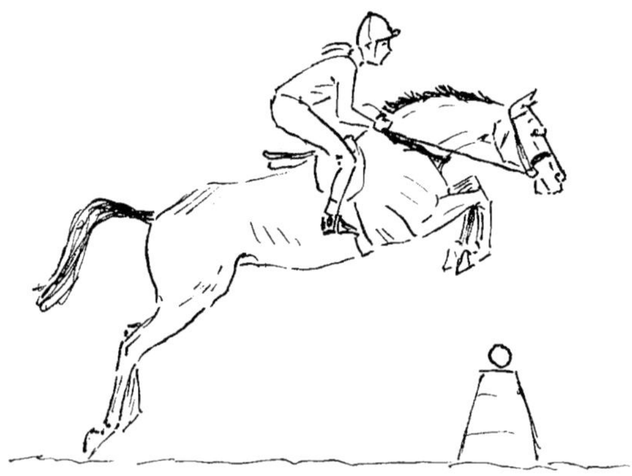

You will now go with the horse as it takes off and your seat will be clear of the saddle.

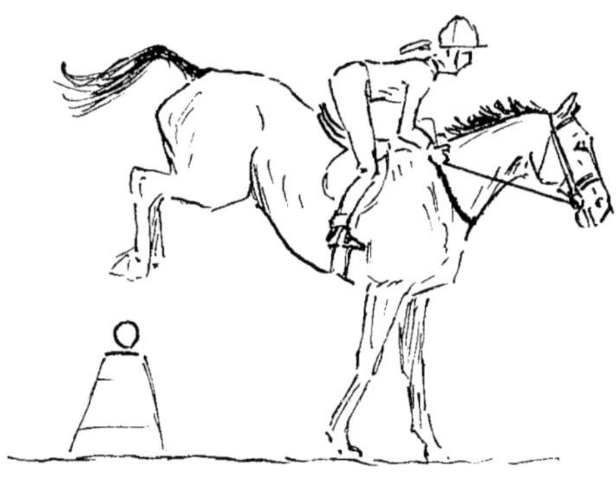

A happy, confidence-giving experience.

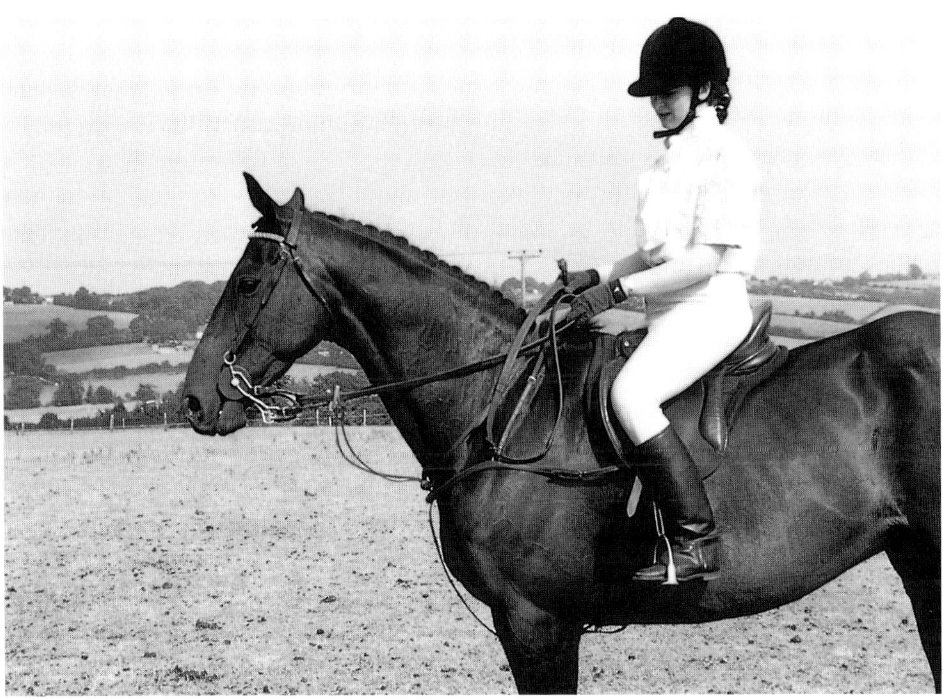

The horse is wearing an American gag bit and breast girth. The rider is sitting in balance, with shortened stirrups, ready for jumping.

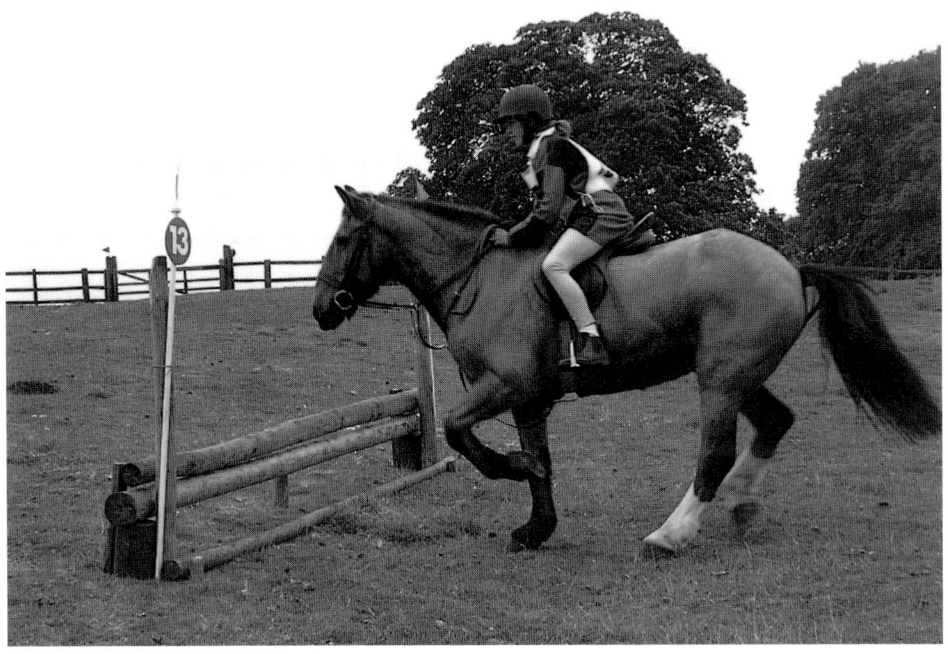

A novice rider on a kind, honest pony which is going straight for the centre of a narrow jump without any wings even through the reins are in loops.

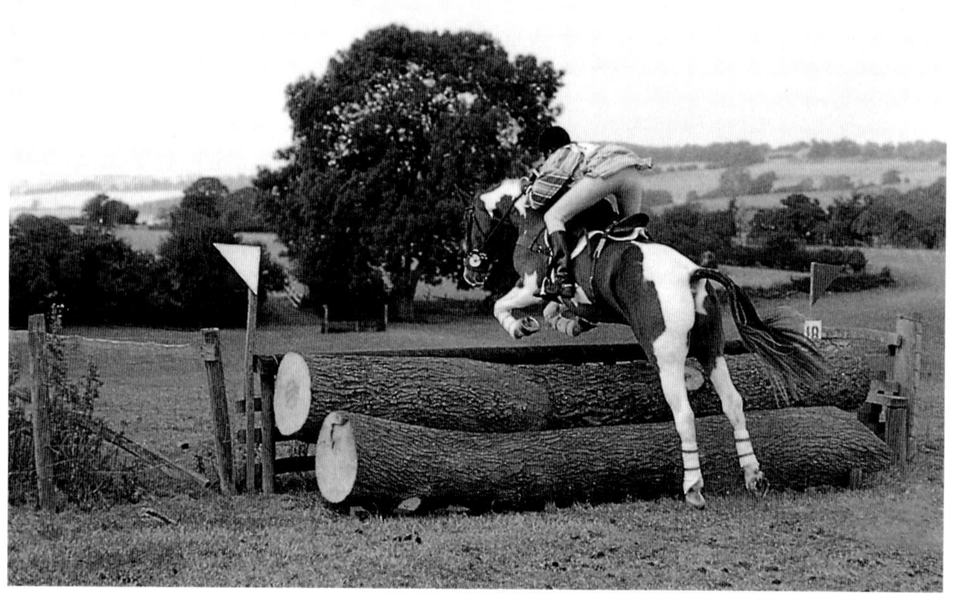

This rider is sitting in balance with his horse.

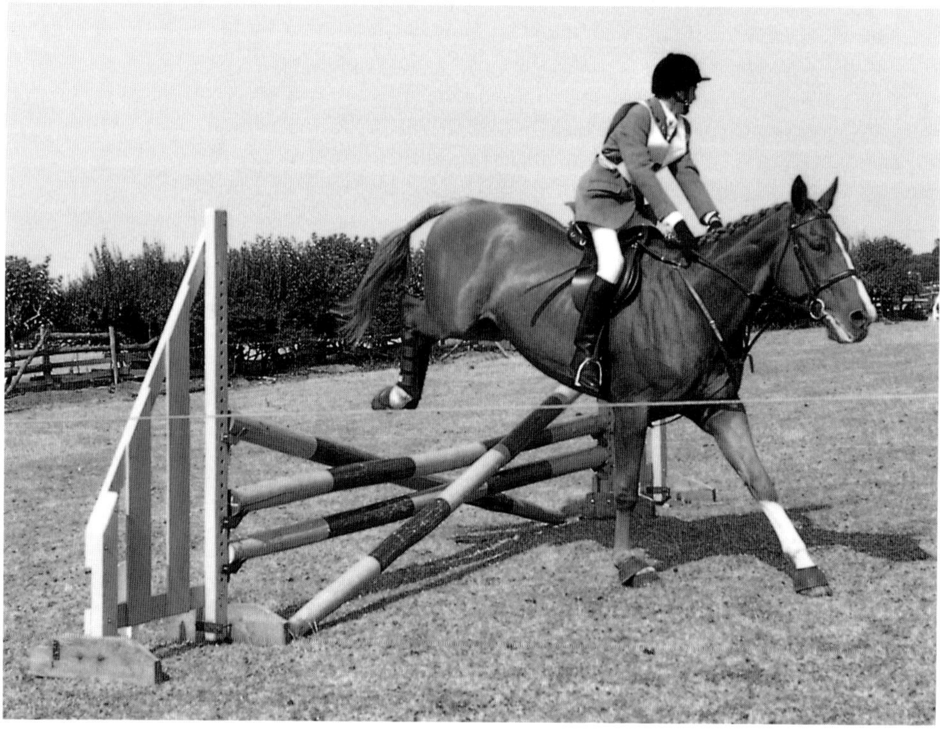

The rider is is looking ahead to the next fence.

Many people will say that you should teach people to ride the approach to a jump sitting in the saddle and tell them to swing forward from their hips at take off. However, a beginner or nervous person has no idea when or where a horse should take off so they usually misjudge the swing, nearly fall off and become even more frightened.

In my opinion, the method of sitting in the saddle in the approach and swinging the upper body forward at take off should be taught much, much later. The rider must feel safe and confident enough to go effortlessly with the horse, to ride it on at the jump if necessary and to know where and when it should take off before this method is taught.

The very basic instructions: 'put your stirrups up two holes, lean forward and hold the mane, now cock your bottom up in the air and stay like that until after you land' have, on hundreds of occasions, produced a look of amazement from novice riders when they discover they have now negotiated the jump in comfort and safety, followed by a huge grin as they began to enjoy jumping. The horses are usually a lot happier too.

Rider problems which upset the horse

- Being out of balance with the horse.
- Using a too severe bit.
- Being so nervous that you really don't want to jump.
- Holding the reins so tight that the horse can't go freely forward.
- Not pushing the hands forward towards the horse's mouth to allow it to stretch out and use its head and neck to jump freely.

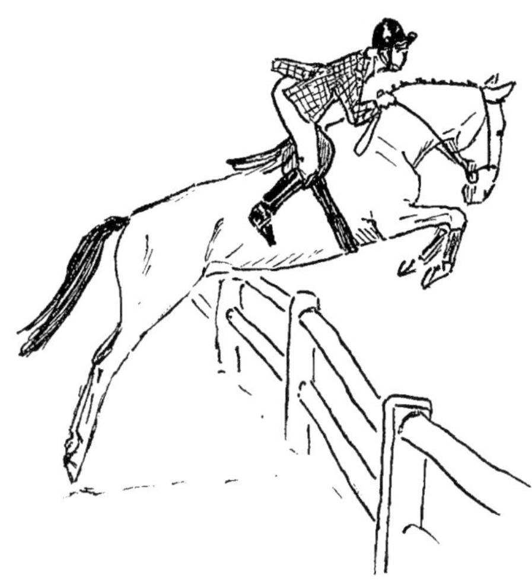

The rider is in front of the movement and not in balance with the horse.

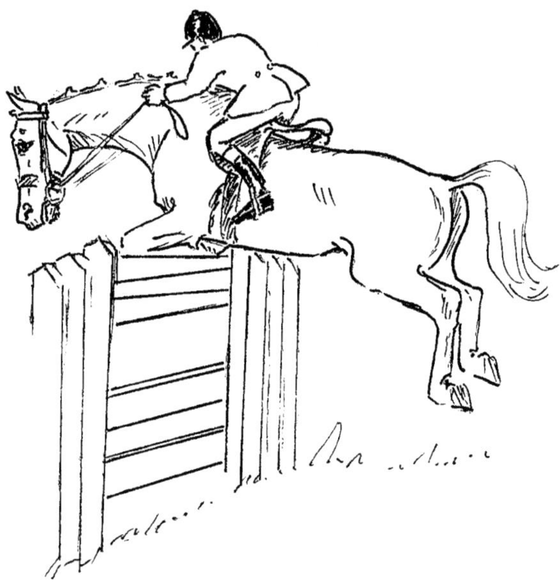

The rider is not in balance and is leaning out to the left. The horse is unlikely to pick up its near hind foot as high as the right hind and may knock the fence.

- Sitting nearly upright at take off so that the upper body and hands go back, giving the horse a jab in the mouth when it jumps.
- Approaching so slowly that the horse does not have enough impulsion to jump.
- Going so fast that the horse becomes out of balance and/or flustered and runs out instead of jumping.
- Approaching at such an acute angle that the gap beside the jump is what is in front of the horse, not the jump, so the horse runs out.
- Being so behind the horse's balance – sitting leaning back with lower leg forward – that when the horse does jump the thrust of its hindquarters catapults the rider up in the air and off. The rider is literally 'jumped off'.

TINY CHILD RIDERS

Losing stirrups

The stirrups must be the correct size for the child's feet. To prevent a small child constantly losing its stirrups, find two small, thin elastic bands and stretch one across the base of each stirrup, about 13 mm (¼ in) up the sides. The back part of the elastic goes under the child's foot. The front part is lifted up over its toes and lies across its foot. This also gives a child the correct feeling of having the stirrup iron under the ball of its foot.

The elastic band will break very easily if the child should fall off.

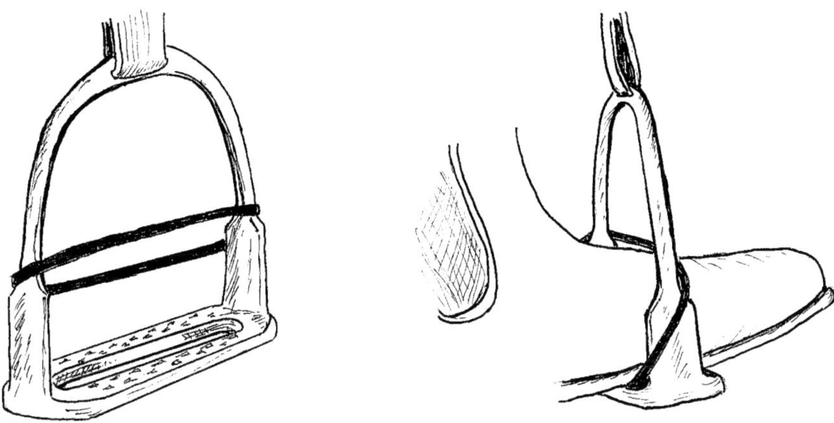

Elastic bands to help a small child to keep their foot in the stirrup.

Keeping the reins the correct length

Put a coloured elastic band on each rein. When the child is on and holding the reins at the correct length, adjust the elastic bands so that they are hidden by the child's hands.

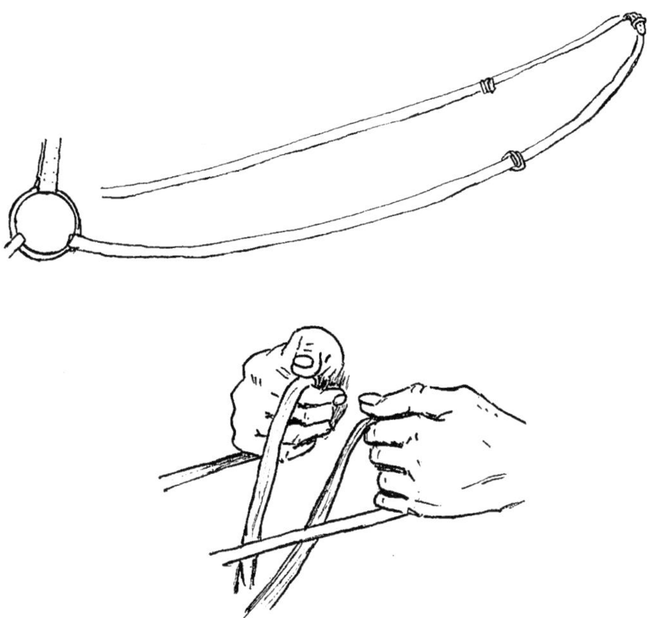

Elastic bands can be placed on the reins to ensure that a child/beginner holds them at the correct length; when held they are out of sight in the hands.

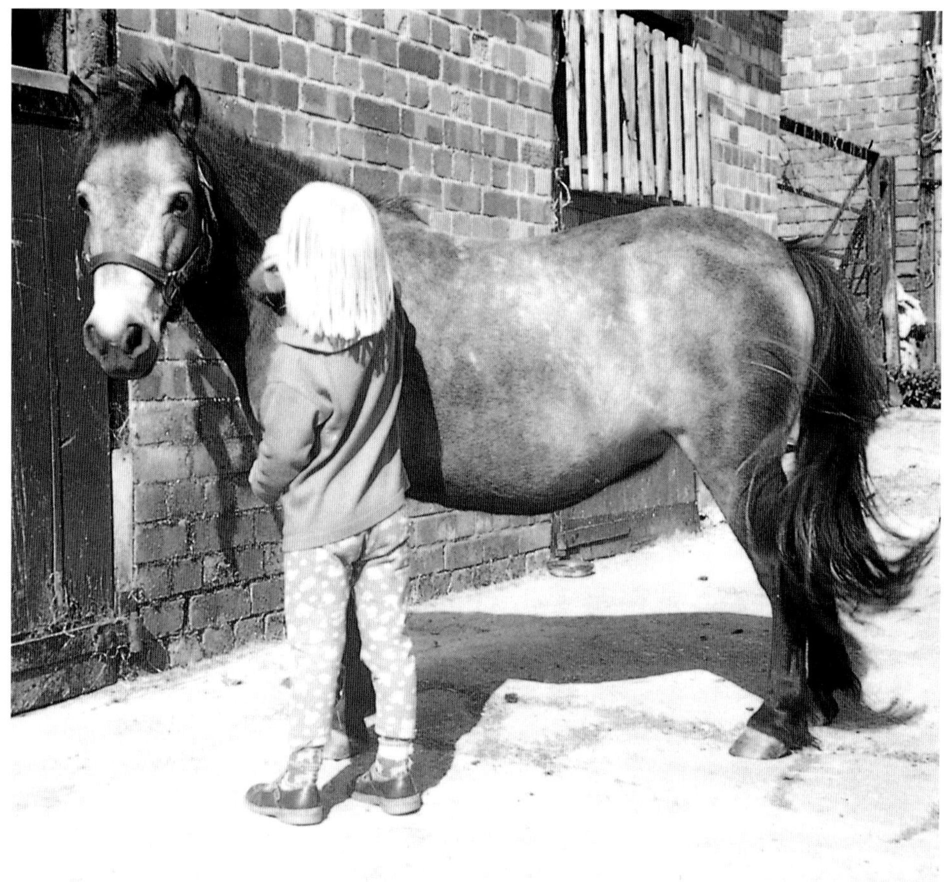

A small child's pony must be trustworthy and kind.

Showing – double-bridle reins or two reins on a Pelham

Put one elastic band round both reins on each side. When the child is on, adjust the elastic bands so that they are hidden by the child's hands and adjust the length of the curb reins so that both reins are the same length and so that the child cannot use too much curb rein. The reins can be held in the normal way with the fingers dividing them.

Felt saddles

A felt saddle is soft and not slippery but it does not give the rider's seat any support and the child tends to sit towards the back of the saddle with its legs stuck forward. Take two sleeves from an old jersey and put one inside the other so that there is a cuff at each end. Stuff them firmly with anything soft so that most of the stuffing is in the centre and it gradually tapers off at each end. Sew up the ends then sew your stuffed crescent shape underneath the back of the felt saddle so that the back is lifted up and there is a place for the child to sit correctly, where it will feel safely supported and be far more secure.

Leather saddles

No one, child or adult, can sit correctly on a saddle which slopes to the back and is up in front. The rider's bottom will slide downhill and they will be forced to sit on the back of the saddle with their legs stuck forward. If possible, have the saddle restuffed so that it rests level on the pony's back with the lowest point in the centre quite close to the stirrup bars.

Temporary improvement can be made by turning the saddle over and examining the underside. If there are pockets at each side that you can push your fingers into, cut pieces of foam rubber and push them into these pockets at the back of the saddle. This will raise the back of the saddle and make it more level on the pony's back. Make sure you put exactly the same amount of foam on each side and that the underneath of the saddle at the back looks the same shape on both sides. Make sure there are no humps or bumps. Check the front of the saddle when it is on the pony and make sure it is not coming down on the withers because when you raise the back of the saddle you may lower the position of the front.

Make a pocket in the part of the back of the numnah nearest to the saddle and put a wedge-shaped pad of foam or stuffing in the pocket so that the thickest part, towards the rear, will raise the back of the saddle.

12 EMERGENCIES

EMERGENCY CONTROL

You discover that a horse has escaped from its field or stable or you meet a loose horse on the road. The horse is not wearing a headcollar so what can you do?

- If you are wearing a belt, put this round the horse's neck, holding it with your right hand. Put your left hand on the bone of its nose above its nostrils.
- If you are wearing a jersey or an anorak, roll up the body part leaving the sleeves free, put the body part on top of the horse's neck easing it forward to just behind its ears, cross the top of the sleeves under its throat and wrap one arm round its nose. Hold on to the cuffs. If the sleeves are long enough, you can knot them behind the horse's chin.

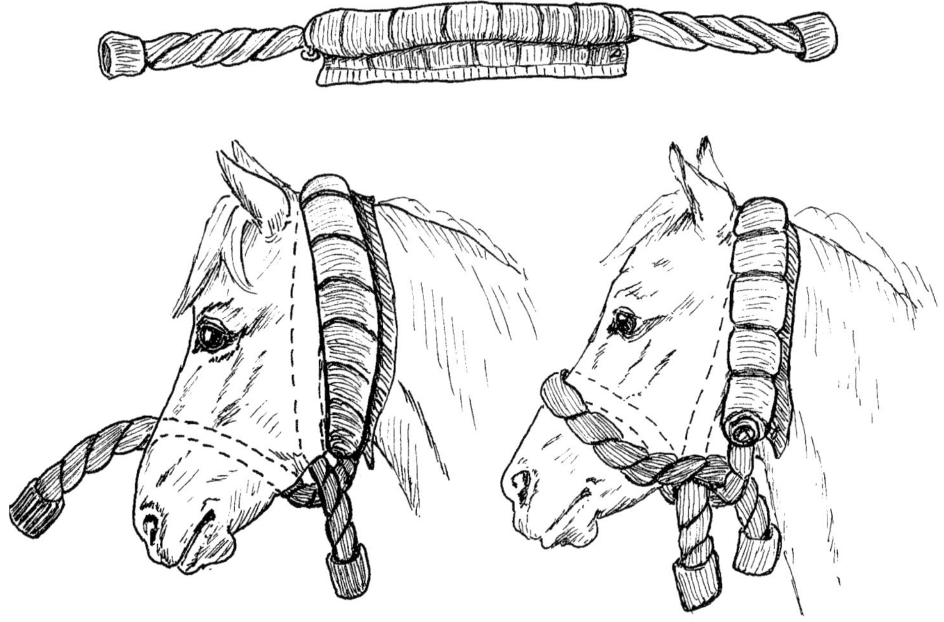

An emergency halter made from a jumper or anorak.

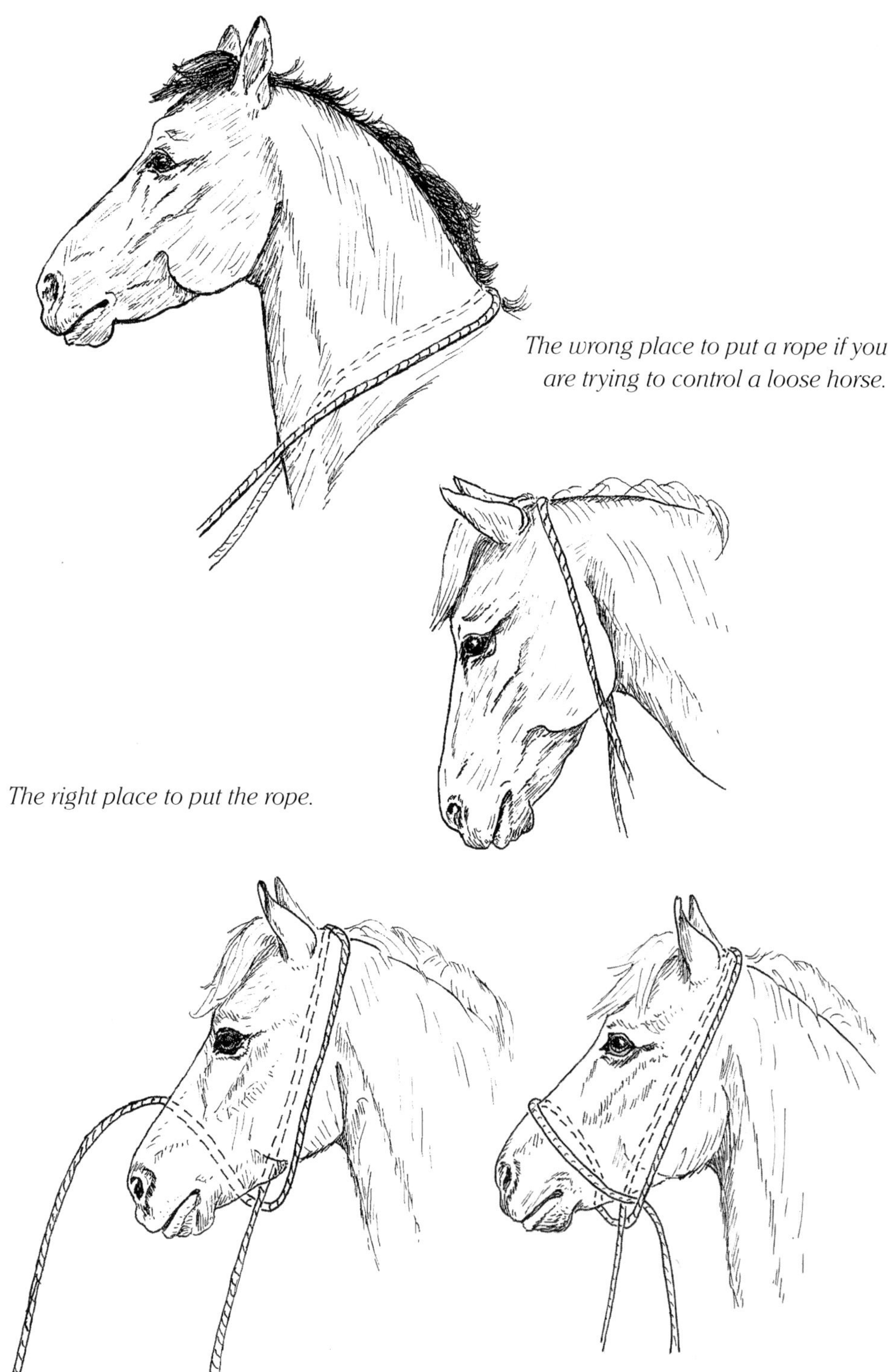

The wrong place to put a rope if you are trying to control a loose horse.

The right place to put the rope.

Making an emergency halter out of a simple rope.

- A length of thick rope (*not* baling twine – if the horse pulls away or you get a finger caught up you can both be badly cut) can be put over the horse's neck behind its ears, twisted in the throatlash area, then one end put round its nose and back through the loop encircling its neck. Hold both ends of the rope.
- If there is time and you have a long enough rope, tie a secure loop to form the noseband. Open up the fibres in the noseband on the opposite side to your knot and pass the end of the rope through the gap you have made. You now have a respectable halter which, when adjusted to size, can be knotted to the noseband to prevent it overtightening on the horse's nose if it pulls back.

Warning: look at the horse's expression as you approach. Having been loose it may be overexcited and may kick out or strike out at you with a foreleg. Try to have something for it even if it is only a bunch of nice grass.

Some horses may be terrified of a jersey or anorak near their heads. Watch their eye and head carriage to see how they are reacting.

You cannot hold a horse which really wants to get away by any of these methods but most calm horses who are used to being handled will believe that you are now in control and allow you to lead them to safety.

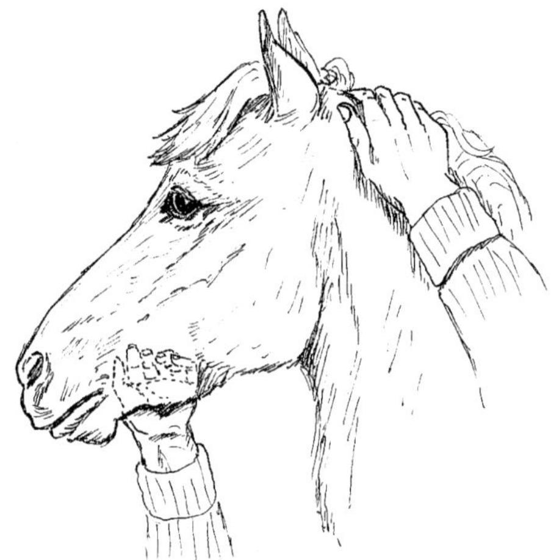

When trying to hold a little pony, it is a good idea to cup your hand under the pony's chin to prevent it from ducking its head down to evade a hand on the nose.

- If you have nothing with which to control the horse, try putting your right hand on top of its head behind its ears and your left hand on the bone of its nose above the nostrils. Some horses will meekly accept this form of control. Little ponies will often duck their heads to escape your hand on their nose. It can be easier to control them by putting your left hand under the chin (where a curb chain would go) and using this hand to keep the head up quite high by cupping it round the lower jaw.

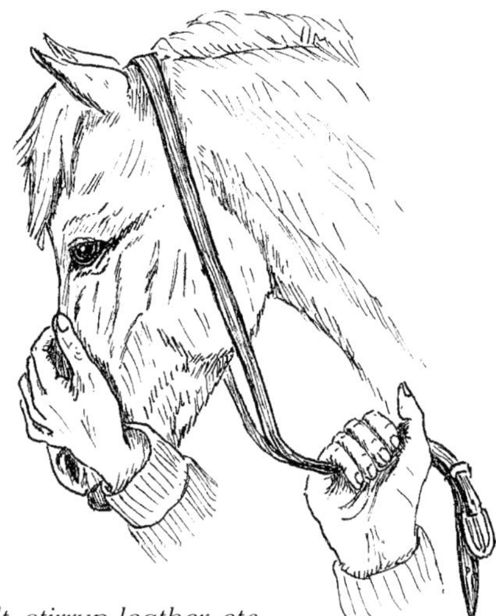

A makeshift halter made out of a belt, stirrup leather, etc.

Very few animals accept being led by their forelock so I do not advise trying this method.

- If the horse has a saddle on but no bridle (the rider having either pulled the bridle off in falling or the horse having broken it by treading on it) use one of the stirrup leathers placed round its neck behind its ears then crossed in the throatlash area, drawn on round its nose where the buckle can be done up and the end passed down through the gap below the spike to secure it or knotted to prevent it from coming undone.

BROKEN BRIDLES

A broken bridle headpiece

If the headpiece of your bridle breaks at the top hole on the near side, you can attach the cheekpiece buckle to the strap of your throatlash or to the strap of your noseband headpiece. It may be necessary to undo the throatlash or noseband headpiece and attach the cheekpiece buckle before you attach their own buckles. To make the bit sit level in the mouth it may be necessary to put the offside cheekpiece up or down a few holes.

If the headpiece breaks at the top hole on the off side, remove the noseband and turn it round, back to front, so that the noseband headpiece does up on the off side, and use its strap to attach to the cheekpiece of your bridle.

A shoelace kept in your pocket can be used as an emergency repair.

A broken bridle cheekpiece

The noseband can be threaded through the bit rings on one or, preferably, both sides to keep the bit level. The noseband may have to be raised or lowered to keep the bit at the correct height in the horse's mouth.

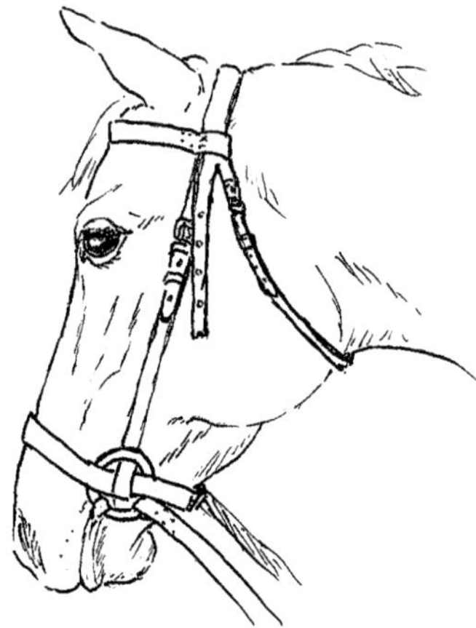

If the cheekpiece breaks, thread the headpiece and the cheekpiece of the noseband through the rings of the bit and adjust this to a comfortable level to hold the bit in the horse's mouth.

Broken reins

Reins broken at the centre buckle can be knotted together. Reins broken near the stud billet (or buckle near the bit) can also be tied. Pass the broken end through the bit, then back to form a circle round the rein. Pass the end up through the circle and pull tight from both directions. If possible then tie the broken end to the rein with string or a shoelace.

A martingale can be used as reins, the neckstrap forming one rein, the main part of the martingale forming the other rein.

One stirrup leather can replace a broken rein. If both reins are broken use two stirrup leathers, threading the tip through the bit ring and then through its own buckle. The tips can be kept together by threading string or a shoelace through the first hole in each.

SADDLE PRESSING DOWN ON THE HORSE'S WITHERS

Tuck your fingers under the front arch of your saddle then lean forwards and stand up in your stirrups. If your fingers get pinched, the saddle is too low on your horse's back and will, at least, be painful for it and make it behave or perform badly and, at worst, damage its spine. Do not ride a horse if the saddle is pressing on its spine. Use a folded jersey or anorak, a towel, blanket or even a pair of gloves to prevent damage for the moment. Take the saddle to be restuffed to fit the horse.

The backs of young horses alter shape as they grow so saddles will need restuffing or even changing to ensure a good fit.

Horses which are round and fat in the summer after lots of grass may lose weight and have a far more prominent wither in the winter. Their saddles may need restuffing. Check the fit of a saddle frequently.

GIRTH TOO LONG

The old-fashioned nylon girths can be shortened by opening a gap in the strands nearest to each buckle and passing the buckle through the gap as many times as possible.

Most of the girths in use today cannot be shortened so an extra numnah, a folded jersey, a folded anorak (be careful where the zip comes), a folded towel or a folded blanket can all be used under the saddle to make the girth fit more snugly and to hold the saddle safely in place.

Never ride with a loose girth as you are likely to have a bad fall if the saddle slips.

TYING A HORSE UP WHEN OUT RIDING

Never tie your horse up by the reins when they are attached to the bit. Your horse's mouth may be badly damaged if it tries to break loose.

A *quiet* horse can be tied up by detaching both reins from the bit and attaching one end of the reins to the noseband while using the other end to tie the horse up.

SHOEING EMERGENCIES

Risen clench

You want to go to a PC rally or competition but on the morning you notice that your horse has a risen clench on the inside of its shoe. (The clench is the bent over end of the nail which secures it in place on the wall of the hoof. It is hammered down and rasped smooth.) As the shoe and nail wear, the clench is sometimes pushed up and sticks out beyond the wall. If it is on the outside it is unlikely to cause any damage but on the inside a sharp piece of nail sticking out can severely cut the opposite leg. It must be dealt with immediately.

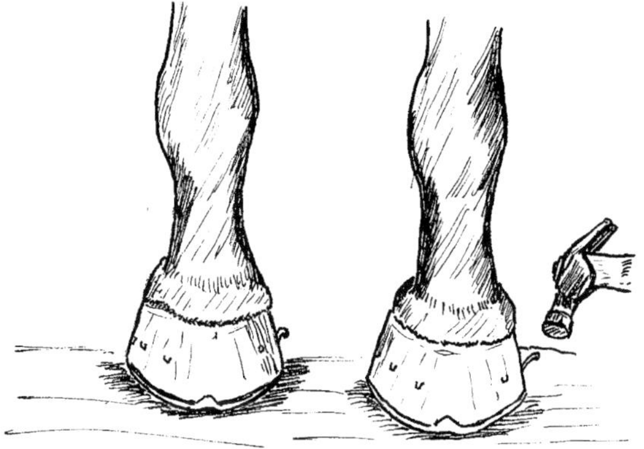

Stand the horse on a hard, smooth surface to hammer down a risen clench.

Stand the horse on hard, level ground such as concrete. While the foot with the risen clench is on the ground, tap the top of the clench with a small hammer, attempt to roll and bend the end over to tighten the nail, then hammer it inwards and, if you have a file or rasp, smooth down any rough edges. Do not take so much off that there is nothing to hold the nail in place. Asking someone to lift up the opposite leg will help to ensure that the horse keeps its full weight on the foot on which you are working.

A risen clench is usually a sign that the horse needs shoeing.

Loose shoe

Several risen clenches mean that the nails are no longer holding the shoe firmly in place. Treat all the risen clenches as suggested in Risen Clench (see page 331) and you may be able to secure the shoe sufficiently to be able to get one more day's use. If the shoe is twisted and sticking out on the inside, it is not safe to ride as the opposite leg can be cut. The horse will need the urgent attention of your farrier. On the day on which your farrier has visited, you should note the visit on a calendar, immediately count six weeks ahead and write the name of the horse which has been shod and 'six weeks'.

It is very easy to forget exactly when a horse was shod and the writing on the calendar jogs your memory.

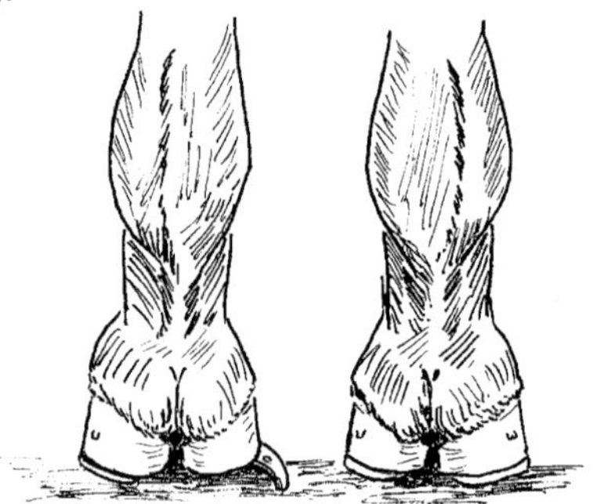

A spread shoe is dangerous.

Shoe twisted and half off

Front

When stumbling, perhaps in heavy ground, a horse can tread on the heel of the front shoe with the toe of a hind shoe and bend the shoe so that most of the nails come out on one side and the heel of the shoe on that side is badly bent and sticking out.

This is dangerous for three reasons.

- The heel of the shoe can cut the horse's opposite leg.
- If the horse treads on the half-off shoe, any nails still in the bent part can be forced into the sensitive sole and may lame the horse.
- The horse can trip because of the angle of the shoe or a hind shoe can tread on the bent heel.

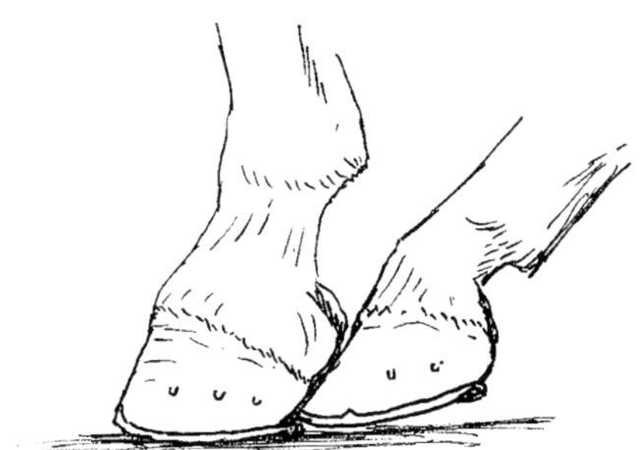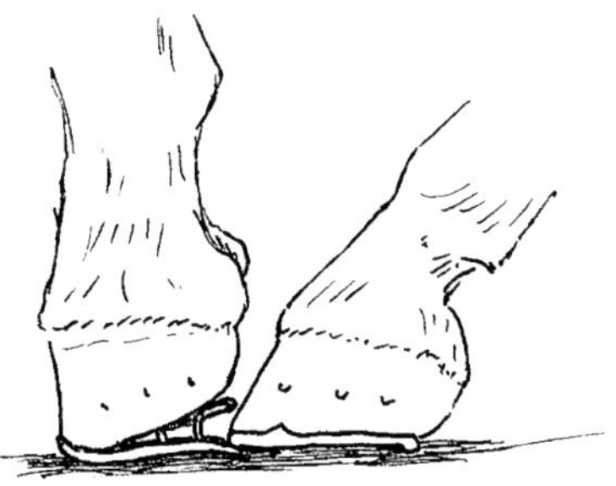

How a front shoe is pulled off by the toe of the hind shoe.

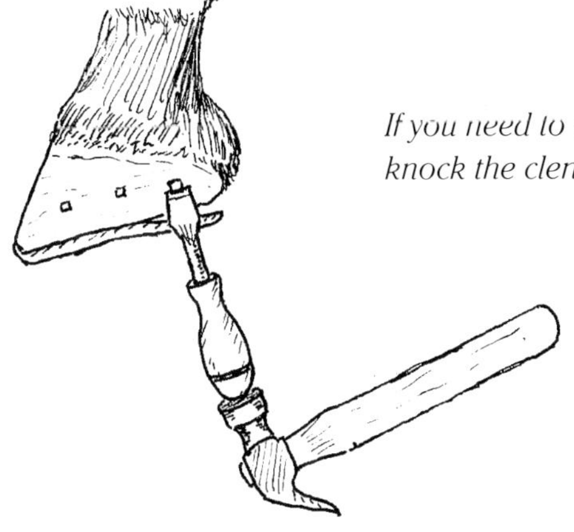

If you need to remove a shoe without the proper tools, knock the clenches up with a screwdriver and hammer.

Put the head of the pincers under the straightened clench. Hit the shoe on each side of the nail head with the hammer while pressing hard on the head of the pincers. The nail head will rise up above the shoe and can now be removed with a forward and inward movement of the pincers.

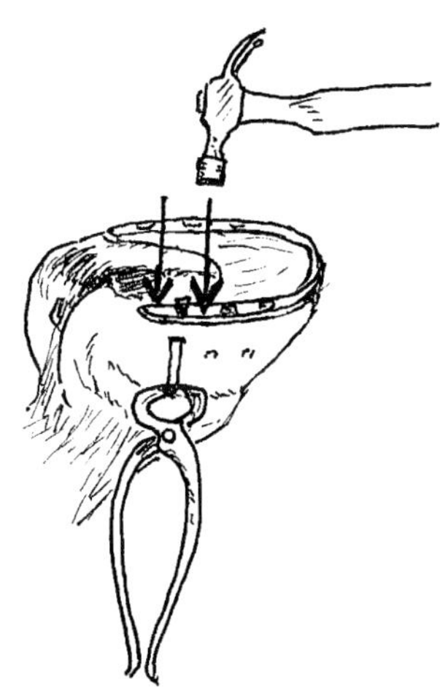

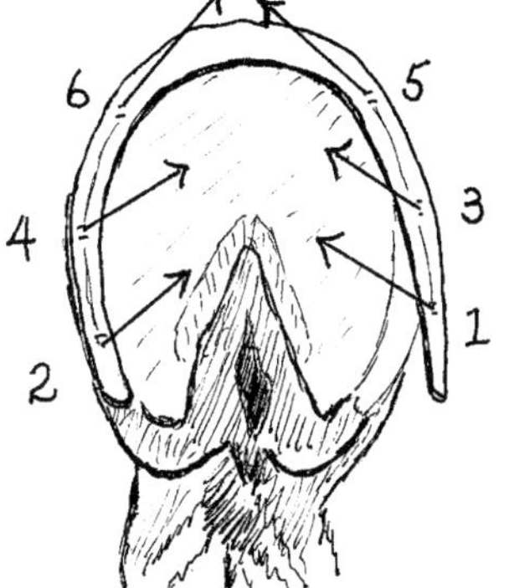

Pull each nail out in numerical order as shown in the illustration.

If there is a slightly bent heel on a front shoe but the nails have not been pulled out of place, it is safe to lead the horse home if it will walk quietly. It is, however, safer to remove the shoe, either by getting a strong man to pull the shoe off if it is really loose and can be removed without badly breaking the walls of the foot, or by finding a screwdriver or chisel to lift the clenches and straighten them, and something to use as a hammer. Pincers or pliers can be used to pull the nails out one at a time. Motorists sometimes carry suitable tools. Pick the foot up, put the head of the pincers or pliers under the clench you have lifted and straightened and tap on the shoe with your hammer on each side of the head of the nail. This will have the effect of making the head rise above the level of the shoe so that pincers or pliers can grasp it to pull it out. Think of the angle at which the nail was driven in and try to pull it out at the same angle, inwards and forwards towards the tip of the frog (the V-shaped leathery piece under the foot).

Hind

A hind shoe can open up if the toe has been weakened by being worn thin or if the horse suddenly screw sideways, for instance when shying or whipping round, and puts all the pressure at an angle on one side of the shoe. If the shoe opens up so that the inside heel has spread and is now sticking out, it can badly damage the opposite leg.

If the hind shoe is loose enough it may be possible to pull it off or to bend it one way then the other, if the toe is weak enough, until it breaks at the toe, leaving half the shoe in place.

If it is essential to remove the shoe, proceed as suggested above when removing a front shoe.

When leading or riding a horse home with half a shoe or a shoe off, keep it on the grass as much as possible to avoid breaking the foot.

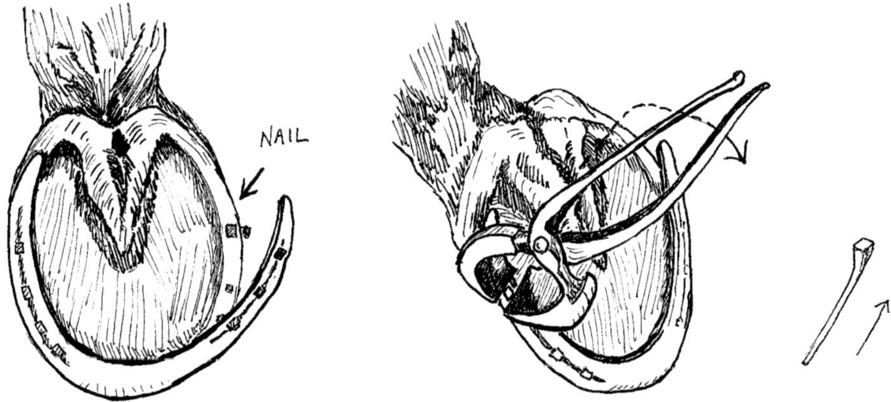

A shoe that is badly spread on the inside is very dangerous for the opposite leg. Take the nails out by pulling inwards and towards the toe.

INDEX